Current Topics in Pathology

87

E. Vollmer A. Roessner (Eds.)

Recent Progress in Atherosclerosis Research

Contributors

M. Althaus · E. Betz · W. Böcker · A. Dobrian
H. Heinle · E. Jaeger · D. Kling · M. Kumamoto
J. Rauterberg · H. Robenek · A. Roessner · H. Sakuda
N. J. Severs · A. Sima · M. Simionescu · N. Simionescu
K. Sueishi · K. Tanaka · D. Tirziu · E. Vollmer

Springer-Verlag
Berlin Heidelberg New York
London Paris Tokyo
Hong Kong Barcelona
Budapest

A. Roessner, Professor Dr.
Institut für Pathologie
der Otto-von-Guericke-Universität
Leipziger Straße 44
39120 Magdeburg, Germany

E. Vollmer, Professor Dr. Dr.
Pathologie, Forschungsinstitut Borstel
Institut für experimentelle Biologie und Medizin
Parkalle 40
23845 Borstel, Germany

With 75 Figures and 9 Tables

ISBN 3-540-54394-5 Springer-Verlag Berlin Heidelberg New York
ISBN 0-387-54394-5 Springer-Verlag New York Berlin Heidelberg

Library of Congress Cataloging-in-Publication Data
Recent progress in atherosclerosis research / E. Vollmer and A. Roessner, eds.: contributors, M. Althaus... [et al.]. p. cm. – (Current topics in pathology: 87)
Includes bibliographical references and index.
ISBN 3-540-54394-5. – ISBN 0-387-54394-5
1. Atherosclerosis – Pathophysiology. I. Vollmer, E. (Ekkehard), 1950– II. Roessner, Albert. III. Althaus, M. IV. Series: Current topics in pathology: v. 87.
[DNLM: 1. Atherosclerosis -- metabolism. 2. Atherosclerosis-physiopathology.
W1 CU821H v. 87 1993 / WG 550] RB1.E6 vol. 87 [RC692] 616.07 s -- dc20
[616.1'3607] DNLM/DLC 93-31211

Typesetting: Thomson Press (India) Ltd., New Delhi
Printing: Saladruck, Steinkopf & Sohn, Berlin, Binding: Lüderitz & Bauer, Berlin
25/3130/SPS – 5 4 3 2 1 0 – Printed on acid-free paper

List of Contributors

Althaus, M., Dr.	Institut für Arterioskleroseforschung Universität Münster Domagkstraße 3 48149 Münster, Germany
Betz, E., Prof. Dr.	Physiologisches Institut I Eberhard-Karls-Universität Tübingen Gmelinstraße 5 72076 Tübingen, Germany
Böcker, W., Prof. Dr.	Gerhard-Domagk-Institut für Pathologie Universität Münster Domagkstraße 17 48149 Münster, Germany
Dobrian, A., Dr.	Institute of Cellular Biology and Pathology 8, B.P. Hasdeu Street R-79691 Bucharest Romania
Heinle, H., Prof. Dr.	Physiologisches Institut I Eberhard-Karls-Universität Tübingen Gmelinstraße 5 72076 Tübingen, Germany
Jaeger, E., Dr.	Institut für Arterioskleroseforschung Universität Münster Domagkstraße 3 48149 Münster, Germany
Kling, D., Dr.	Physiologisches Institut I Eberhard-Karls-Universität Tübingen Gmelinstraße 5 72076 Tübingen, Germany

KUMAMOTO, M., Dr.
Department of Pathology
Faculty of Medicine
Kyushu University
3-1-1 Maidashi, Higashi-ku
Fukuoka 812
Japan

RAUTERBERG, J., Prof. Dr.
Institut für Arterioskleroseforschung
Universität Münster
Domagkstraße 3
48149 Münster, Germany

ROBENEK, H., Prof. Dr.
Institut für Arterioskleroseforschung
Universität Münster
Domagkstraße 3
48149 Münster, Germany

ROESSNER, A., Prof. Dr.
Institut für Pathologie
der Otto-von-Guericke-Universität
Leipziger Straße 44
39120 Magdeburg, Germany

SAKUDA, H., Dr.
Department of Pathology
Faculty of Medicine
Kyushu University
3-1-1 Maidashi Higashi-ku,
Fukuoka 812 Japan

SEVERS, N.J., Dr.
National Heart and Lung Institute
University of London
Dovehouse Street
London SW3 6LY, UK

SIMA, A., Dr.
Institute of Cellular Biology and
Pathology
8, B.P. Hasdeu Street
R-79691 Bucharest
Romania

SIMIONESCU, M., Prof. Dr.
Institute of Cellular Biology and
Pathology
8, B.P. Hasdeu Street
R-79691 Bucharest
Romania

SIMIONESCU, N., Prof. Dr.
Institute of Cellular Biology and Pathology
8, B.P. Hasdeu Street
R-79691 Bucharest
Romania

SUEISHI, K., Prof. Dr.
Department of Pathology
Faculty of Medicine
Kyushu University
3-1-1 Maidashi, Higashi-ku
Fukuoka 812
Japan

TANAKA, K., Prof. Dr.
Department of Pathology
Faculty of Medicine
Kyushu University
3-1-1 Maidashi, Higashi-ku
Fukuoka 812
Japan

TIRZIU, D., Dr.
Institute of Cellular Biology and Pathology
8, B.P. Hasdeu Street
R-79691 Bucharest
Romania

VOLLMER, E., Prof. Dr. Dr.
Pathologie Forschungsinstitut Borstel
Institut für experimentelle Biologie und Medizin
Parkallee 40
23845 Borstel, Germany

Preface

During the past years a considerable number of books have been published on atherosclerosis research. Much attention has been focused on the biochemical properties of lipoproteins and the involvement of lipoprotein metabolism in the atherogenic process. The monograph presented here focuses on morphologic studies of atherosclerotic plaque.

One chapter deals with the pathobiochemical changes in the arterial wall at the inception of atherosclerosis. Recently the specific role of macrophages in atherogenesis has been the object of much interest. A morphological study of their role and differentiation is the topic of another chapter. This is complemented by a study of lipoprotein receptors on macrophages and smooth muscle cells both in cell culture and in situ, based on electron microscopic investigations. An immunohistological study on the in situ localization promotes our understanding of lipoprotein metabolism in the arterial wall. The morphologic aspects of more advanced lesions are presented in studies of collagens and angiogenic processes in the atherosclerotic vessel wall. Experimental investigations have also been useful for understanding the pathogenetic aspects of atherosclerosis; one chapter concentrates on the metabolism of fibromuscular and atheromatous plaques in an experimental model. A final chapter deals with transplant arteriopathy and its possible parallels with conventional atherosclerosis. The widespread discussion of atherogenesis is focused on the arterial wall and its morphological alterations, emphasizing once again the importance of morphological research for understanding the pathological basis of disease.

Borstel and Magdeburg
October 1993

E. Vollmer and A. Roessner

Contents

Pathobiochemical Changes of the Arterial Wall at the Inception of Atherosclerosis

N. SIMIONESCU, A. SIMA, A. DOBRIAN, D. TIRZIU, and M. SIMIONESCU

Abbreviations used in the text: apo A-I, apolipoprotein A-I; apo B, apolipoprotein B; apo E, apolipoprotein E; ALp, aggregated lipoproteins; CETP, cholesteryl ester transfer protein; CSPG, chondroitin sulfate-proteoglycan; ECs, endothelial cells; EDRF, endothelial-derived relaxing factor; ELAM, endothelial leukocyte adhesion molecules; ELs, extracellular liposomes; FLp, fused lipoproteins; FN, fibronectin; HDL, high-density lipoproteins; ICAM, intercellular adhesion molecules; IDL, intermediate-density lipoproteins; LDL, low-density lipoproteins; Lp(a), lipoprotein a; MCP-1, monocyte chemotactic protein 1; MLp, monomeric lipoproteins; MM-LDL, minimally modified LDL; MRLp, modified and reassembled lipoproteins; OTO, osmium–thiocarbohydrazide–osmium; PAGE, polyacrylamide gel electrophoresis; TA-PDA, tannic acid–paraphenylenediamine; VCAM, vascular cell adhesion molecules; VLDL, very low-density lipoprotein; VLp, vesiculated lipoproteins; WHHL, Watanabe heritable hyperlipidemic

Current Topics in Pathology
Volume 87, Vollmer/Roessner (Eds.)

1 Introduction

The pathogenesis and molecular mechanism of atherosclerosis are still an intriguing and challenging puzzle for cardiovascular research. The potential therapeutic implications of decoding this disease fully justify the efforts to understand the subtle processes which may underlie atherogenesis. Present knowledge does not allow a comprehensive picture of the multiplicity of factors and the sequence of molecular and cellular events which lead to the alterations of the artery wall that generate myocardial and cerebral infarction. Valuable contributions from several laboratories, especially in the last decade, have led to several hypotheses regarding the mechanisms by which elevated serum cholesterol induces atherosclerosis. Among these theories, particularly seminal have been the revised "response-to-injury" (Ross 1986) and the "lipid infiltration" hypotheses, the latter focusing primarily on the role of oxidized low-density lipoprotein (LDL) (Steinberg et al. 1989). Important contributions have also emerged from the laboratories of A. Fogelman, R. Mahley, and others, not to mention the pioneering work on LDL metabolism and LDL receptors, by M. Brown and J. Goldstein. However, focusing the interpretation on a single pathogenic factor can only inadvertently obscure the data accumulate on other lines of investigation and delay the formulation of a coherent theory of atherosclerosis based on generally accepted factual evidence.

If one considers, on the one hand, the marked heterogeneity of human atherosclerotic lesions, among which about 50% are virtually devoid of lipid infiltration (Velican and Velican 1986), and, on the other hand, the fact that most cases of experimentally induced atherosclerosis are based on a single pathogenic factor, i.e., diet-induced hypercholesterolemia, it appears very likely that we are dealing not only with a multifactorial disease entity but also with a variety of pathogenic pathways leading eventually to different or similar lesions.

In recent years, the impact of cell biology on research into atherosclerosis has been obvious. However, the otherwise valuable information obtained by in vitro observations should be interpreted cautiously until in vivo studies or studies on ex vivo explants of artery wall are performed. As compared to cancer research, our knowledge of the genetic aspects of atherogenesis is still restricted, although relevant achievements have been accomplished, especially by the identification of the genes coding for the four proteins [i.e., apo B, apo E, Lp (a), and LDL receptor] which have well-established links to inherited atherosclerosis. As in other diseases, the molecular biology approach, which has strongly reinforced the link between hypercholesterolemia and coronary artery disease, is justifiably expected to add new dimensions to our understanding of autherogenesis.

Despite the aforementioned advances, numerous unanswered questions remain. A substantial new body of data and a more open conceptual approach are required to clarify which of the registered changes (such as LDL oxidation) represent a cause of the disease and which are just a beneficial local defense reaction (SIMIONESCU 1990, 1992b).

If we accept to exercise the stoic will to live with the uncertainty, one should admit that we are still at the stage of investigating and elucidating the likely segments from which the immensely complex atherosclerotic process is constructed. One such segment which, though little explored, is certainly important, comprises the minute pathobiochemical modifications which occur in the artery wall at the inception of atherogenesis. This review article is an attempt to collate some of the observations regarding these prelesional events (SIMIONESCU et al. 1986, 1990) which have to date been detected at the onset of hypercholesterolemic experimental atherosclerosis. Furthermore, we present some data based on the work conducted in our laboratory. For the sake of simplicity we do not discuss a series of factors which are known to play or which may play a role in atherosclerosis (e.g., viral pathogenesis) (HAJJAR 1991) but for which the changes associated with the development of the disease are insufficiently defined.

2 LDL Transport and Metabolism by the Normal Artery Wall

The interaction of LDL with arteries is a complex multistep and multifactorial process largely dependent on the organization and physiologic properties of various components of the vessel wall. As a general pattern, the following steps may be distinguished (Fig. 1):

- LDL influx into the artery wall
- Intramural LDL metabolism and interstitial circulation
- LDL efflux from the artery wall via the local lymphatics to reenter the blood

2.1 LDL Influx into the Artery Wall

Based on transmural concentration profiles of ^{125}I-LDL perfused in rabbits, it has been estimated that in the thoracic aorta about two-thirds of LDL penetrates through the arterial luminal surface and about one-third via the vasa vasorum (BRATZLER et al. 1977). As shown immunocytochemically, upon binding to the endothelial cell surface, by a largely reversible process, LDL particles can be either (a) taken up by coated pits—coated vesicles and delivered to endosomes and lysosomes for hydrolytic catabolism (endocytosis) or (b) ingested by plasmalemmal vesicles to be translocated across the cell (usually bypassing the lysosomal compartment) and discharged into the subendothelial space (transcytosis) (VASILE et al. 1983, 1985; SIMIONESCU et al. 1986, 1991a, b; SMELTING-HAVINGA et al. 1989). Normally LDL do not penetrate endothelial junctions (VASILE et al. 1983; SMELTING-HAVINGA et al. 1989). Upon direct contact or

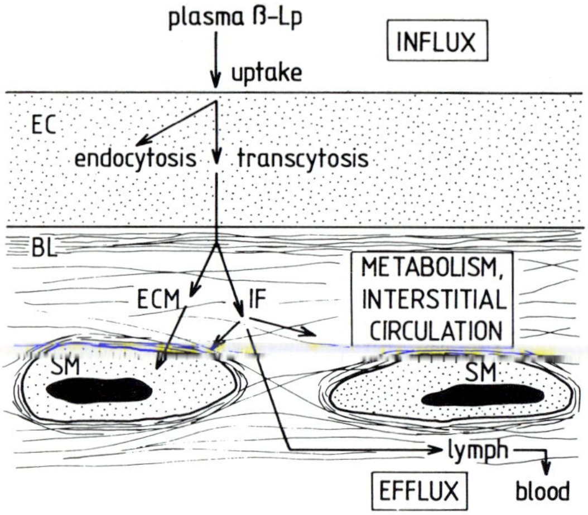

Fig. 1. Schematic representation of the plasma β-lipoprotein (β-*Lp*) transport by the normal artery wall. The β-Lp *influx* is initiated upon interaction with the luminal plasmalemma of endothelial cells (*EC*). The subsequent endocytosis is largely mediated by the cognate receptors, whereas transytosis is predominantly, if not entirely, a receptor-independent process. The transcytosed lipoprotein particles cross and interact successively with endothelial basal lamina (*BL*) and extracellular matrix (*ECM*); the reactions with the components of the BL and ECM are reversible and no significant trapping of lipoproteins normally occurs. Being transported by the interstitial fluid (*IF*), some of the lipoproteins are taken up and metabolized by the intima cells, i.e., EC and smooth muscle cells (*SM*), while the rest of the β-Lp enter the local lymphatics through which the lymph returns them to the blood circulation (*efflux*)

LDL binding to luminal plasmalemma or to the membrane of plasmalemmal vesicles, the two partners can affect each other's properties and interchange cholesterol. While LDL endocytosis seems to be receptor mediated, transcytosis has been shown to be largely receptor independent (VASILE et al. 1983, 1985; WIKLUND et al. 1985) or at least in part mediated by low-affinity binding sites (so far poorly characterized) (VASILE et al. 1983; SIMIONESCU and SIMIONESCU 1991a). It is assumed, but not yet proven, that a fraction of plasmalemmal vesicles can internalize LDL by fluid-phase endocytosis and deliver it to lysosomes (SIMIONESCU and SIMIONESCU 1991a). At present, there are insufficient data on the contribution of the normal artery walls to the plasma clearance of LDL, which is dominated ($\sim$ 70%–80%) by the liver receptor-mediated uptake. As an exception, a nonreceptor mechanism is predominant in receptor-deficient FH homozygotes and Watanabe heritable hyperlipidemic (WHHL) rabbits, in which virtually all plasma LDL are degraded in the liver and some extrahepatic tissues by a receptor-independent process (SPADY et al. 1987). Studies on human aortic tissue have shown that, considering the concentrations in plasma, infflux of cholesteryl ester from high-density lipoproteins (HDL) is greater than that from LDL (STENDER and HJELMS 1988). In vivo measurements in genetically hyperlipidemic rabbits suggest that at elevated plasma levels, the arterial influx of LDL, intermediate-density lipoprotein (IDL), and very low-density lipoprotein (VLDL) cholesterol is linearly dependent on plasma concentration, regardless of the lesion size (NORDESTGAARD et al. 1992).

2.2 Intramural LDL Metabolism and Interstitial Circulation

There is marked variation in the arterial wall permeability to LDL, as shown in normal rabbit (STEMERMAN et al. 1986) and squirrel monkey aorta (TOMPKINS et al. 1989). However, no consistent correlation could be established between the foci of high permeability and areas of inception of atherosclerotic lesions. The presence of LDL in the normal arterial intima was demonstrated immunohistochemically or biochemically. Studies on normal human aortas revealed that the LDL concentration in the intima is about twice as high as that in plasma and is freely diffusible, suggesting that lipoproteins are not complexed with components of the extracellular matrix (SMITH 1986; SMITH and STAPLES 1982). Intimal deposition of albumin is only a quarter of the plasma concentration. The amount of lipoprotein influx into the intima was found to be correlated with the plasma cholesterol level. No measurable quantities of LDL were detected in the media. Both cholesteryl ester hydrolysis and esterification of free cholesterol (BROWN et al. 1979) were demonstrated to occur in normal human aortic tissue (STENDER and HJELMS 1984; STEIN and STEIN 1973). The overall rates of irreversible LDL degradation in the normal rabbit aorta in vivo, assessed by radioiodinated thyramine cellobiose-labeled LDL, revealed that about 40% of all the degradation can be ascribed to a receptor-mediated process within the intima (presumably involving the endothelial cells). To a certain extent, smooth muscle cells of the media also may be involved in this process (STEINBERG et al. 1985).

Within the interstitial fluid of the normal human aortic wall, LDL, although displaying a slight decrease in its negative charge (SMITH and ASHALL 1983), circulates freely, unlike other plasma macromolecules such as fibronectin, which binds to extracellular matrix components (SMITH 1986). Thus, it appears that under normal conditions there is a very dynamic, continuous, and well-balanced flux of LDL into and out of the normal aortic wall, without significant "trapping" by extracellular matrix components.

2.3 LDL Efflux from the Artery Wall

Because of the technical difficulties involved in collecting samples of interstitial fluid from normal arteries, most of our knowledge about the interstitial fluid lipoproteins has derived from lymph collection studies. Emerging data reveal that all density classes of plasma lipoproteins, including LDL, are present in the lymph, and that they are generally more heterogeneous in size than their plasma counterparts. Although most information on cholesterol efflux and transfer has emerged from in culture studies, by extrapolation to other cell systems it may be assumed that within the artery wall the efflux of cholesterol can occur as (a) unesterified cholesterol (after intracellular de-esterification of the endocytosed cholesteryl esters), (b) cholesteryl ester, mediated by cholesteryl ester transfer protein (CETP), and/or (c) lipoprotein particles. Lymph LDL is enriched in free cholesterol; this is considered by some investigators an indication of either de novo formation and/or peripheral LDL modification, thus suggesting a possible role of LDL in reverse cholesterol transport (SLOOP et al. 1987). It has been shown that HDL (KHOO et al. 1990) and CETP might play an important role in promoting cholesteryl ester efflux from aortic interstitium in both normal and pathologic conditions (STEIN et al. 1985). Some investigators consider that in the "round trip" of cholesterol through the arterial intima, virtually the sole outbound carrier is HDL (KOVANEN 1990). According to KLEIN and RUDEL (1983), the primary effect of increased dietary cholesterol level in nonhuman primates is augmentation of the cholesteryl ester content of all lymph lipoproteins without an increase in a specific lipoprotein class. There are significant differences in the lymph/plasma ratio of lipoproteins among animal species (JULIEN et al. 1981) and among various tissues (e.g., the ratio is generally higher in cardiac lymph than in peripheral lymph). It has been speculated that the propensity of the coronary vessels to develop atherosclerosis may be a function of the concentration and composition of the interstitial lipoproteins as compared to their plasma counterparts. Although not trapped in the extracellular matrix, the lipoproteins, including LDL, undergo some modifications in the interstitia (faster electrophoretic mobility, decrease in net negative charge, etc.); thus it can be assumed that, as reflected by lymph, each interstitial compartment has a characteristic mixture of lipoproteins that can be altered by a high cholesterol diet in a fashion particular to each tissue (JULIEN et al. 1984). In atherogenesis, the lipid accumulation within the arterial or valvular wall can be expressed as an imbalance between the inflow and outflow of lipoproteins or their modified components, but this is only one parameter of a more complex multifactorial process.

3 The Prelesional Events in Atherogenesis: A Tentative General Picture

There is an almost general consensus that in certain laboratory animals diet-induced hypercholesterolemia can produce arterial lesions similar to some of those observed in humans (JOKINEN et al. 1985; WISSLER and VESSELINOVITCH 1977). The high levels of dietary fat used can generate accelerated hyperlipoproteinemic atherosclerosis (MAHLEY 1983; FAGGIOTO et al. 1984; SIMIONESCU et al. 1986; JORIS et al. 1983). A virtually identical lesion, but with slower development, can be produced in nonhuman primates by low-level hypercholesterolemia

(200–400 mg/dl—values closer to those found in humans) (MASUDA and ROSS 1990).

There is now substantial evidence, both in humans and from animal models, that the initiation of atherosclerosis does not require endothelial denudation or platelet involvement. The earliest cellular event so far reported has been the focal adherence of monocytes to arterial endothelium. Most of the present data on atherogenesis concern the modifications which follow the recruitment of the monocytes and their migration through the arterial endothelium ("*lesional stage*"). Very little is known on the subtle biochemical and ultrastructural changes which appear in the lesion-prone areas of the artery wall at the onset of atherosclerosis, before monocyte adhesion, i.e., during the "*prelesional stage*" (SIMIONESCU et al. 1986; for review see SIMIONESCU 1988, 1992b). In recent years, most of our work has been aimed at the characterization of the pathobiochemical changes which hypercholesterolemia induces in the arterial lesion-prone regions before detectable bona fide atherosclerotic lesions occur. As animal models, we have used fat-fed rabbits and hamsters in which the aortic arch and the aortic valve were examined at 4, 7, 14 and 30 days; in our experimental conditions, the first 2 weeks of diet corresponded to the prelesional stage. A spectrum of investigations have addressed such issues as: (a) changes in endothelial cell surface charge and chemistry, (b) modification in some endothelial biosynthetic activities, (c) changes in endothelial transport of lipoproteins, (d) detection of early intimal accumulation of lipoprotein-derived material, and (e) isolation and characterization of the intimal lipid deposits. The prelesional modifications detected were correlated with the results of plasma lipid analysis and with the subsequent monocyte emigration in the areas examined.

The results of our studies, corroborated by the findings of other investigators, may be tentatively collated to provide a general picture of what might be some of the chief events taking place at the earliest stages of hypercholesterolemic atherogenesis (or at least, the way it occurs in rabbits and hamsters). At present, our interpretation merely represents a working hypothesis that has been only partially substantiated by the factual evidence briefly presented later in this chapter.

Figure 2 is a diagrammatic representation of the main pathobiochemical events which hypercholesterolemia appears to induce in the arterial and valvular intima (some of the illustrated events have already been demonstrated; others remain to be proven). Although pronounced hypercholesterolemia is already present during the first 2 weeks of diet, it does not produce physical damage to endothelium, which appears morphologically intact with no significant changes in the luminal surface net electrical charge and general chemistry. No platelet adhesion to endothelium can be visualized. However, hypercholesterolemia seems to alter several functional activities of endothelial cells (ECs). The high concentrations of plasma LDL (hamster) or β-VLDL (rabbit) induce a concentration gradient that generates enhanced endothelial transport (especially transcytosis) of lipoproteins. Upon interaction with ECs (the exact site of action is unkown) or after arrival in the subendothelial compartment, lipoproteins are

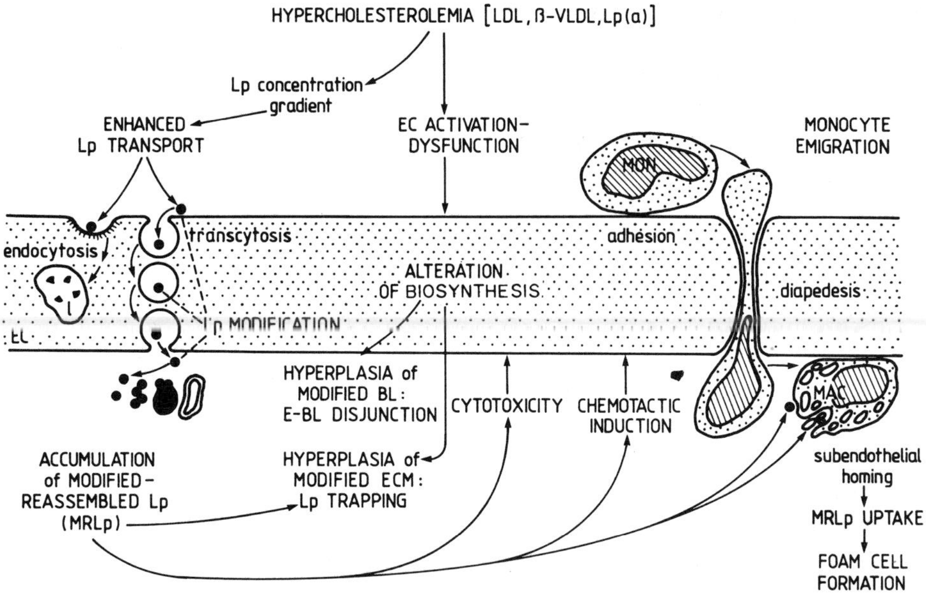

Fig. 2. Schematic illustration of a hypothetical sequence of the main pathobiochemical events occurring at the inception of the experimentally induced atherogenesis. Hypercholesterolemia generated by elevated levels of plasma LDL, *β*-VLDL, and/or Lp(a) is associated with a morphologically intact endothelium devoid of relevant changes in the general nonspecific chemistry of its surface; no adherent platelets are seen at this stage. Due to a concentration gradient, the transport of excess lipoproteins (*Lp*) is markedly enhanced. Some lipoprotein particles are endocytosed chiefly by a receptor-mediated mechanism involving coated pits and vesicles which deliver lipoproteins to the lysosomal compartment (*l*). A larger fraction of lipoprotein particles undergo nonspecific transcytosis via plasmalemmal vesicles and their transiently derived transendothelial channels. Lipoproteins are chemically modified presumably either at the EC surface, within transcytotic vesicles, or in a perturbed microenvironment of the subendothelial space and/or extracellular matrix. The physico-chemically altered lipoproteins undergo self-aggregation, fusion, and/or vesiculation, generating abnormal features (which were detected in vivo and in the lipid fractions extracted from aortic intima). Such modified and reassembled lipoproteins (*MRLp*) can appear as aggregated lipoproteins, fused micelles of lipoproteins, or vesiculated lipoproteins (extracellular liposomes). Concomitantly, ECs undergo activation and can enter a dysfunctional state expressed, among other ways, in alteration of some biosynthetic activities. These may be directly or indirectly responsible for prominent hyperplasia of modified basal lamina (*BL*) accompanied by EC-BL disjunction. Progressive hyperplasia and reorganization of a chemically modified extracellular matrix (*ECM*) appear to be at least in part involved in the local trapping of the MRLp. The latter generate both cytotoxic and chemotactic induction effects on ECs which produce chemoattractants for leukocytes (some of them specific for monocytes) and express, on luminal plasmalemma, newly induced monocyte adhesion molecules such as "ATHERO-ELAM." Following their adherence to ECs, recruited monocytes undergo transjunctional migration (diapedesis) followed by subendothelial homing. In this location, the activated macrophages ingest particulate or reassembled lipoproteins (via scavenger receptor or phagocytosis) and become foam cells

chemically modified. This is marked by lipid peroxidation, followed by particle self-aggregation, fusion, and/or vesiculation, leading to a progressive accumulation of modified and reassembled lipoproteins (MRLp). The formation and presence of the latter is associated with some local defence reactions.

At the same time, ECs gain some ultrastructural features of activation and there is dysfunction of several biosynthetic activities. Among the latter, a prominent alteration is expressed by the overproduction of successive layers of basal lamina-like material accompanied by large areas of endothelial–basal lamina disjunction. In parallel with the accumulation of MRLp and hyperplasic basal lamina, the proliferation of different components of the intimal extracellular matrix becomes increasingly obvious. As a result of these alterations in the composition and geometry of the arterial extracellular compartment, most of lipid deposits, complexed or not with elements of extracellular matrix, are eventually trapped, rendering the lipoprotein efflux much lower than the lipoprotein influx.

At this stage, ECs are concomitantly exposed to two injurious conditions: hypercholesterolemia, acting on their luminal front, and the MRLp with their soluble factors, acting on the abluminal front. The MRLp, present in large numbers, exert cytotoxic effects and cause indirect chemotactic induction. The luminal plasmalemma expresses newly induced, more or less specific, monocyte adhesion molecules. The latter mediate monocyte adhesion followed by transjunctional emigration, subendothelial homing, and activation as macrophages, which by taking up MRLp become foam cells. The evidence that partially backs up this possible sequence of events is presented in the following section.

4 Factual Evidence and Unanswered Questions

4.1 Hypercholesterolemia

Within the first 2 weeks of the cholesterol diet, corresponding to the prelesional stage of diet-induced hyperlipidemia, rabbit plasma cholesterol increased from ~40 mg/dl to 250–500 mg/dl, β-VLDL being the major cholesterol carrier (Simionescu et al. 1986; Mora et al. 1987, 1989). In the hamster, serum cholesterol, carried chiefly by LDL, almost doubled within 2–3 weeks following initiation of the diet (Nistor et al. 1987; Filip et al. 1987; Sima et al. 1990). The excess plasma cholesterol seems to be confined to native β-lipoproteins. Any oxidized lipoproteins generated within the plasma are very rapidly taken up and degraded in the liver, especially by the sinusoidal liver cells; thus, the half-life of oxidatively modified LDL in the circulation is extremely short (Henriksen et al. 1982; Nagelkerke et al. 1984). Plasma is endowed with a very potent antioxidant activity secured by several of its components. Such a natural defense system seems to be critically involved in preventing the free radical-mediated lipid peroxidation occurring in a large spectrum of disease states and aging (Frei et al. 1988). Moreover, the presence of the serum itself inhibits LDL oxidation in cell culture because of the natural antioxidant plasma molecules such as albumin, ceruloplasmin, and α-tocopherol (Halliwell 1987). In addition to liver, another important tissue potentially capable of degrading large amounts of native or oxidized LDL is vascular endothelium, the aggregate mass of which has been estimated at about 1 kg, almost equal to that of the liver. Given that (a) in vitro studies show that all cell types of the vessel walls (ECs, smooth muscle cells, and macrophages) are capable of oxidizing LDL (STEINBERG et al. 1989), and (b) oxidized LDL is detected in atherosclerotic lesions (HABERLAND et al. 1988; PALINSKI et al. 1989; YLA-HERTTUALA et al. 1989; ROSENFELD et al. 1990), it has been postulated that LDL oxidative modification takes place in the intima (STEINBERG et al. 1989). However, the site and mechanism(s) of such oxidation remain to be demonstrated, and several candidates currently can be envisaged, i.e. endothelial luminal plasmalemma, plasmalemmal vesicle membrane (during LDL transcytosis), and the subendothelial or another intimal microcompartment. As a methodological point, one should bear in mind the following two facts: (a) when using human LDL, preparations from different subjects have varying susceptibility to oxidative modification (JIALAL et al. 1991), and (b) the denser LDL subfractions, i.e., LDL_2 and LDL_3 (DE GRAAF et al. 1991) and the small, more electronegative LDL (AVOGARO et al. 1991) are more susceptible to oxidation than are the other subfractions.

4.2 Endothelium in the Prelesional Stage

During the first 2–3 weeks of experimental hypercholesterolemia, in both lesion-prone and non-lesion-prone areas the endothelial lining appeared morphologically intact and no adherent platelets could be detected (JORIS et al. 1983, 1984; SIMIONESCU et al. 1986; REIDY 1985; HANSSON and BONDJERS 1980). Our studies showed that in the prelesional stage, the endothelial luminal glycocalyx is very resistant to very high levels of plasma cholesterol; no relevant alterations were observed in the distribution and density of anionic, cationic, sialyl, and oligosaccharide moieties. The first detectable alterations in the general chemistry of the EC surface appear when monocytes begin to adhere to endothelium. However, more subtle changes even before that stage cannot be ruled out (GHINEA et al. 1987).

As hypercholesterolemia and intimal lipid deposition advance, atherosclerotic tendencies were associated with focal endothelial functional modifications such as increased thymidine uptake, enhanced permeability to plasma proteins, accumulation of IgG by ECs, and certain ultrastructural modifications, i.e., reduction in ruthenium red and concanavalin A binding, and increase in the number of plasmalemmal vesicles, transendothelial channels, and Weibel-Palade bodies (TRILLO and PRICHARD 1979; SCHWARTZ et al. 1991).

It has been shown that LDL incubation with cultured ECs, smooth muscle cells, or macrophages results in oxidative modification of LDL that renders them recognizable by the acetyl LDL or scavenger receptor (HENRIKSEN et al. 1982; QUINN et al. 1985; STEINBRECHER et al. 1984). The oxidized LDL or β-VLDL is toxic for cultured ECs (see Sect. 4.10), but the sites, and mechanism(s) of this effect in vivo are still unclear.

Through this physically intact endothelium, prior to the first wave of monocyte recruitment and migration, in the lesion-prone areas of the aortic arch and aortic valve, there is commonly an enhanced transport of lipoproteins that are progressively modified and accumulated in the intima, mostly as MRLp.

During all these prelesional events, EC properties and function pass from the stage of modulation to dysfunction, but only in advanced lesions may ECs show physical injury (SIMIONESCU 1992a).

4.3 Enhanced Transport of Lipoproteins

Substantial evidence is emerging from both in vitro and in vivo experiments that LDL and β-VLDL interactions with vascular endothelium are only to a limited extent comparable to those with fibroblasts, macrophages, smooth muscle cells, or hepatocytes. Because of their special position as a selective barrier between blood and surrounding tissues, ECs are endowed with a dual mechanism for monitoring and handling the circulating lipoproteins, i.e., endocytosis and transcytosis. These mechanisms operate both in normal and in hyperlipoproteinemic animals. Taking up lipoproteins by receptor-mediated endocytosis, ECs secure cholesterol for their own metabolic needs—a process common to most cells. In addition, ECs also transport the lipoprotein cholesterol to other cells by transcytosis, which is largely a receptor-independent or a low-affinity, nonsaturable process involving plasmalemmal vesicles (see Sect. 2.1). The transcytotic route is the same for LDL, β-VLDL, their oxidized forms, and apoprotein B alone. The process is an important means of monitoring excess plasma lipoproteins, as occur in the case of diet-induced hypercholesterolemia. In this abnormal condition, during the prelesional stage the lipoprotein transport pathways are the same as in control animals. During plaque development, lipoprotein influx and intimal deposition largely reflect the plasma lipoprotein composition (ROSENFELD et al. 1988). In advanced lesions, abnormal opening of endothelial junctions may add a connective passage, while in areas with endothelial denudation, the largely exposed subendothelial compartments may allow a mass influx of all plasma components (ROSS 1986; FAGGIOTTO et al. 1984; ROSENFELD et al. 1987). This may explain, at least in part, the higher number of native LDL particles, more or less modified, which can be extracted from advanced human atheroma.

Experiments of β-VLDL uptake and transport in normal and hypercholesterolemic rabbits (based on artery wall incorporation of dietary [^{3}H]cholesterol, or β-VLDL conjugates with ^{125}I, DiI, or gold) showed that in the early stages of hypercholesterolemia the main means of transport of β-VLDL is transcytosis by plasmalemmal vesicles, endocytosis being generally less pronounced [SIMIONESCU et al. 1986; VASILE et al. 1989). In general, the uptake and intimal deposition of lipoproteins are markedly enhanced in the aorta, coronary arteries, and cardiac valves of both hypercholesterolemic rabbits and hyperlipidemic hamsters

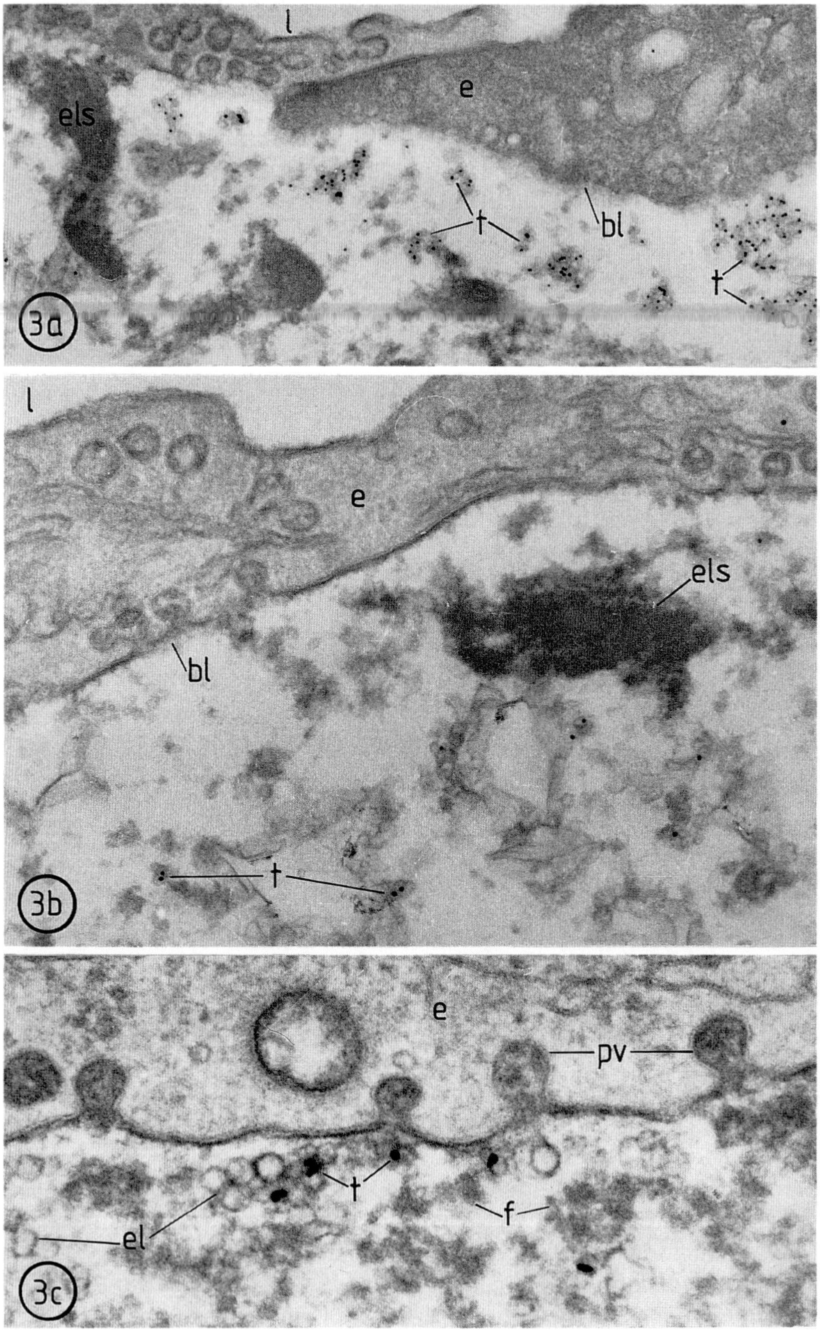
l
e
els
t
bl
t
3a
l
e
els
bl
t
3b
e
pv
t
el
f
3c

(Fig. 3). The extent of lipoprotein transport differs among various regions of aortic, coronary, and valvular intima (SIMIONESCU 1988; STEMERMAN et al. 1986).

Repeating the experimental models used by other investigators, SCHWENKE and CAREW (1989) confirmed that in cholesterol-fed rabbits the lesion-prone areas of the aortic arch showed an increased concentration of LDL up to 16 days after commencement of the diet.

In normal adult human intima, virtually all plasma macromolecules are present in relatively high concentrations (SMITH and STAPLES 1982). During the initial phases of atherogenesis, the protein composition of the human aortic intima shows alterations, the most predominant being in the concentrations of albumin α_1-antitrypsin, transferrin, and apolipoprotein A-I (STASTNY et al. 1986). Among plasma proteins, a special attention was focused on its major component albumin, endowed with multiple important functions including that of a very potent antioxidant. Experiments performed both in vivo and in vitro to measure the steady-state uptake of labeled albumin and chromium ethylenediamine-tetracetate by various blood vessels in the rabbit indicated that the walls of the pulmonary artery and the vena cava have much greater distribution volumes for albumin than do systemic arteries, including the aorta. These observations were considered to explain in part the differences between vessels in terms of their susceptibility to atherosclerosis (LEVER and JAY 1990). The antiatherogenic effect of calcium antagonists such as nicardipine and verapamil was ascribed to their capacity to increase the albumin uptake across the media without altering the overall endothelial permeability (TEDGUI et al. 1987). By protein A-gold immunocytochemistry it was demonstrated that under steady-state conditions, endogenous albumin is present in endothelial plasmalemmal vesicles and is unevenly distributed over the interstitial spaces of normal rat aorta, appearing preferentially associated with collagen fibers (LONDONO and BENDAYAN 1989). In hyperlipidemic rabbits, this heterogeneous distribution is generally maintained and pronounced (MORA et al., unpublished observations). Recently, LIN et al. (1990) have postulated that dying or dead ECs can make a significant contribution to local enhancement of aortic endothelial permeability. Studies with monoclonal antibodies have indicated that, while in human aortas fibrin (ogen) degradation products are not seen in early atherosclerotic lesions, increased fibrin formation and degradation do appear to be associated with progression of atheroma (BINI et al. 1989), being responsible for immobilization of LDL or Lp(a) in the extracellular matrix (SMITH 1990).

Lipoproteins which are endocytosed by ECs are subjected to degradation along a pathway and by a mechanism similar to that described in other cell

Fig. 3a–c. Intimal accumulation of LDL-gold conjugate perfused through the aorta of a hyperlipidemic hamster at 3 weeks of cholesterol-rich diet. After 10 min of perfusion, tracer particles (*t*) can be seen in high concentration in the subendothelium of the aortic arch, with a tendency to form aggregates (**a**) or associated with fibrillar material (**b**). In coronary artery, the tracer particles appear associated with extracellular liposomes (*el*) and fibrillar material (*f*) of the subendothelial space. *bl*, basal lamina; *l*, lumen; *e*, endothelial cell; *els*, elastic elements; *pv*, plasmalemmal vesicles. **a** × 50000; **b** × 76500; **c** × 113000

types, endothelium being a major site for LDL hydrolysis and cholesterol esterification in the artery wall (STEINBERG et al. 1985). In early hypercholesterolemia, ECs may begin to display lipid deposits the number of which can increase markedly in more advanced lesions, so that ECs may be transformed into true foam cells (LUPU et al. 1987; SIMIONESCU 1988, 1992b). At later stages, these endothelial foam cells can detach from their basal lamina, exposing the subendothelial structures. Lipid accumulation is particularly rapid and prominent in the endothelium of the aortic valve of hypercholesterolemic hamsters.

4.4 Modification of β-Lipoproteins

It is still unknown whether, during transcytosis, lipoproteins undergo chemical modifications by direct interaction with either EC luminal plasma membrane or with some enzymatic machinery (as yet unidentified) of the plasmalemmal vesicle membrane, which reportedly has a different chemistry to the plasmalemma proper (SIMIONESCU and SIMIONESCU 1991a, b). When detected in the intima of hyperlipidemic animals, transcytosed lipoproteins are to a large extent modified and reassembled, and until new data become available it is to be considered that modification of lipoproteins, including their lipid peroxidation, takes place in the intima (STEINBERG et al. 1989).

There are numerous reports that under culture conditions ECs can induce relevant modifications of β-lipoproteins, characteristically associated with the formation of lipid peroxides: increased negative charge and buoyant density, decreased content of cholesterol and phospholipids, and fragmentation of apolipoprotein B. Similar alterations may be produced in a cell-free system by incubating LDL with high concentrations of Cu^{2+} or Fe^{3+}. In vitro oxidation can be produced to both LDL and β-VLDL (PARTHASARATHY et al. 1989). Such modifications are inhibited by antioxidants (MOREL et al. 1984; PARTHASARATHY et al. 1985, 1989). The oxidized LDL is taken up by the acetyl-LDL receptor of macrophages up to tenfold more avidly than native LDL (STEINBRECHER et al. 1984; PARTHASARATHY et al. 1985). Monocytes and neutrophils in vitro can also oxidize LDL, making it cytotoxic (CATHCART et al. 1985).

Exposure of freshly prepared LDL to an oxygen-saturated buffer (ESTERBAUER et al. 1987) or directly to air (MORA et al., unpublished observations) leads to loss of polyunsaturated fatty acids and the generation of malondialdehyde or 4-hydroxynonenal (ESTERBAUER et al. 1987), as well as increased amounts of lysophosphatidylcholine (ZHANG et al. 1989).

Since LDL oxidation seems to be a prerequisite for macrophage uptake of the excess lipoproteins transcytosed in the intima, one cannot conclude that there is a strict causative relation between atherogenesis and LDL modification—such a process may be just a component of a complex local defense mechanism of the vessel wall. Factors other than lipid peroxidation may also play a crucial role in atherogenesis and its complications (WITZTUM and STEINBERG

1991). Once they are accumulated within the subendothelial compartments, oxidized LDL and the various forms taken in vivo by the MRLp can exert a dual effect: (a) by virtue of their cytotoxicity they can alter the overlying endothelium, and (b) by inducing chemoattractant production by ECs and smooth muscle cells, they can have a beneficial effect. A number of other modifications can convert LDL to forms taken up more extensively and rapidly by macrophages and foam cells; among these modifications are self-aggregation, formation of complexes (with proteoglycans, elastin, collagens, fibrin, immune complexes, and heparin), and nonenzymatic glycation of apolipoprotein B.

Unlike LDL, β-VLDL can be ingested by macrophages to generate foam cells even in the absence of any modification.

4.5 Intimal Accumulation of Modified and Reassembled Lipoproteins

4.5.1 In Vivo Observations

To determine the state of lipoproteins transcytosed in the intima during the prelesional stages, we examined the lesion-prone areas of the aortic arch and cardiac and aortic valves in hamsters and rabbits fed for 1–2 weeks with a cholesterol-rich diet. While no relevant lesions could be detected at this early period, at the ultrastructural level we observed a progressive deposition of extracellular heterogeneous lipid material appearing as monomeric Lp (MLp) in the size range of LDL and VLDL, aggregated Lp (ALp), fused Lp (FLp) in the form of micelles of compact lipid droplets, or vesiculated Lp (VLp) (Fig. 4). The last-mentioned (100–300 nm in diameter) were called "extracellular liposomes" (ELs) (SIMIONESCU et al. 1986) and were shown to consist chiefly of phospholipid lamellae (one or more concentric layers). As demonstrated by incubation with filipin followed by freeze-fracture, ELs are rich in unesterified cholesterol (SIMIONESCU et al. 1986; FILIP et al. 1987) and display on their outer contour immunoreactive apolipoprotein B (MORA et al. 1987, 1989). The accumulation of these MRLp started very rapidly (within 3–4 days of commencement of the diet) on the arterial aspect of the cardiac valves and was prominent on the inner lesser curvature of the aortic arch after 7 days of diet. Commonly, the most visible were lipid droplets (FLp) and vesicles (VLp), whose appearance in the subendothelium was concurrent with the proliferation of successive layers of basal lamina-like material (Figs. 4, 5). In deeper regions of the intima, one could detect a progressive proliferation of microfibrils, elastin bundles, collagen, and proteoglycans [visualized with safranin O, ruthenium red, or cuprolinic blue (as described by SIMIONESCU et al. 1989)]. At this early stage of atherogenesis, MRLp deposition occurred in cell-free subendothelial zones devoid of signs of cellular lysis.

In tissue fragments reacted successively with an anti-apolipoprotein B–horseradish peroxidase (anti-apo B-HRP) conjugate and tomatin (reportedly

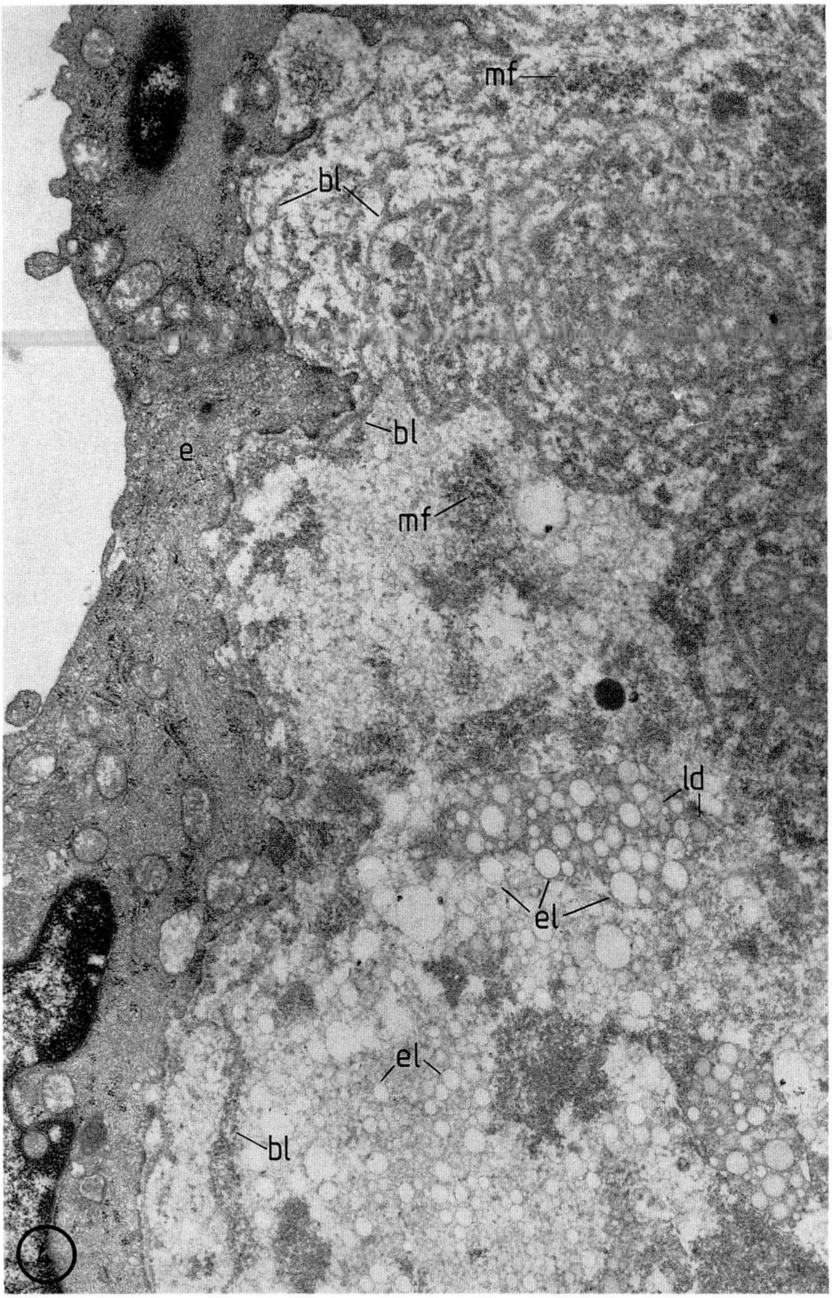

Fig. 4. Arterial region of the aortic valve of a hamster fed a cholesterol-rich diet for 4 days. Beneath a morphologically intact endothelium (*e*), a cell-free intima displays substantial extracellular accumulation of lipidic material appearing mostly as compact lipid droplets (*ld*) or extracellular liposomes (*el*) interspersed with proliferated basal lamina-like material (*bl*) and groups of proliferated microfibrils (*mf*). × 21 000

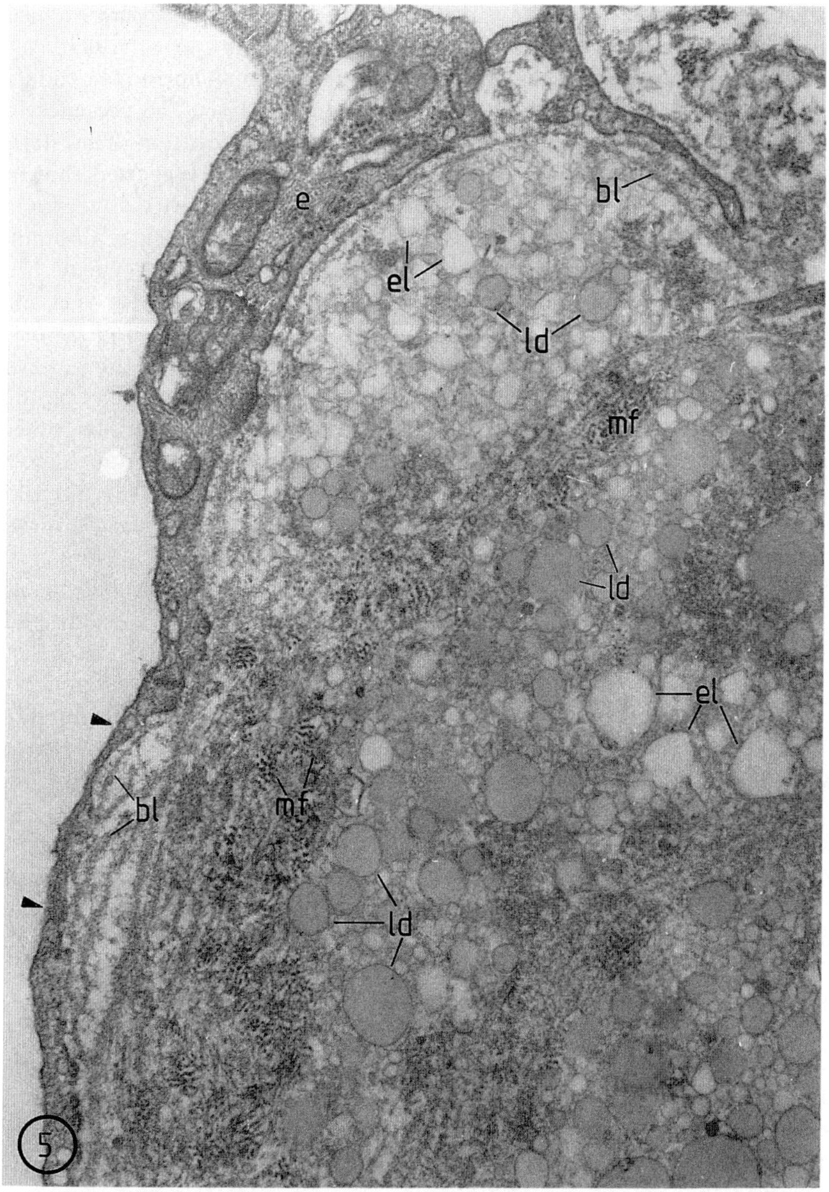

Fig. 5. Region similar to that in Fig. 4, but collected from an animal that had been on a fat-rich diet for 2 weeks. Note an intact, continuous endothelium (*e*) but with areas of visible attenuation (*arrowheads*). In subendothelial intima, there is characteristic extracellular accumulation of MRLp, mostly present as compact lipid droplets (*ld*) and extracellular liposomes (*el*) organized in clusters or alternating with hyperplasic basal lamina (*bl*) or bundles of proliferated microfibrils (*mf*). Specimen prepared by the osmium–tannic acid–paraphenylenediamine technique (see Sects. 4.5.1.1 and 4.5.1.2). × 25 300

specific for free cholesterol), we have demonstrated that apo B and unesterified cholesterol colocalize in close association with EL (MORA et al. 1987). We examined specimens of intimal regions containing a serous–fibrinous exudate that had been incubated with tomatin and anti-apo B-HRP. The presence in these areas of characteristic tomatin spicules (indicating the location of unesterified cholesterol) and the absence of apo B reaction product suggested that in such zones the unesterified cholesterol may have been transported by carriers other than lipoproteins; the most probable candidate for such a role is albumin, which is known to have the capability to carry cholesterol and which has recently been detected immunocytochemically in such areas (MORA et al., unpublished observations). Vesicle-like features similar to ELs have been reported previously and are usually considered the result of cellular lysis (for review, see SIMIONESCU 1988). We assume that the prelesional EL deposits may be the ultrastructural equivalent of the filipin-positive particles visualized by other investigators by fluorescence microscopy (KRUTH 1984). Apo B and apo A have been visualized in human aortic fibrinoid lesions (BOCAN et al. 1988) and apo B fragments have been shown to mediate the LDL interactions with arterial proteoglycans (CAMEJO et al. 1988).

The existence in vivo, in early stages of atherogenesis, of various forms of MRLp raises questions as to the atherogenicity of each class of these altered lipoproteins. These questions concern the degree of oxidation and/or other physicochemical modifications, the formation of complexes with different components of the extracellular matrix, cytotoxicity, chemotactic induction, uptake by macrophages, smooth muscle cells, and ECs, etc. Although incomplete, there is growing information on each of the forms of MRLp.

4.5.1.1 Aggregated Lipoproteins (*ALp*). Incubation of human plasma LDL with phosphatidylcholine vesicles resulted in particle aggregation and formation of vesicles. Pretreatment of LDL with trypsin prevented aggregate formation, indicating the participation of apolipoprotein B in this process (HUNTER et al. 1982). LDL subjected to brief (30 s) vortexing at room temperature form self-aggregates that are rapidly ingested (by phagocytosis or by LDL receptor) by macrophages which become cholesteryl ester-rich foam cells (KHOO et al. 1988). A similar effect could be obtained by incubating LDL with phospholipase C (SUITS et al. 1989); the aggregation could be inhibited by addition of HDL or apolipoproteins A-I only (KHOO et al. 1990). In an elegant study using ultrarapid freezing and rotary shadow freeze-etching, FRANK and FOGELMAN (1989) showed that in cell-free aortic regions of the WHHL rabbit and after only 10 days of cholesterol feeding, lipoprotein-derived clusters of vesicles appeared enmeshed in the network of extracellular matrix. In a similar inquiry employing deep-etching and immunocytochemistry on ultrarapidly frozen rabbit aortic tissue, it was demonstrated that clustering and interaction with extracellular matrix of LDL-size particles occurred in the intima within 2 h after bolus infusion of LDL (NIEVELSTEIN et al. 1991). Electron microscopic examination using alternatively the osmium–tannic acid–paraphenylenediamine (TA–PDA) and osmium–thiocarbohydrazide–osmium (OTO) techniques revealed that aggregation of LDL by vortexing or prolonged storage results in the formation of droplets and vesicles (GUYTON et al. 1991). It was also shown that both oxidized LDL and LDL extracted from human atherosclerotic plaques have a marked tendency to form aggregates, leading to enhanced phagocytosis and degradation by macrophages (HOFF and O'NEIL 1991).

4.5.1.2 Fused Lipoproteins (*FLp*). As discussed above, LDL self-aggregation in vitro is frequently associated with particle fusion and the formation of compact lipid droplets. In vivo, lipoprotein-derived droplets have frequently been observed both at the prelesional stage (SIMIONESCU 1988, 1992b) and in atherosclerotic lesions (GUYTON and his collaborators, using the TA–PDA or OTO techniques). The latter procedures indicated that unlike vesicles [formed mainly by phospholipids and unesterified cholesterol (SIMIONESCU et al. 1986)], lipid droplets contain in their core neutral lipids, i.e., cholesteryl ester (GUYTON and KLEMP 1988, 1989). The same laboratory demonstrated that in human aortic fibrolipid lesions, the lipid deposits of the core region of the fibrous plaques are almost entirely extracellular (GUYTON et al. 1990).

4.5.1.3 Vesiculated Lipoproteins (*VLp*). Under this term, we understand those fused LDL or β-VLDL which have become vesicles, either directly or after passing through a stage of compact lipid droplet, a likely process that is not yet proven. In the prelesional stage of atherogenesis, the presence of extracellular uni- or multilamellar, 100- to 300-nm phospholipid vesicles rich in unesterified cholesterol was first described in the aortic arch and aortic valve of hypercholesterolemic rabbits (SIMIONESCU et al. 1986). Similar structures have also been identified in the aorta of WHHL or cholesterol-fed rabbits, either by standard electron microscopy (ROSENFELD et al. 1987) or by rapid freezing and freeze-etching (AMANUMA et al. 1986; TAKANO and MINEO 1990; FRANK and FOGELMAN 1989; NIEVELSTEIN et al. 1991; MASUDA and ROSS 1990). Extracellular liposome-like structures appear very early after LDL infusion (NIEVELSTEIN et al. 1991) during high-level as well as low-level hypercholesterolemia in nonhuman primates (MASUDA and ROSS 1990). Similar lipid deposits have also been found in atherosclerotic human aortas (GUYTON et al. 1990; CHAO et al. 1990). Abnormal human serum lipoproteins appearing as flattened lamellar vesicles have been reported in cholestasis (HAMILTON et al. 1971).

Recently, by electron microscopic examination of human aortas that were grossly normal or showed minimal intimal thickening and had been taken from yound individuals killed in accidents, we identified the subendothelial presence of lipid droplets and extracellular liposomes morphologically identical to those discovered in hypercholesterolemic rabbits and hamsters (TIRZIU et al., manuscript in preparation). These novel findings revealed that: (a) at least some of the so-called intimal thickening is not produced initially by smooth muscle proliferation but rather by concurrent hyperplasia of the extracellular matrix and deposition of MRLp, especially lipid droplets and extracellular liposomes; and

(b) there is a close resemblance between the features that arise during the prelesional stage in the lesion-prone aortic and valvular areas in cholesterol-fed rabbits and those observed in human aortas appearing grossly normal or with minimal intimal thickening, suggesting, at least for some cases, similar atherogenic mechanisms and processes.

4.5.2 Isolation and Characterization of Lipid Deposits Extracted from Rabbit and Human Aortas in the Prelesional Stage of Atherogenesis

Several laboratories have succeeded in isolating and partially characterizing the lipid phases of advanced human or animal atherosclerotic lesions. The focus of these studies has chiefly been to define the chemical modifications of the extracted aortic β-lipoproteins (HOFF and GAUBATZ 1982; HOFF and MORTON 1985; HOLLANDER et al. 1979; KATZ and SMALL 1980; MORTON et al. 1986; SHAIKH et al. 1988; ROSENFELD et al. 1988; SMITH and STAPLES 1980; CHAO et al. 1990). Isolation and chemical analysis of lesion-free aortic tissue from children and adults have also been concentrated on the immunologic characterization of apolipoproteins B and E and their interactions with intimal glycosaminoglycans (YLA-HERTTUALA et al. 1987, 1988).

Extraction and characterization of lipid deposits from early, prelesional stages of atherogenesis have not been reported so far. Recently, we have developed a four-step procedure for the isolation, purification, and chemical analysis of MRLp from the aortas of cholesterol-fed rabbits at the prelesional (2 weeks) and lesional (16 weeks of diet) stages of atherogenesis (MORA et al. 1990). Briefly, isotonic saline extracts of aortic intima were subjected to gel filtration followed by density gradient ultracentrifugation to obtain a crude MRLp-enriched fraction which also contained albumin. The particulate β-lipoprotein and apo B fragments were removed by affinity chromatography on an anti-apo B–Sepharose column, and albumin was retained on an anti-albumin–Sepharose immunoadsorbent. The final purified fraction consisted of extracellular liposomes (ELs) (or "vesiculated lipoproteins"). Each step of the procedure was monitored by negative staining and assays for lipids, lipid peroxides (expressed as thiobarbituric acid reactive substances), protein (SDS-PAGE, electroblotting, autoradiography), and uronic acid. The results showed that, compared to serum LDL and β-VLDL, the crude MRLp fraction was characterized by a higher relative percentage mass of unesterified cholesterol, phospholipids, apo B, and albumin. These differences were more pronounced in the lesional stage. The purified EL fraction contained almost exclusively (~97%) unesterified cholesterol and phospholipids and only small traces (~3%) of cholesteryl esters, triglycerides, and (unexpectedly) albumin. Since the albumin was not adsorbed on the anti-albumin column, we subjected aliquots of the purified EL fraction to delipidation or pronase digestion followed by dot-blot immunolabeling and autoradiography which revealed that albumin was located within the aqueous core of ELs. Lipid peroxides were present in relatively high amounts in the crude MRLp fraction, from which they eluted mainly with the immunoadsorbed β-lipoproteins.

Lipid deposits isolated from human aortas that were grossly normal or showed minimal intimal thickening were purified and analyzed using the same four-step procedure as described above for rabbit aorta (TIRZIU et al., manuscript in preparation). Two liposome-enriched fractions were separated: one consisting mostly of multilamellar liposomes (EL_1) and another represented chiefly by unilamellar liposomes (EL_2). As compared with human serum LDL, the esterified/unesterified cholesterol ratio was ~15 times lower for the EL_2 fraction and 6 times lower for the EL_1 fraction.

These observations indicate that in both experimental animals and humans, MRLp represent chemically altered lipoproteins reassembled extracellularly. The vesiculated forms of these MRLp (ELs) carry the attestor of two local defense reactions: (a) the reputedly sclerogenic cholesterol (ADAMS and MORGAN 1967) is rendered inoffensive by reassembly into a phospholipid lamellar liquid crystalline phase (SMALL and SHIPLEY 1974; SIMIONESCU et al. 1986), and (b) in their core the ELs trap albumin, a potent natural antioxidant (HALLIWELL 1988; PIRISINO et al. 1988), presumably upon interaction with lysophosphatidylcholine produced by lipid peroxidation (KUMAR et al. 1989).

4.5.3 In Vitro Formation of Oxidatively Modified and Reassembled Lipoproteins

To explore in more depth the molecular mechanisms involved in the formation, interactions, and atherogenic properties of each form of MRLp detected in vivo, we tried to reproduce such altered lipoproteins in vitro.

Native, freshly isolated human LDL (d = 1.019–1.063 g/l) were subjected to oxidative conditions by maintaining the probes in loosely capped glass tubes in the dark at 37°C in the absence or presence of 5 μM copper ions, for time intervals varying from 24 to 96 h. The presence and relative proportions of different forms of MRLp, e.g., ALp, FLp, VLp, and MLp, were determined by examination of negatively stained probes in electron microscopy (Fig. 6). The appearance of MRLp was paralleled by extensive peroxidation (expressed as thiobarbituric acid reactive substances), lipid peroxide formation, progressive degradation of apo B, and modification of the lipid moiety of lipoproteins. After 96 h of peroxidation, a mixture containing all the major types of MRLp was obtained. This was subjected to centrifugation at 12000 *g* for 30 min; the pellet containing ALp was analyzed by negative staining and assessed for lipid and protein composition. On SDS-PAGE, ALp revealed high-molecular-weight components which could not penetrate the 5% gel. Supernatant was subsequently separated either by FPLC chromatography or affinity chromatography on an anti-apo B column; after elution, the retained fraction contained a homogeneous population of monomeric LDL-like particles. The unretained fraction was a mixture of compact lipid droplets (composed of FLp), 40- to 100-nm

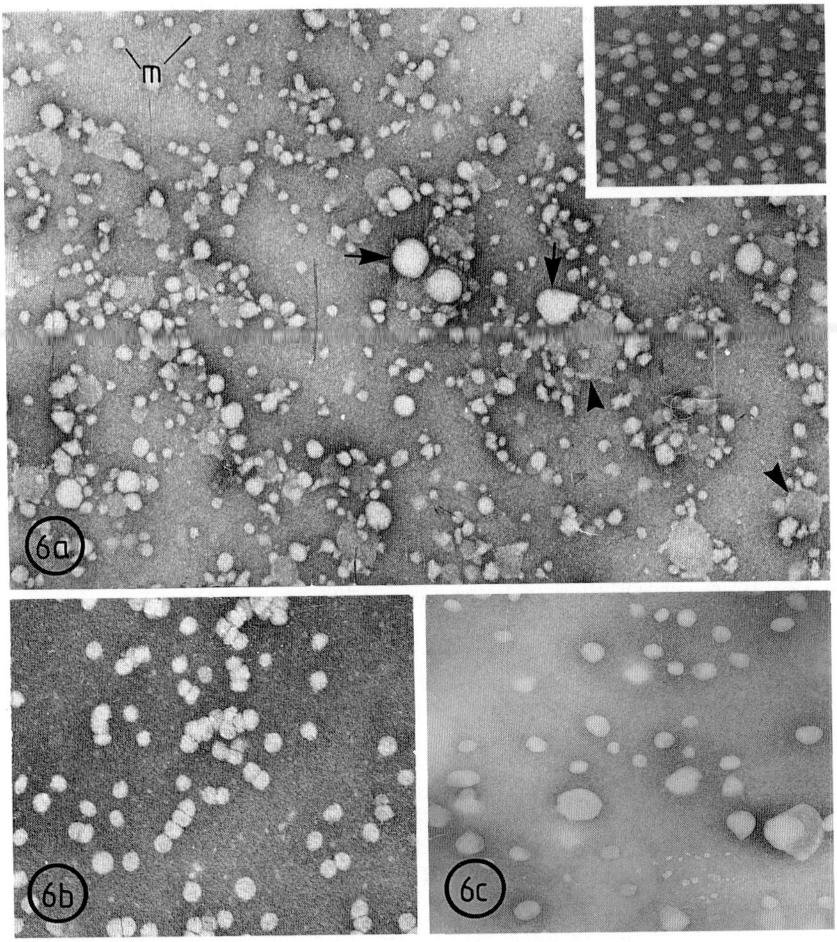

Fig. 6a–c. Electron micrographs of negatively stained MRLp. **a** Human LDL after 96 h of incubation at 37°C in the presence of 5 μM $CuSO_4$; the presence of fused lipoproteins (FLp) (arrows), vesiculated particles (VLp) (*arrowhead*), and monomeric LDL particles (MLp; *m*) can be observed. *Insert* represents native, freshly isolated LDL. **b** MLp, slightly aggregated, separated from the incubation mixture by affinity chromatography on an anti-apo B column. **c** The FLp-enriched fraction after the three-step purification procedure; the seperated particles were 40–110 nm in size. **a,c** × 74 000; *insert*, × 93 000; **b** × 94 000

liposome-like vesicles (VLp), and a small number of monomeric particles. Finally, this fraction was subjected to density gradient ultracentrifugation at 150 000 *g* for 6 h: two bands were collected, one at d < 1.012 g/ml (containing mostly FLp), and the other at d = 1.012–1.019 g/ml (corresponding to the VLp-enriched fraction). After oxidation, as a result of apo B degradation the monomeric particles displayed high-molecular-weight bands which cross-reacted with the anti-apo B column. The FLp as well as the VLp-enriched fractions also showed a fragmented apo B pattern with a major band of 69 kDa.

The cholesterol/protein ratio was increased in the VLp, FLp, and MLp fractions and markedly decreased in the ALp fraction. The unesterified cholesterol content was augmented especially in the VLp fraction, while the cholesteryl ester content was increased in samples containing ALp. The atherogenic properties of each class of MRLp which appear during in vitro peroxidation of lipoproteins are under investigation.

4.6 Endothelial Cell Activation and Dysfunction

While the involvement of endothelium in atherogenesis has been recognized since the time of Rokitansky and Virchow, its complexity—including the elaborate mechanisms through which ECs may react to an altered plasma composition such as occurs in hypercholesterolemia—has only recently been appreciated. Put in a very simplified manner, one can consider that vascular endothelium responds to an abnormal stimulus such as elevated levels of plasma β-lipoproteins by adjusting, within a physiologic range, its constitutive functions (e.g., permeability, maintenance of nonthrombogenic surface, biosynthesis, integration and transduction of blood-borne signals, regulation of vascular tone, and metabolism of vasoactive mediators and hormones). During this process and the stage of modulation there are no significant perturbations in EC structures and interactions with blood cells (SIMIONESCU 1992a). The following can be considered expressions of such functional modulation: enhanced transport of the excess plasma β-lipoproteins, increased secretion of prostacyclin and endothelial-derived relaxing factor (EDRF), and endothelial adaptation according to modification of blood flow parameters (ZAND et al. 1988; MAJNO et al. 1988). In physiopathologic and clinical terms, there is no clear delimitation between endothelial modulation and dysfunction. The latter, when expressed as an impaired ability to produce EDRF, was considered to be significantly linked to coronary disease by HEALEY (1990).

Extended endothelial exposure to hyperbetalipoproteinemia may affect the expression of some constitutive functions or may induce new properties reflected in perturbed cell activities and interactions. Such a dysfunction appears as a localized alteration of endothelium brought up temporarily to a nonadaptive functional state bearing on a reversible phenotypic change (GIMBRONE and BEVILACQUA 1988; GIMBRONE 1989; GORDON and PEARSON 1982; SIMIONESCU 1992a). Endothelial dysfunction is commonly associated with the increased production of cytokines, especially interleukin-1, and tissue necrotic factor (CAVENDER et al. 1989). An example of dysfunction is "endothelial activation", a term extrapolated from comparable macrophage and lymphocyte activation. Endothelial activation, which has been demonstrated both in vitro and in vivo (COTRAN and POBER 1988), has a morphologic correlate in hypertrophic cuboidal cells with large ovoid nuclei and increased copies of organelles involved in biosynthesis (COTRAN et al. 1989). The concept of EC activation has been seminal for cardiovascular research, although further characterization of both the stimuli responsible and the signal transduction mechanisms is required, as is quantitation of the resulting phenotype (RYAN 1987).

Prolonged and excessive adverse influences of hypercholesterolemia, concurrent with the cytotoxic effects produced by the subendothelial MRLp, may result in physical damage of ECs overlying an advanced fatty streak or fibrolipid plaque; such damage characterizes an "*injury*" (SIMIONESCU 1992a). Some authors use the term *injury* in a broader sense that includes the whole spectrum of endothelial perturbations from functional to structural alterations leading eventually to endothelial denudation (ROSS 1986). In hypercholesterolemia, EC injury may be final or reversible, either through a repair process taking place within the damaged cell or by its replacement by local nondenuding regeneration of the endothelial lining (REIDY 1985).

4.7 Alteration of Biosynthetic Activities

During its modulation or dysfunctional state, vascular endothelium can undergo significant changes in the nature and quantity of its constitutive secretory products or, under appropriate stimuli, can acquire the capability to express newly induced molecules (the latter will be discussed in Sect. 4.12).

Like all other cells involved in the development of atherosclerotic lesions, ECs have the capacity to produce growth-regulatory molecules which can stimulate or inhibit the proliferation and activity of each of the cells located in the forming plaque. Mediated by cytokines, ECs can express a surface-associated tissue factor-like procoagulant activity and also secrete interleukin-1 and tumor necrosis factor (TNF), while an increased production of plasminogen activator inhibitor parallels the decrease in the production of tissue plasminogen activator (GIMBRONE 1989). Transforming growth factor beta (TGF-β) can act as a potent inhibitor of EC proliferation, while the fibroblast growth factors, both acidic and basic, are endothelial mitogens (ROSS 1992).

Work in our laboratory demonstrated that cultured bovine ECs incubated with either native β-VLDL or acetyl-β-VLDL or with hydroxynonenal showed modified production of prostacyclin: its production was stimulated by the native β-VLDL and inhibited by acetyl-β-VLDL and hydroxynonenal, probably due to their lipid peroxides. Native β-VLDL can also increase the thromboxane A_2 production (TASCA et al., unpublished observations). In the intimal areas rich in MRLp, the overlying ECs are frequently hypertrophic with elaborate rough and smooth endoplasmic reticulum, a well-developed perinuclear Golgi complex, and relatively large vacuoles containing an amorphous material. This shift to a secretory phenotype resembles the activated ECs described in immune reactions and inflammation (COTRAN et al. 1989). The ultrastructural modulations of ECs in lesion-prone areas usually coexist with a remarkable hyperplasia of basal lamina-like material.

4.8 Hyperplasia of Modified Basal Lamina: Endothelial–Basal Lamina Disjunction

Starting as early as 3–4 days after commencement of a fat-rich diet, the lesion-prone areas of the cardiac aortic valve (the arterial aspect) and aortic arch (inner lesser curvature) become the site of progressive accumulation of successive layers of basal lamina-like material. As seen especially often in the hamster cardiac and aortic valves, a fibrillar network composed of as many as 15–20 layers is thereby formed (Fig. 7). Frequently, extracellular liposomes and lipid droplets are interspersed between these hyperplastic layers of basal lamina (HAJJAR et al. 1980; SIMIONESCU et al. 1986, 1990). One salient feature is the extensive detachment of the innermost basal lamina layer from the abluminal front of

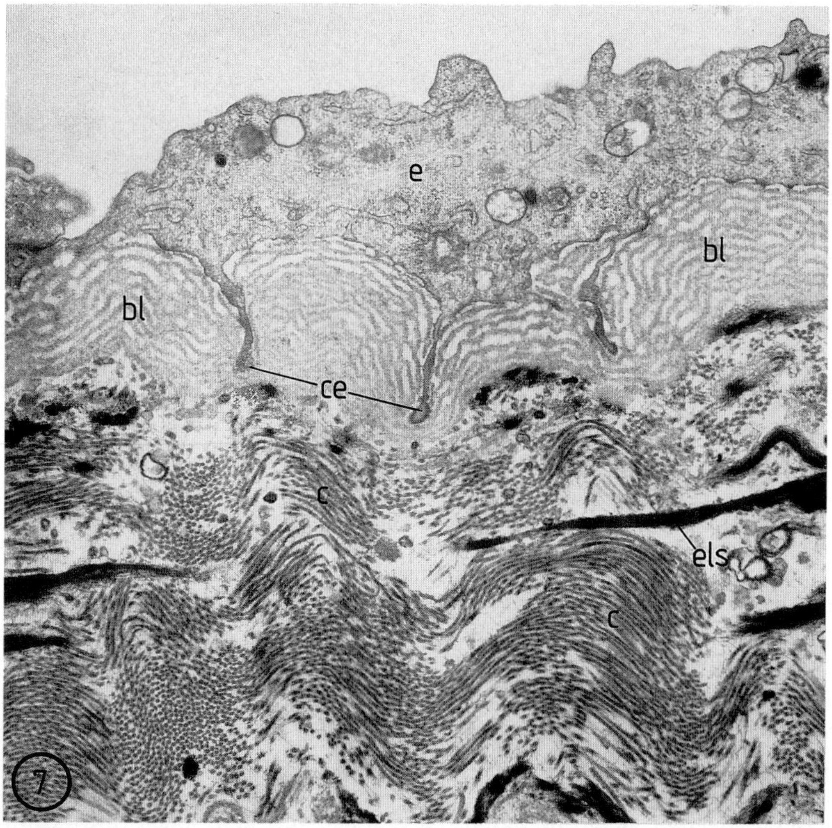

Fig. 7. Aortic valve (arterial region) of a hamster that had been on a fat-rich diet for 7 days. Area with pronounced hyperplasia of basal lamina-like material (*bl*) display up to ten superimposed and partially anastomosed layers. The laminae are separated in subzones by abluminal cytoplasmic extensions (*ce*) of ECs (*e*) apparently rich in cytoskeletal elements. In the deeper regions, bundles of proliferated collagens (*c*) and elastin (*els*) are present. × 14 800

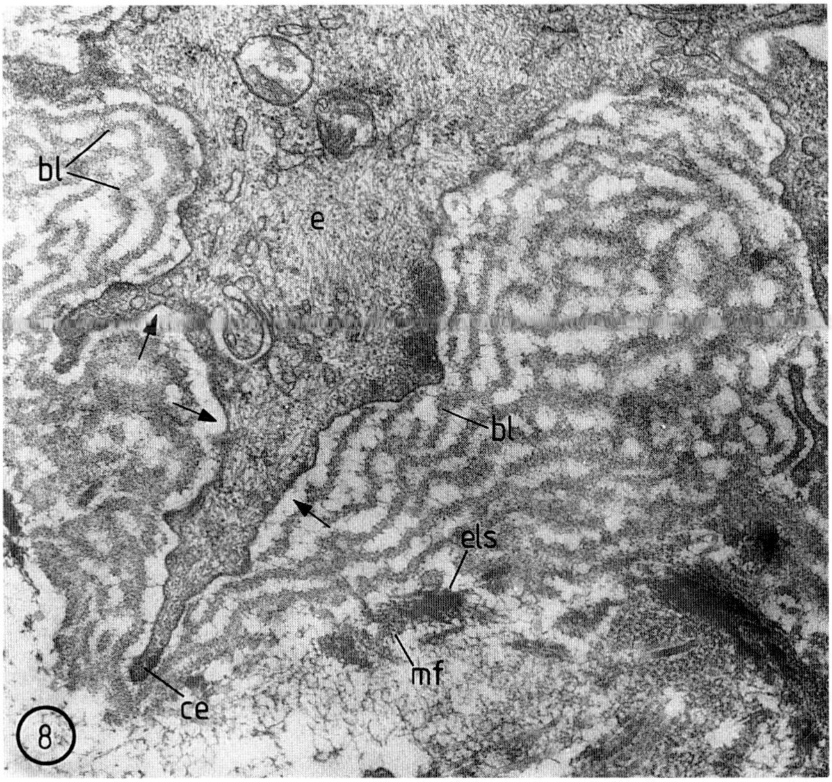

Fig. 8. A detail from a region similar to that in Fig. 7, showing zones of endothelial-basal lamina disjunction (*arrows*). *e*, endothelium; *bl*, basal laminae; *ce*, endothelial cytoplasmic extension, *mf*, microfibrils; *els*, elastin. × 25 300

endothelium, on which only rare spots of attachment can be seen. At their level, ECs extend tiny pseudopods with a condensed bundle of microfilaments (Fig. 8). The endothelial–basal lamina disjunction is marked by regions of apparently edematous subendothelial space. Sometimes even this space can display small lipid droplets and/or extracellular liposomes. Often the ECs overlying intimal regions with hyperplastic basal lamina show features of secretory shift. It is still unknown whether the excessive production of basal lamina is associated with significant qualitative alterations in its chemistry. It has recently been shown that in cultured porcine aortic ECs, high levels of LDL decrease basement membrane-associated heparan sulfate proteoglycans and affect fibronectin synthesis only slightly (OLGEMOLLER et al. 1990). Given their crucial role in the cell–matrix attachment, study of the state of abluminal endothelial integrins at sites of endothelial–basal lamina disjunction may elucidate the molecular mechanism responsible for this altered EC–extracellular matrix interaction.

4.9 Hyperplasia of Modified Extracellular Matrix: Trapping of Modified and Reassembled Lipoproteins

In this context, we understand by extracellular matrix the macromolecular complexes that form the intercellular mass of the vessel wall beyond the basal lamina, which in a broader sense can be considered part of the extracellular matrix. The components of these assemblies are synthesized by ECs and smooth muscle cells which also produce their own basal lamina. Some constituents of the types found in extracellular matrix (e.g., proteoglycans) are also associated with the luminal EC surface, where they are directly involved in important functions such as permeability, lipid metabolism, hemostasis, and thrombosis. Extracellular matrix is percolated by the interstitial fluid.

In our experiments, hypercholesterolemia is associated at a very early stage with hyperplasia of modified intimal extracellular matrix, generating a dense and chemically altered three-dimensional network of elements. This network comprises safranin O-positive and cuprolinic blue-positive fibers, compact bundles of banded collagens, and areas with a high density of microfibrils which alternate with irregular elastin elements difficult to identify as reflecting either elastogenesis or elastolysis. Some restricted areas may contain distinct zones of a serofibrinous insudate. Regions with an altered extracellular matrix are very often the site for MRLp in which heteromorphic large lipid droplets and extracellular liposomes appear trapped and linked to the matrix filaments (Fig. 9) (SIMIONESCU 1988; FRANK and FOGELMAN 1989).

The role played in the retention of MRLp within the arterial wall has been well documented for proteoglycans, collagens, elastin, and fibronectin.

4.9.1 Proteoglycans

It is generally believed that amounts of sulfated glycosaminoglycans increase with age and with the cholesterol content of the human aorta, as does the ratio of chondroitin sulfate to dermatan sulfate, whereas the corresponding amounts of heparan sulfate decrease. Although proteoglycans are only minor components ($\sim 5\%$) of arterial extracellular matrix, it has been demonstrated that in plaque formation, lipid infiltration and proteoglycan alterations are related events. Despite some conflicting results, dermatan sulfate and chondroitin-6-sulfate proteoglycans fairly consistently increase in accordance with the extensiveness of fatty streaks and fibrous plaques (BERENSON et al. 1985; for reviews see VOLKER et al. 1990; CHERCHI et al. 1990).

A particularly potent LDL-binding subfraction of chondroitin sulfate proteoglycan could be extracted from bovine aorta (SRINIVASAN et al. 1989). Also, Lp(a) was shown to have a high reactivity with proteoglycans, that may account for its atherogenicity (KOSTNER and BIHARI-VARGA 1990).

Interactions of LDL with arterial proteoglycans have been extensively studied by several laboratories. Although a general consensus has not yet been

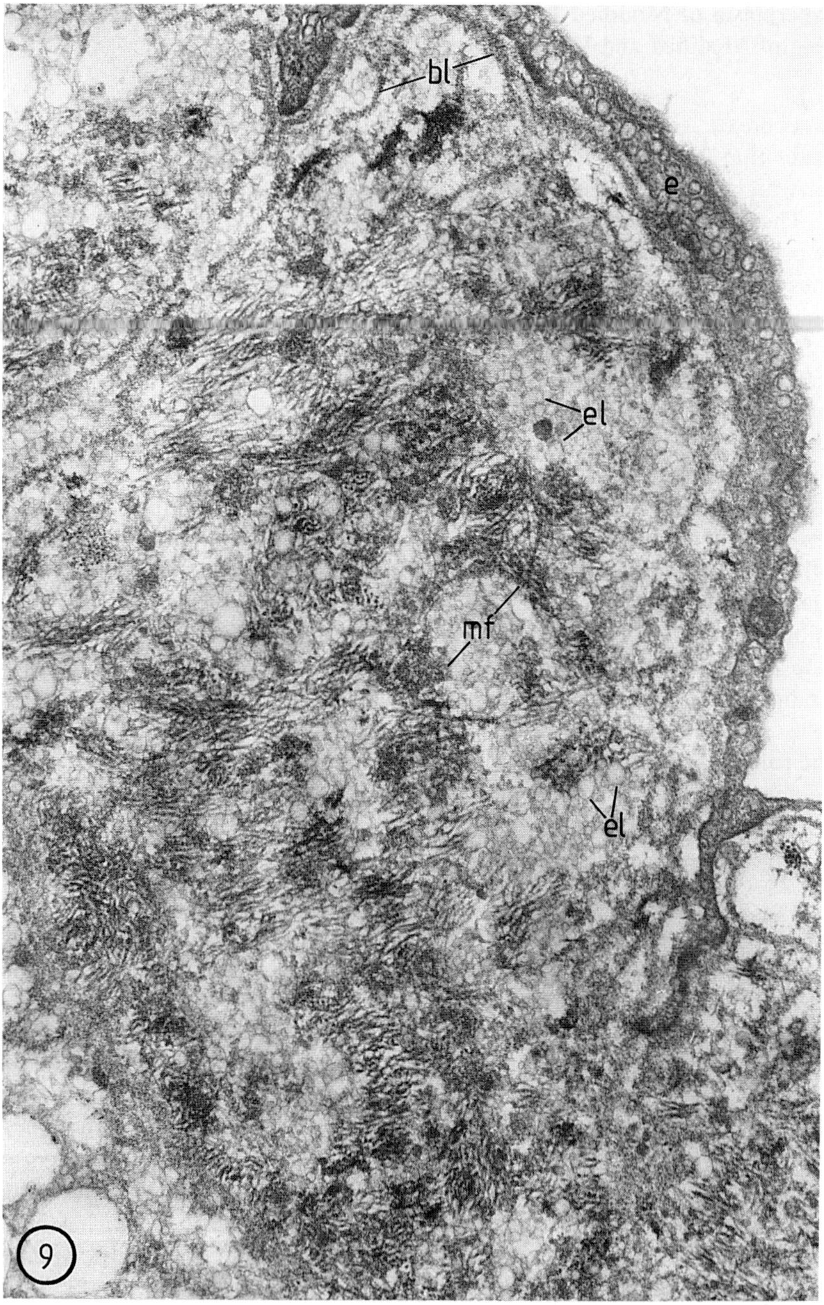

Fig. 9. Region of aortic intima from a hypercholesterolemic rabbit after 2 weeks on a cholesterol-rich diet. A relatively large part of the subendothelial region is occupied by a heteromorphic combination of extracellular liposomes (*el*), highly proliferated microfibrils (*mf*), and a few layers of basal lamina (*bl*). × 32 200

reached, some data are worth mentioning because of their potential relevance for the initiation and development of lipid accumulation within extracellular matrix modified by hypercholesterolemia. Reportedly, LDL have a higher affinity for chondroitin sulfate proteoglycan (CSPG) than VLDL, whereas HDL do not bind CSPG. The apo B regions rich in positively charged side chains (arginine and lysine probably located on the lipoprotein surface) are among the structures responsible for β-lipoprotein association with proteoglycans (CAMEJO et al. 1988, 1991). There are special subpopulations of LDL which are particularly sensitive to proteoglycan complexing and uptake by macrophages (HURT-CAMEJO et al. 1990). The LDL-proteoglycan uptake is mediated by the LDL receptor and possibly also by another nonspecific pathway (HURT et al. 1990; VIJAYAGOPAL et al. 1991). It has been postulated that LDL treatment with CSPG causes enhanced access of Cu^{2+} to LDL hydrophobic regions (CAMEJO et al. 1991). SAMBANDAM et al. (1991) showed that the degree (and not the position) of sulfation determines CSPG affinity for LDL. Recent immunochemical findings suggest that both normal and atherosclerotic pigeon aortas contain one or more keratan sulfate proteoglycan, the sulfation of which is greater in the plaque (ROBBINS et al. 1992).

4.9.2 Collagens

Although data in the literature are controversial, it was in the past generally considered that the unaffected human aorta contains ~70% type III collagen and ~30% type I collagen. In the atherosclerotic intimal plaques a shift in this distribution was observed, collagen type III accounting for only 35% (MCCULLAGH and BALIAN 1975). More recent estimates have claimed that in both normal and diseased arterial intima, 50%–75% of collagen is of type I (MURATA et al. 1986). In vitro studies have demonstrated that LDL particles bind more markedly to collagen type III than to type I. The increase in high ionic strength and pH reduces the binding, indicating the electrostatic nature of the interaction (ESKENASY et al. 1984). Immunofluorescence microscopy of fatty streaks has located LDL particles along collagen fibers (HOFF et al. 1974). Binding of LDL to collagen is enhanced by oxidative modification and by increasing particle net negative charge (HOOVER et al. 1988).

During the prelesional stage of diet-induced atherogenesis in hamsters and rabbits, in the lesion-prone areas bundles of banded collagen fibers are initially not markedly increased as compared with other elements of the extracellular matrix such as microfibrils and elastin or with the hyperplastic basal lamina. This situation also pertains in the early periods of foam cell formation. Significant proliferation of collagen fibers with reorganization in their spatial distribution becomes visible especially at the stage of transition of the fatty streak into a fibrous or fibrolipid plaque. Given the frequent association of clusters of MRLp with collagen fibers, a potential role of these proteins in lipid trapping in the extracellular matrix of arterial intima cannot be ruled out (HOOVER et al. 1988).

4.9.3 Elastin and Microfibrils

In cholesterol-fed animals (rabbits and hamsters), hypercholesterolemia is rapidly (within 4–7 days) associated with a proliferative reaction of intimal microfibrils and elastic elements. The process is particularly prominent in the aortic valve, where a true internal lamina elastica is missing. In arteries (coronary and aorta) the internal lamina elastica is generally intact for an extended period of time, while small elastic bundles appear scattered within the intima. In advanced lesions, cellular proliferation and migration from both directions, involving subendothelial macrophages and media smooth muscle cells, disrupt the continuity of elastic lamellae. Often native LDL, as well as MRLp, display a tendency to reside adjacent to or apparently within elastic fibers (GUYTON et al. 1985; SIMIONESCU 1988). As compared to normal, human atherosclerotic elastin exhibits a two- to fourfold higher capacity for binding LDL (PODET et al. 1991). This may be due to the degradation of elastin (ROBERT et al. 1984), which is known to have affinity for β-lipoproteins (SRINIVASAN et al. 1981).

4.9.4 Fibronectin

Fibronectin is a large glycoprotein that is present in small amounts in the intima of normal aorta; it is closely associated with endothelium and subendothelium, and accumulates markedly in cushion-like thickenings (JENSEN et al. 1983). Macrophages incubated with complexes of LDL-fibronectin, heparin, and gelatin accumulate cholesteryl esters (FALCONE et al. 1984). The apo(a) portion of Lp(a) binds to the carboxy-terminal heparin binding domain of fibronectin, which can be cleaved proteolytically by incubation with apo(a) or Lp(a). This effect means that the potential role of Lp(a) in atherogenesis is still unclear (EHNHOLM et al. 1990), but fibronectin degradation may significantly alter the integrity of the arterial extracellular matrix.

4.10 Cytotoxicity

As mentioned above, during the early stages of hypercholesterolemia, arterial endothelium is concomitantly exposed on the luminal front to elevated levels of plasma β-lipoproteins, and on the abluminal front to the subendothelial accumulation of oxidatively modified and reassembled lipoproteins (MRLp). The virtual absence of oxidized LDL in the circulation can be explained in two ways: either such modification does not occur in plasma, or, if oxidized LDL are produced, they are rapidly taken up and degraded by the liver sinusoid ECs (NAGELKERKE et al. 1984) and Kupffer cells (VAN BERKEL et al. 1991). Since LDL-like lipoproteins extracted from atherosclerotic aortas of humans and animals have properties similar to LDL oxidized in vitro (HABERLAND et al. 1988; PALINSKI et al. 1989; YLA-HERTTUALA et al. 1989; MORTON et al. 1986), it is assumed that an oxidative modification of β-lipoproteins also takes place in vivo, either at the level of the endothelium during transcytosis (SIMIONESCU 1988, 1990, 1992b) or in the intima (STEINBERG et al. 1989). Within the latter, β-lipoproteins can undergo autoxidation either by mechanisms similar to those demonstrated in cell-free systems (ESTERBAUER et al. 1987) or by interaction with a microenvironment altered by hypercholesterolemia, especially through the free radicals liberated by the intimal cells (ESTERBAUER et al. 1987; WITZTUM and STEINBERG 1991).

In vitro, it has been demonstrated that LDL can be modified by all cell types of the vessel wall, including ECs (HENRIKSEN et al. 1982; MOREL et al. 1984; STEINBRECHER et al. 1984). On the other hand, some cells, i.e., ECs and macrophages, recognize and internalize oxidized LDL via a scavenger receptor (for review, see WITZTUM and STEINBERG 1991; LUC and FRUCHART 1991; STEINBERG et al. 1989). Recently, CUSHING et al. (1990) have demonstrated that minimally modified LDL is not recognized by the EC scavenger receptor and is not distinguished from native LDL by the LDL receptor; unlike native LDL, it induces the production of monocyte chemotactic protein 1 (MCP-1) in cultured ECs. Whether a similar process takes place in vivo remains to be demonstrated. The existence of an EC receptor specific for oxidized LDL is still being debated; the most recent evidence indicates the absence of such additional specific sites (KUME et al. 1991). At any rate, it seems that ECs have constitutively the machinery to interact more or less specifically with different levels of modified LDL.

The effect of high levels of plasma native β-lipoproteins on ECs has been insufficiently explored and most of the data have come from in vitro studies. It has been shown that prolonged exposure of cultured human venous ECs to atherogenic concentrations of LDL does not alter EC viability but does increase their prostacyclin production (HOLLAND et al. 1988; TRIAN et al. 1988). Incubation of cultured swine aortic ECs with rabbit β-VLDL and macrophages produced a synergistic adverse effect leading to (time- and dose-dependent) EC damage as estimated by $[^3H]$adenine release; the effect could be prevented by antioxidants (TANIMURA et al. 1990). Treatment of rabbit aortic ECs for 3 days with either β-VLDL or malondialdehyde-LDL, but not native LDL, caused a 50%–100% increase in total cell unesterified cholesterol localized mostly in plasma membrane, which may be functionally altered by this condition (KIM et al. 1991). H_2O_2 was shown to alter the fluidity and leakiness of EC membrane (BLOCK 1991) by liberating unesterified fatty acids (DUANE et al. 1991). Aortic ECs from swine fed cholesterol for 3 days displayed a two- to threefold increase in $[^3H]$thymidine incorporation (FLORENTIN et al. 1969).

Because of the virtual absence of oxidized LDL from the circulation, one can assume that such effects can operate in vivo, being due to the action of the oxidatively modified LDL or its derivatives (the MRLp) on the abluminal front of the overlying endothelium. The effects of oxidized LDL on ECs have been investigated mostly under culture conditions.

Among various biologic properties of oxidized LDL (e.g., immunogenicity with autoantibody formation, perturbation of vasomotoricity of coronary arteries, and alteration of gene expression of neighboring cells such as induction of MCP-1 and colony-stimulating factors), the following are of special physiopathologic relevance for prelesional atherogenesis: cytotoxicity for ECs, chemotactic activity, perturbation of coagulation pathways, and enhanced uptake by macrophages leading to cholesteryl ester loading and foam cell formation.

Oxidized LDL, including minimally modified LDL, is cytotoxic to ECs and smooth muscle cells in culture (MOREL et al. 1984), probably via the generation of reactive oxygen species (LUC and FRUCHART 1991; WITZTUM and STEINBERG 1991; MOREL et al. 1983; SHATOS et al. 1991). ECs are targets for free radicals in a broad array of pathobiologic conditions, including inflammation and ischemia/reperfusion injury to various tissues and organs (HALLIWELL 1987). There are numerous examples of deleterious changes in various cell types being brought about by products known to be released by LDL oxidation such as lysophosphatidylcholine, fatty acids, and their oxidized derivatives (for review, see ESTERBAUER et al. 1987). Cells appear to be more susceptible to oxidized LDL during their proliferation, apo B not being required for the cytotoxic effect. Oxidants can reversibly enhance the EC permeability to ions and macromolecules (WILSON et al. 1990), but reduce the pinocytic activity (BORSUM et al. 1985). Common cholesterol autoxidation products such as the isomeric cholesterol-5,6-epoxides are also cytotoxic to ECs (SEVANIAN et al. 1991).

At the ultrastructural level, during subendothelial accumulation of MRLp the endothelial lining is intact. Progressively, however, it becomes heterogeneous with a tendency for local flattenings to occur; nevertheless, marked attenuation can be seen only after macrophage-derived foam cells start to develop immediately beneath the endothelium (see Sect. 4.14).

4.11 Chemotactic Induction by Modified β-Lipoproteins

Unlike native β-lipoproteins, modified LDL can play an important role in mediating the recruitment of monocytes and their migration into the artery wall. While highly oxidized LDL is a potent chemoattractant (QUINN et al. 1985), minimally modified LDL (MM-LDL) is itself not chemotactic, but can induce the expression by ECs of MCP-1, a 14-kDa monomeric cationic peptide produced by ECs and smooth muscle cells (BERLINER et al. 1990). By in situ hybridization it was demonstrated that MCP-1 mRNA is present in macrophage-rich regions of aortic plaques of humans and rabbits (YLA-HERTTUALA et al. 1991). By immunocytochemistry, it was revealed that the early cholesterol accumulation in the aortic intima of hypercholesterolemic rabbits coincides with deposition of C5b-9 complement, which is known to be chemotactic for monocytes (SEIFERT et al. 1989). Human atherosclerotic lesions have been shown to contain C5b-9 complexes (NICULESCU et al. 1987; RUS et al. 1986; VLAICU et al. 1985); after lesion ulceration, plaque components can activate complement intravascularly.

As for the various forms of MRLp detected in vivo, it remains to be determined which of them are particularly active in cytotoxicity, chemotactic induction (direct or indirect), immunogenicity with immune complex formation, adduct formation with matrix proteins and/or cellular proteins, complement activation, etc.

4.12 Monocyte Recruitment and Adhesion to Endothelium

Two types of leukocytes are commonly encountered in the forming atherosclerotic plaque, monocytes (the predominant class) and T lymphocytes (LIBBY and HANSSON 1991). Their presence has been well documented with monoclonal antibody technology (AQEL et al. 1985; JONASSON et al. 1986; GOWN et al. 1986; VAN DER WAL 1989; HANSSON et al. 1991). Their appearance in the lesion-prone areas marks the transition from the prelesional to the lesional stage of atherogenesis with the formation of fatty streaks.

At the onset of atherogenesis, the elevated levels of plasma β-lipoproteins, concurrent with the subendothelial accumulation of oxidatively modified LDL and β-VLDL, may alter the endothelial interactions with the circulating blood cells. Further in depth investigations are still required into the effects of hypercholesterolemia on the minute chemistry of different classes of blood cells, especially leukocytes. Hypercholesterolemia may alter the cell surface, which displays a general tendency toward procoagulant activity (RODGERS et al. 1988; WEIS et al. 1991; HAJJAR et al. 1989) and, more importantly, expresses newly induced adhesion molecules, some of them specific for monocytes.

Monocyte interaction with arterial endothelium in hypercholesterolemic animals can be described as comprising four successive phases presumably governed, at least in part, by different mechanisms: recruitment, adhesion, diapedesis, and subendothelial homing.

4.12.1 Recruitment

The biochemical changes which render some populations of circulating monocytes more susceptible to attachment to endothelium are still poorly understood. Our observations on cholesterol-fed rabbits did not reveal significant changes in the surface charge and major glycoconjugates of circulating monocytes or endothelium of aortic lesion-prone areas (GHINEA et al. 1987). However, it has been reported that monocyte margination to arterial endothelium is more pronounced in hyperlipoproteinemic animals than in controls (although no correlation between the severity of this process and plasma β-VLDL or HDL concentrations could be established) (for review, see SIMIONESCU 1988). The possible role of the

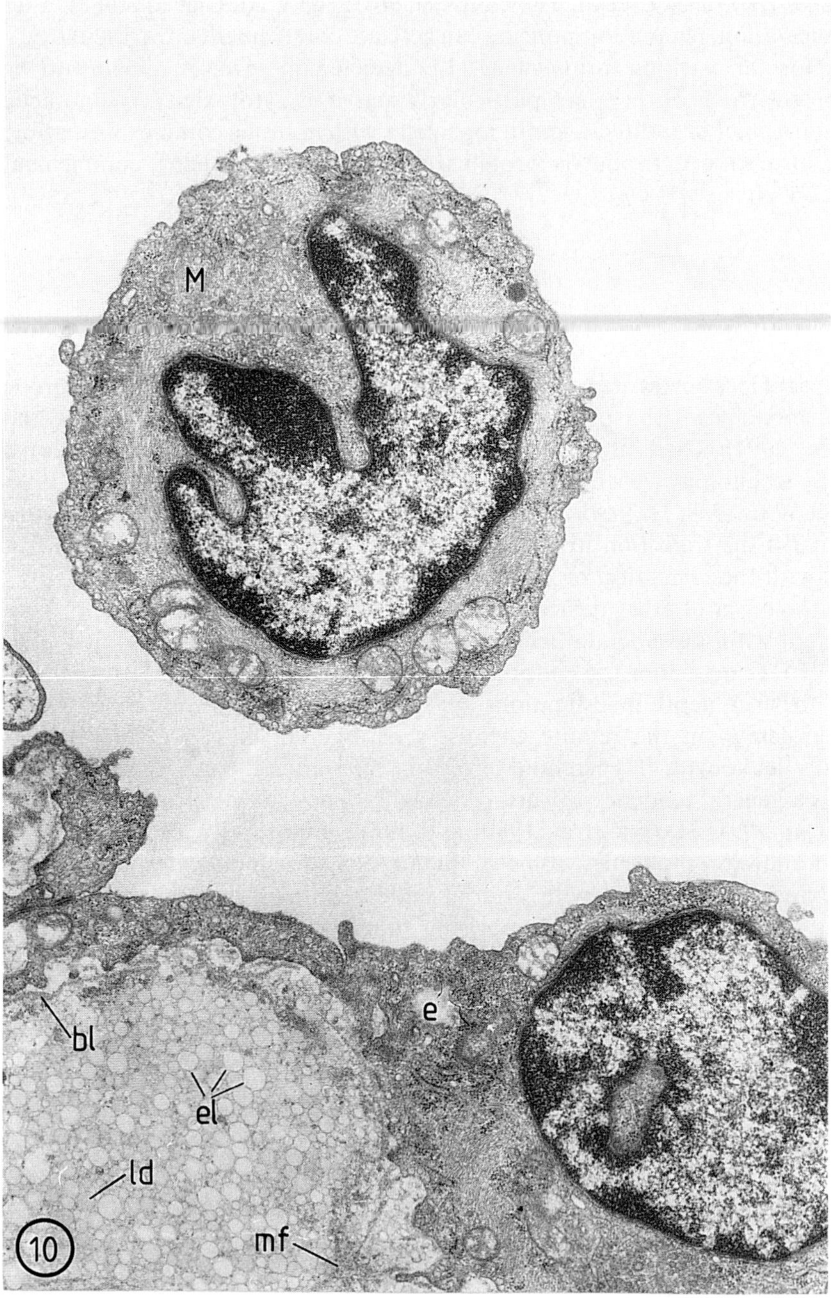

Fig. 10. Rabbit aortic intima after 2 weeks on a cholesterol-rich diet. Monocyte (*M*) found close to a region rich in extracellular liposomes (*el*) and lipid droplets (*ld*). *e*, endothelium; *bl*, basal lamina; *mf*, microfibrils. × 14 800

chemoattractants secreted by the cells of the artery wall has been discussed previously. However, in vivo, chemotactic factors released by tissues should be rapidly washed away by the bloodstream. Moreover, a generalized stimulation by circulating chemoattractants cannot account for the focal nature of leukocyte adhesion. Chemotactic factors may act more potently after monocytes have been attached to the endothelial surface. In our experiments, we found that in lesion-prone areas, mononuclear leukocytes are preferentially attracted to regions rich in MRLp, especially extracellular liposomes (Fig. 10) (SIMIONESCU 1990, 1992b).

In partial agreement with some results reported by Rodgers's laboratory, in preliminary studies we found that in culture or ex vivo exposure of ECs to atherogenic concentrations of β-VLDL resulted in decreased protein C activation and a significant switch to procoagulant activity expressed by surface exposure of anionic phospholipids, increased binding of factors IXa and Xa, and augmented prothrombinase activity. Concomitantly, a stimulation of tissue plasminogen activator activity was paralleled by a slight reduction in PAI-1 expression (LUPU et al., manuscript in preparation).

4.12.2 Adhesion

It is conceivable that monocyte attachment to the endothelium of lesion-prone areas is regulated by a multiplicity of molecules such as cytokines, integrins and selectins, specific attractants (e.g., MCP-1), and leukocyte adhesion molecules of the ELAM and ICAM types. Emerging from a very elaborate and fruitful area of research, current knowledge of the molecular partners involved in monocyte–endothelial interaction is focused on the existence of a network of multiple monocyte receptors and EC ligands of a relatively large combinatorial diversity. There is a time course of expression of the EC ligands for various leukocytes, including monocytes, but in the case of the latter, the exact involvement of the pair molecules in the sequence adhesion–diapedesis–homing is still obscure. The existence of a basal (nonstimulated) monocyte adherence to ECs is not surprising, given the continuous physiologic need for monocyte migration into tissues to provide for the renewing population of local macrophages.

The integrin receptors of the monocytes are represented by VLA-4 (α, CD49d/β1, CD29), LFA.1 (αL, CD11a/β2, CD18), CD18 complexes (panleukocyte integrins, mostly acting through cytokines), and Mac-1 (αM, CD11a/β2, CD18), which have as counterparts, in a network fashion, the EC ligands VCAM-1, ICAM-1, and ICAM-2. The inducible selective endothelial leukocyte adhesion molecule-1 (ELAM-1) is expressed by cultured ECs upon stimulation by various inflammatory/immune mediators such as interleukin-1, tumor necrosis factor, and lymphotoxin (BEVILACQUA et al. 1987). ELAM-1 was demonstrated immunohistochemically to be transiently expressed by human microvascular endothelium during certain pathologic processes (COTRAN et al. 1986). More recently, CYBULSKI and GIMBRONE (1990, 1991) have reported that cultured ECs as well as activated ECs overlying forming atheroma in cholesterolfed or WHHL rabbits express an "athero-ELAM" antigen that may be, at least in part, instrumental in monocyte adhesion in the initial phases of atherogenesis.

The interactions responsible for T lymphocyte recruitment and penetration into the atherosclerotic artery wall are less defined in molecular terms. Several factors have so far been implicated, such as interferon-γ, interleukin-1, interleukin-6, interleukin-8, and tumor necrosis factor, but much work is required to promote the understanding of this process.

4.13 Monocyte Emigration and Subendothelial Homing

A clear picture does not exist of the molecular pairs [monocyte receptor(s)–endothelial ligand(s)] and the mechanisms by which a monocyte, once attached to the endothelial luminal surface, is translated towards the endothelial junction. Likewise, we lack an estimate of the number of adhered monocytes which eventually penetrate the intima, but the process continues during all phases of fatty streak formation and to a certain extent even later, during conversion of the lesion into a fibrous plaque. The extent of chemoattractant gradients in the intima, their nature, and their topography require clarification. During *trans-junctional diapedesis*, the monocyte plasma membrane maintains tight apposition with the plasmalemma of the adjacent EC. The intercellular space in not permeable to tracers such as LDL-gold, β-VLDL-gold and albumin-gold. At more advanced stages, during foam cell formation, junctional permeability is increased, notably for albumin-gold. Often, such zones with high permeability are also marked by a serofibrinous insudate focally developed in regions devoid of ELs (SIMIONESCU 1988).

One striking aspect of the monocyte–endothelial interaction is the continuous close attachment between the two cell types, at the end of which the monocyte enters (or dissects) the subendothelial space already opened by the endothelial–basal lamina disjunction. This special kind of *homing* can be seen even later, when foam cells occupy most of the intima. The subendothelial location of monocyte-derived macrophages was also detected in spontaneously hypertensive rats (CLOZEL et al. 1991).

4.14 Uptake of Modified and Reassembled Lipoproteins: Foam Cell Formation

In their subendothelial location, monocytes are activated and the macrophages start ingesting MRLp to becomes foam cells. Even at the lipid-laden cells stage, the basal lamina is largely present around the abluminal aspect of the monocyte-macrophage-derived foam cell. This may indirectly suggest that part of the ingested lipidic material may come directly through the overlying endothelium.

It is likely that the transcytosed β-lipoproteins can undergo oxidative modification, either during transendothelial vectorial passage or by exposure to the free radicals released by the ECs or the macrophages within the sequestrated subendothelial space.

It has to be noted that the EC-attached monocytes do not exhibit the morphologic characteristics of activation/differentiation to macrophages (in particular the extensive cytoplasmic pseudopods or lamellae, large cell body vacuoles, and pinocytic vesicles) (SCHWARTZ et al. 1991). It appears that such activation/differentiation occurs in the intima, being triggered and/or mediated by a very complex interplay of factors including cytokines, interferons, complement C5a, and polyanions. Concomitantly, macrophages, once activated, exhibit enhanced superoxide anion generation and increased secretion of several enzymes (collagenase, elastase, lipoprotein lipase, plasminogen activator, etc.) which play relevant roles in plaque formation, remodeling, and complication (or regression). Activated macrophages undergo a crucial phenotypic modulation by expressing LDL receptors and scavenger receptors (or a family of such receptors) which are instrumental in the uptake and degradation of oxidized LDL (QUINN et al. 1985; HOFF and COLE 1991) and modified β-VLDL (MAZZONE et al. 1987), and presumably in the phagocytosis of various forms of MRLp (SIMIONESCU 1988, 1990, 1992b; SUITS et al. 1989; KHOO et al. 1988). LDL complexes with other proteins (e.g., heparin, proteoglycans, collagen, fibronectin) are also taken up by macrophages and cause accumulation of cholesteryl esters by a poorly regulated or unregulated uptake.

It remains to be established whether the subendothelial macrophage-derived foam cells digest the detached endothelial innermost basal lamina to migrate deeper into the intima and transiently vacate the subendothelial space for another wave of monocytes.

References

Adams CWM, Morgan RS (1967) The effect of saturated and polyunsaturated lecithins on the resorption of 4–^{14}C-cholesterol from subcutaneous implants. J Pathol Bacteriol 94:73–76

Amanuma K, Kanaseki T, Ikeuchi Y, Ohkuma S, Takano T (1986) Studies on fine structure and location of lipids in quick-freeze replicas of atherosclerosis aorta of WHHL rabbits. Virchows Arch [A] 410:231–238

Aqel NM, Ball RY, Waldmann H, Mitchinson MJ (1985) Identification of macrophages and smooth muscle cells in human atherosclerosis using monoclonal antibodies. J Pathol 146:197–205

Avogaro P, Cazzolato G, Bittolo-Bon G (1991) Some questions concerning a small, more electronegative LDL circulating in human plasma. Atherosclerosis 91:163–171

Berenson GS, Radhakrishnamurthy B, Srinivasan SR, Vijayagopal P, Dalferes ER (1985) Proteoglycans and potential mechanisms related to atherosclerosis. Ann NY Acad Sci 454:69–78

Berliner JA, Territo MC, Sevanian A, et al. (1990) Minimally modified low density lipoprotein stimulates monocyte endothelial interactions. J Clin Invest 85:1260–1266

Bevilacqua MP, Pober JS, Mendrick DL, Cotran RS, Gimbrone MA Jr (1987) Identification of an inducible endothelial-leukocyte adhesion molecule. Proc Natl Acad Sci USA 84:9238–9242

Bini A, Fenoglio JJ Jr, Mesa-Tejada R, Kudryk B, Kaplan KL (1989) Identification and distribution of fibrinogen, fibrin and fibrin(ogen) degradation products in atherosclerosis. Use monoclonal antibodies. Arteriosclerosis 9:109–121

Block ER (1991) Hydrogen peroxide alters the physical state and function of the plasma membrane of pulmonary artery endothelial cells. J Cell Physiol 146:362–369

Bocan TMA, Brown SA, Guyton JR (1988) Human aortic fibrolipid lesions. Immunochemical localization of apolipoprotein B and apolipoprotein A. Arteriosclerosis 8:499–508

Borsum T, Henriksen T, Reisvaag A (1985) Oxidized low density lipoprotein can reduce the pinocytic activity in cultured human endothelial cells as measured by cellular uptake of [^{14}C] sucrose. Atherosclerosis 58:81–96

Bratzler RL, Chisolm GM, Colton CK, Smith KA, Lees RS (1977) The distribution of labeled low-density lipoproteins across the rabbit thoracic aorta in vivo. Atherosclerosis 28:289–307

Brown MS, Goldstein JL, Krieger M, Ho YK, Anderson RGW (1979) Reversible accumulation of cholesteryl esters in macrophages incubated with acetylated lipoproteins. J Cell Biol 82:597–613

Camejo G, Olofsson SO, Lopez F, Carlsson P, Bondjers G (1988) Identification of apo B-100 segments mediating the interaction of low density lipoproteins with arterial proteoglycans. Arteriosclerosis 8:368–377

Camejo G, Hurt-Camejo E, Rosengren B, Wiklund O, Lopez F, Bondjers G (1991) Modification of copper-catalyzed of low density lipoprotein by proteoglycans and glycosaminoglycans. J Lipid Res 32:1983–1991

Carew TE, Pittman RC, Marchaud ER, Steinberg D (1984) Measurement in vivo of irreversible degradation of low density lipoprotein in the rabbit aorta. Arteriosclerosis 4:214–224

Cathcart MK, Morel DW, Chisolm GM (1985) Monocytes and neutrophils oxidize low density lipoproteins making it cytotoxic. J Leukocyte Biol 38:341–350

Cavender DE, Edelbaum D, Ziff M (1989) Endothelial cell activation induced by tumor necrosis factor and lymphotoxin. Am J Pathol 134:551–560

Chao FF, Blanchette-Mackie J, Chen Y-J, et al. (1990) Characterization of two unique cholesterol-rich lipid particles isolated from human atherosclerotic lesions. Am J Pathol 136:169–179

Cherchi GM, Coinu R, Demuro P, et al. (1990) Structural and functional modifications of human aorta proteoglycans in atherosclerosis. Matrix 10:362–372

Clozel M, Kuhn H, Hefti F, Baumgartner HR (1991) Endothelial dysfunction and subendothelial monocyte macrophages in hypertension. Effect of angiotensin converting enzyme inhibition. Hypertension 18:132–141

Cotran RS (1987) New roles for the endothelium in inflammation and immunity. Am J Pathol 129:407–413

Cotran RS, Pober JS (1988) Endothelial activation: its role in inflammatory and immune reactions. In: Simionescu N, Simionescu M (eds) Endothelial cell biology in health and disease. Plenum, New York, pp 335–347

Cotran RS, Gimbrone MA Jr, Bevilacqua MP, Mendrick DL, Pober JS (1986) Induction and detection of a human endothelial activation antigen in vivo. J Exp Med 164:661–666

Cotran RS, Kumar V, Robbins SL (1989) Pathologic basis of disease. WB Saunders, Philadelphia, pp 1–38

Cushing SD, Berliner JA, Valente AJ, et al. (1990) Minimally modified low density lipoprotein induces monocyte chemotactic protein 1 in human endothelial cells and smooth muscle cells. Proc Natl Acad Sci USA 87:5134–5138

Cybulski MI, Gimbrone MA Jr (1990) Endothelial cells express a monocyte adhesion molecule during atherogenesis. FASEB J 4:A1135–A1142

Cybulski MI, Gimbrone MA Jr (1991) Endothelial expression of a mononuclear leukocyte adhesion molecule during atherogenesis. Science 251:788–791

Cybulski MI, Gimbrone MA Jr (1992) Endothelial leukocyte adhesion molecules in acute inflammation and atherogenesis. In: Simionescu N, Simionescu M (eds) Endothelial cell dysfunctions. Plenum, New York, pp 129–140

de Graaf J, Hak-Lemmers HLM, Hectors MPC, Deinacker PNM, Hendrisk JCM, Stalenhoef AFH (1991) Enhanced susceptibility to in vitro oxidation of the dense low density liporpotein subfraction in healthy subjects. Arteriosclerosis Thromb 11:298–306

Deliconstantinos G, Tsopanakis C, Karayiannakos P, Skalkeas G (1986) Evidence for the existence of non-esterified cholesterol carried by albumin in rat serum. Atherosclerosis 61:67–75

Duane PG, Rice KL, Charbonean DE, King MB, Gilboe DP, Niewoehner DE (1991) Relationship of oxidant-mediated cytotoxicity to phospholipid metabolism in endothelial cells. Am J Respir Cell Mol Biol 4:408–416

Ehnholm C, Jauhiainen M, Metso J (1990) Interaction of lipoprotein (a) with fibronectin and its potential role in atherogenesis. Eur Heart J 11 [Suppl E]: 190–195

Eskenasy M, Mora R, Simionescu N (1984) In vitro study of low density lipoprotein-collagen interaction. Morphol Embryol 30:147–152

Esterbauer H, Jurgens G, Quchenberger O, Koller E (1987) Autoxidation of human low density lipoprotein: loss of polyunsaturated fatty acids and vitamin E, and generation of aldehydes. J Lipid Res 28:495–509

Faggiotto A, Ross R (1984) Studies on hypercholesterolemia in the nonhuman primate. II. Fatty streak conversion to fibrous plaque. Arteriosclerosis 4:341–356

Faggiotto A, Ross R, Harker L (1984) Studies on hypercholesterolemia in the nonhuman primate. I. Changes that lead to fatty streak formation. Arteriosclerosis 4:323–340

Falcone DJ, Mated N, Shio H, Minick CR, Fowler SD (1984) Lipoprotein-heparin-fibronectin-denaturated collagen complexes enhance cholesteryl ester accumulation in macrophages. J Cell Biol 99:1266–1274

Filip DA, Nistor A, Bulla A, Radu A, Lupu F, Simionescu M (1987) Cellular events in the development of valvular atherosclerotic lesions induced by experimental hypercholesterolemia. Atherosclerosis 67:199–214

Florentin RA, Nam SC, Lee KT, Thomas WA (1969) Increased ^{3}H-thymidine incorporation into endothelial cells of swine fed cholesterol for 3 days. Exp Mol Pathol 10:250–255

Frank JS, Fogelman AM (1989) Ultrastructure of intima of WHHL and cholesterol fed rabbit aorta prepared by ultrarapid freezing and freeze etching. J Lipid Res 30:967–978

Frei B, Stocker R, Ames BN (1988) Antioxidant defenses and lipid peroxidation in human blood plasma. Proc Natl Acad Sci USA 85:9748–9752

Ghinea N, Leabu M, Hasu M, Muresan V, Colceag J, Simionescu N (1987) Prelesional events in atherogenesis: changes induced by hypercholesterolemia in the cell surface chemistry of arterial endothelium and blood monocytes in rabbit. J Submicrosc Cytol 19:209–227

Gimbrone MA Jr (1989) Endothelial dysfunction and atherosclerosis. J Cardiac Surg 4:180–183

Gimbrone MA Jr, Bevilacqua MP (1988) Vascular endothelium: functional modulation at the blood interface. In: Simionescu N, Simionescu M (eds) Endothelial cell biology in health and disease. Plenum, New York, pp 255–273

Gordon JL, Pearson JD (1982) Responses of endothelial cells to injury. In: HL Nossel, HJ Vogel (eds) Pathobiology of the endothelial cell. Academic, New York, pp 433–454

Gown AM, Tsukada T, Ross R (1986) Human atherosclerosis. II. Immunohistochemical analysis of the cellular composition of human atherosclerotic lesions. Am J Pathol 125:191–198

Guyton JR, Klemp KF (1988) Ultrastructural discrimination of lipid droplets and vesicles in atherosclerosis: value of osmium-thiocarbohydrazide-osmium and tannic acid-paraphenylendiamine technique. J Histochem Cytochem 36:1319–1328

Guyton JR, Klemp KF (1989) The lipid-rich core region of human atherosclerotic fibrous plaques. Prevalence of small lipid droplets and vesicles by electron microscopy. Am J Pathol 134:705–717

Guyton JR, Bocan TMA, Schifani TA (1985) Quantitative ultrastructural analysis of perifibrous lipid and its association with elastin in nonatherosclerotic human aorta. Arteriosclerosis 5:644–652

Guyton JR, Klemp KF, Black BL, Bocan TMA (1990) Extracellular lipid deposition in atherosclerosis. Eur Heart J 11 [Suppl E]: 20–28

Guyton JR, Klemp KF, Mims MP (1991) Altered ultrastructural morphology of self-aggregated low density lipoproteins: coalescence of lipid domains forming droplets and vesicles. J Lipid Res 32:953–962

Haberland ME, Fong D, Cheng L (1988) Malondialdehyde-altered protein occurs in atheroma of Watanabe heritable hyperlipidemic rabbits. Science 241:215–218

Hajjar DP (1991) Warner-Lambert/Parke-Davis Award lecture. Viral pathogenesis of atherosclerosis. Am J Pathol 139:1195–1211

Hajjar DP, Wight TN, Smith SC (1980) Lipid accumulation and ultrastructural change within the aortic wall during early spontaneous atherogenesis. Am J Pathol 100:683–702

Hajjar KA, Gavish D, Breslow JL, Nachman RL (1989) Lipoprotein(a) modulation of endothelial cell surface fibrinolysis and its potential role in atherosclerosis. Nature 339:303–305

Halliwell B (1987) Oxidants and human disease: some new concepts. FASEB J 1:358–364

Halliwell B (1988) Albumin—an important extracellular antioxidant? Biochem Pharmacol 37:569–571

Hallmann J, Schmidt A, van Bassewitz D-B, Buddecke E (1989) Relationship of sulfated glycosaminoglycans and cholesterol content in normal and arteriosclerotic human aorta. Arteriosclerosis 9:154–158

Hamilton RL, Havel RJ, Kane JP, Blaurock AE, Sata T (1971) Cholestasis: lamellar structure of the abnormal human serum lipoprotein, Science 172:475–478
Hammami M, Maume G, Maume BF (1986) Role of albumin for the cholesterol transport and on the steroidogenic pathways in serum—free medium newborn rat adrenocortical cell cultures. Cell Biol Int Rep 10:649–658
Hansson GK, Bondjers G (1980) Endothelial proliferation and atherogenesis in rabbits with moderate hypercholesterolemia. Artery 7:316–329
Hansson GK, Jonasson L, Seifert PS, Stemme S (1989) Immune mechanisms in atherosclerosis. Arteriosclerosis 9:567–578
Hansson GK, Seifert PS, Olsson G, Bondjers G (1991) Immunohistochemical detection of macrophages and T lymphocytes in atherosclerotic lesions of cholesterol-fed rabbits. Arteriosclerosis Thromb 11:745–750
Healey B (1990) Endothelial cell dysfunction: an emerging endocrinopathy linked to coronary disease. J Am Cell Cardiol 16:357–358
Henriksen T, Mahoney EM, Steinberg D (1982) Interactions of plasma lipoproteins with endothelial cells. Ann NY Acad Sci 401:102–116
Hoff HF, Cole TB (1991) Macrophage uptake of low density lipoprotein modified by 4-hydroxynonenal. An ultrastructural study. Lab Invest 64:254–264
Hoff HF, Gaubatz JW (1982) Isolation, purification and characterization of a lipoprotein containing apo B from the human aorta. Atherosclerosis 42:273–291
Hoff HF, Morton RE (1985) Lipoproteins containing apo B extracted from human aortas: structure and function. Ann NY Acad Sci 454:183–194
Hoff HF, O'Neil J (1991) Lesion-derived low density lipoprotein and oxidized low density lipoprotein share a lability for aggregation, leading to enhanced macrophage degradation. Arteriosclerosis Thromb 11:1209–1222
Hoff HF, Jackson RL, Mao SJT, Gotto AM Jr (1974) Localization of low density lipoproteins in atherosclerotic lesions from human normolipemics employing a purified fluorescent-labeled antibody. Biochim Biophys Acta 351:407–415
Holland YA, Pritchard KA, Rogers NY, Stemerman MB (1988) Perturbation of cultured human endothelial cells by atherogenic levels of low density lipoprotein. Am J Pathol 132:474–478
Hollander W, Paddock J, Colombo M (1979) Lipoproteins in human atherosclerotic vessels. Part I. Biochemical properties of arterial low density lipoproteins, very low density lipoproteins and high density lipoproteins. Exp Mol Pathol 30:144–158
Hoover GA, McCormick S, Kalant N (1988) Interaction of native and cell-modified low density lipoprotein with collagen gel. Arteriosclerosis 8:525–534
Hunter JA, Shahrokh Z, Forte TM, Nichols AV (1982) Aggregation of low density lipoproteins with unilamellar phosphatidylcholine vesicles. Biochem Biophys Res Commun 105:824–834
Hurt E, Bondjers G, Camejo G (1990) Interaction of LDL with human arterial proteoglycans stimulates its uptake by human monocyte-derived macrophages. J Lipid Res 31:443–454
Hurt-Camejo E, Camejo G, Rosengren B, Lopez F, Wiklund O, Bondjers G (1990) Differential uptake of proteoglycan-selected subfractions of low density lipoprotein by human macrophages. J Lipid Res 31:1387–1398
Jensen BA, Holund B, Clemmensen I (1983) Demonstration of fibronectin in normal and injured aorta by an indirect immunoperoxidase technique. Histochemistry 77:395–403
Jialal I, Freeman DA, Grundy SM (1991) Varying susceptibility of different low density lipoprotein to oxidative modification. Arteriosclerosis Thromb 11:482–488
Jokinen MP, Clarkson TB, Prichard RW (1985) Recent advances in molecular pathology. Animal models in atherosclerosis research. Exp Mol Pathol 42:1–28
Jonasson L, Hohn J, Skalli O, Bondjers G, Hansson GK (1986) Regional accumulations of T cells, macrophages, and smooth muscle cells in the human atherosclerotic plaque. Arteriosclerosis 6:131–139
Joris I, Zand T, Nunnary JL, Krolikowski FJ, Majno G (1983) Studies on the pathogenesis of atherosclerosis. I. Adhesion and emigration of mononuclear cells in the aorta of hypercholesterolemic rats. Am J Pathol 113:341–358
Joris I, Billingham M-E, Majno G (1984) Human coronary arteries: an ultrastructural search for the early changes of atherosclerosis. Fed Proc 43:710
Julien P, Donwar E, Angel A (1981) Lipoprotein composition and transport in the pig and dog cardiac lymphatic system. Circ Res 49:248–254
Julien P, Fong B, Angel A (1984) Cardiac and peripheral lymph lipoproteins in dogs fed cholesterol and saturated fat. Arteriosclerosis 4:435–442

Katz SS, Small DM (1980) Isolation and partial characterization of the lipid phases of human atherosclerotic plaques. J Biol Chem 255:9553 9758
Khoo JC, Miller E, McLoughlin P, Steinberg D (1988) Enhanced macrophage uptake of low density lipoprotein after self-aggregation. Arteriosclerosis 8:348–358
Khoo JC, Miller E, McLoughlin P, Steinberg D (1990) Prevention of low density lipoprotein aggregation by high density lipoprotein or apolipoprotein A-I. J Lipid Res 31:645–652
Kim JA, Maxwell K, Hajjar DP, Berliner JA (1991) β-VLDL increases endothelial cell plasma membrane cholesterol. J Lipid Res 32:1125–1131
Klein RL, Rudel LL (1983) Effect of dietary cholesterol level on the composition of thoracic duct lymph lipoproteins isolated from nonhuman primates. J Lipid Res 24:357–367
Kostner GM, Bihari-Varga M (1990) Is the atherogenicity of Lp(a) caused by its reactivity with proteoglycans?. Eur Heart J 11 [Suppl E]:184–189
Kovanen PT (1990) Atheroma formation: defective control in the intimal round-trip of cholesterol. Eur Heart J 11:238–246
Kruth HS (1984) Filipin-positive, oil red O negative particles in atherosclerotic lesions induced by cholesterol feeding. Lab Invest 50:87–98
Kumar VV, Malewicz B, Baumann WJ (1989) Lysophosphatidylcholine stabilizes small unilamellar phosphatidylcholine vesicles. Phosphorus-31 NMR evidence for the "wedge" effect. Biophys J 55:789–792
Kume N, Arai H, Kawai C, Kita T (1991) Receptors for modified low-density lipoproteins on human endothelial cells: different recognition for acetylated low density lipoprotein and oxidized low density lipoprotein. Biochim Biophys Acta 1091:63–67
Lever MJ, Jay MT (1990) Albumin and Cr-EDTA uptake by systemic arteries veins and pulmonary artery of rabbit. Arteriosclerosis 10:551–558
Libby P, Hansson GK (1991) Involvement of the immune system in human atherogenesis: current knowledge and unanswered questions. Lab Invest 64:5–15
Lin S-J, Jan K-M, Chien S (1990) Role of dying endothelial cells in transendothelial macromolecular transport. Arteriosclerosis 10:703–709
Londono J, Bendayan M (1989) Distribution of endogenous albumin across the rat aortic wall as revealed by quantitative immunocytochemistry. Am J Anat 186:407–416
Luc G, Fruchart J-C (1991) Oxidation of lipoproteins and atherosclerosis. Am J Clin Nutr 53:206S–209S
Lupu F, Danaricu I, Simionescu N (1987) The development of intracellular lipid deposits in the lipid-laden cells of the atherosclerotic lesions: a cytochemical and ultrastructural study. Arteriosclerosis 67:127–142
Mahley RW (1983) Development of accelerated atherosclerosis: concepts derived from cell biology and animal model studies. Arch Pathol Lab Med 107:393–399
Majno G, Joris J, Zand T (1985) Atherosclerosis: new horizons. Hum Pathol 16:3–5
Majno G, Zand T, Nunnari JJ, Kowala MC, Joris I (1988) Intimal response to shear stress, hypercholesterolemia and hypertension: studies in the rat aorta. In: Simionescu N, Simionescu M (eds) Endothelial cell biology in health and disease. Plenum, New York, pp 349–367
Masuda J, Ross R (1990) Atherogenesis during low level hypercholesterolemia in the nonhuman primate. I. Fatty streak formation. Arteriosclerosis 10:164–177
Mazzone T, Lopez C, Bergstraesser L (1987) Modification of very low density lipoproteins leads to macrophage scavenger receptor uptake and cholesteryl ester deposition. Arteriosclerosis 7:191–196
McCullagh KG, Balian G (1975) Collagen characterization and cell transformation in human atherosclerosis. Nature 258:73–84
Mora R, Lupu F, Simionescu N (1987) Prelesional events in atherogenesis. Colocalization of apolipoprotein B, unesterified cholesterol and extracellular phospholipid liposomes in the aorta of hyperlipidemic rabbit. Atherosclerosis 67:143–154
Mora R, Lupu F, Simionescu N (1989) Cytochemical localization of beta-lipoproteins and their compoents in successive stages of hyperlipidemic atherogenesis of rabbit aorta. Atherosclerosis 79:183–195
Mora R, Simionescu M, Simionescu N (1990) Purification and partial characterization of extracellular liposomes isolated from the hyperlipidemic rabbit aorta. J Lipid Res 31:1793–1807
Morel DW, Hessler JR, Chisolm GM (1983) Low density lipoprotein cytotoxicity induced by free radical peroxidation of lipid. J Lipid Res 24:1070–1078
Morel DW, Di Corleto PE, Chisolm GM (1984) Endothelial and smooth muscle cells alter low density lipoprotein in vitro by free radical oxidation. Arteriosclerosis 4:357–364

Morton RE, West GA, Hoff HF (1986) A low density-lipoprotein-sized particle isolated from human atherosclerotic lesions is internalized by macrophages via a non-scavenger receptor mechanism. J Lipid Res 27:1124–1134

Murata K, Motayama T, Kotake C (1986) Collagen types in various layers of the human aorta and their changes with the atherosclerotic process. Atherosclerosis 60:251–262

Nagelkerke JF, Barto KP, van Berkel TJ (1983) In vivo and in vitro uptake and degradation of acetylated low density lipoprotein by rat liver endothelial, Kupffer, and parenchymal cells. J Biol Chem 258:12221–12227

Nagelkerke JF, Havekes L, van Hinsbergh VWM, van Berkel TJC (1984) In vivo catabolism of biologically modified LDL. Arteriosclerosis 4:256–264

Niculescu F, Hugo F, Rus HG, Vlaicu R, Bhakdi S (1987) Quantitative evaluation of the terminal C5b-9 complement complex by ELISA in human atherosclerotic arteries. Clin Exp Immunol 69:477–486

Nievelstein PFEM, Fogelman AM, Mottino G, Frank JS (1991) Lipid accumulation in rabbit aortic intima two hours after bolus infusion of low density lipoprotein. A deep-etch and immunolocalization study of ultrarapidly frozen tissue. Arteriosclerosis Thromb 11:1795–1805

Nistor A, Bulla A, Filip DA, Radu A (1987) The hyperlipidemic hamster as a model of experimental atherosclerosis. Atherosclerosis 68:159–173

Nordestgaard BG, Tybjaerg-Hansen A, Lewis B (1992) Influx in vivo of low density lipoproteins into aortic intimas of genetically hyperlipidemic rabbits. Roles of plasma concentration, extent of aortic lesion, and lipoprotein particle size as determinants. Arteriosclerosis Thromb 12:6–18

Olgemoller B, Schleicher ED, Schwaabe S, Guretzki H-J, Gerbitz KD (1990) High concentrations of low density lipoprotein basement membrane-associated heparan sulfate proteoglycan in cultured endothelial cells. FEBS Lett 264:37–39

Palinski W, Rosenfeld ME, Yla-Herttuala S, et al. (1989) Low density lipoprotein undergoes oxidative modification in vivo. Proc Natl Acad Sci USA 86:1372–1376

Parthasarathy S, Steinbrecher VP, Barnett J, Witztum JL, Steinberg D (1985) Essential role phospholipase A activity in endothelial cell-induced modification of low density lipoprotein. Proc Natl Acad Sci USA 82:3000–3004

Parthasarathy S, Quinn MT, Schwenke DC, Carew TE, Steinberg D (1989) Oxidative modification of beta-very low density lipoprotein. Potential role in monocyte recruitment and foam cell formation. Arteriosclerosis 9:398–404

Pirisino R, DiSimplicio P, Ignesti G, Bianchi G, Barbera P (1988) Sulfhydryl groups and peroxidase-like activity of albumin as scavenger of organic peroxides. Pharmacol Res Commun 20:545–552

Podet EJ, Shaffer DR, Gianturco SH, Bradley WA, Yang CY, Guyton JR (1991) Interaction of low density lipoproteins with human aortic elastin. Arteriosclerosis Thromb 11:116–122

Quinn MT, Parthasarathy S, Steinberg D (1985) Endothelial cell-derived chemotactic activity for mouse peritoneal macrophages and the effects of modified forms of low density lipoprotein. Proc Natl Acad Sci USA 82:5949–5953

Reidy MA (1985) A reassessment of endothelial injury and arterial lesion formation. Lab Invest 53:513–520

Robbins RA, Wagner WD, Register TC, Caterson B (1992) Demonstration of a keratan sulfate-containing proteoglycan in atherosclerotic aorta. Arteriosclerosis Thromb 12:83–91

Robert L, Jacob MP, Frances C, Godeau G, Hornebeck W (1984) Interaction between elastin and elastases and its role in the aging of the arterial wall, skin and other connective tissues: a review. Mech Ageing Dev 28:155–166

Rodgers GM, Kane WH, Pitas RE (1988) Formation of factor Va by atherosclerotic rabbit aorta mediates factor Xa-catalyzed prothrombin activation. J Clin Invest 81:1911–1919

Rosenfeld ME, Tsukada T, Gown AM, Ross R (1987) Fatty streak initiation in Watanabe heritable hyperlipemic and comparably hypercholesterolemic fat-fed rabbits. Arteriosclerosis 7:9–23

Rosenfeld ME, Chait A, Bierman EL, King W, Goodwin P, Walden CE, Ross R (1988) Lipid composition determines aortic lipid composition of aorta of Watanabe heritable hyperlipemic and comparably hypercholesterolemic fat-fed rabbits. Plasma liqid composition of hypercholesterolemic rabbits. Arteriosclerosis 8:338–347

Rosenfeld ME, Palinski W, Yla-Herttuala S, Butler S, Witztum JL (1990) Distribution of oxidation specific lipid-protein adducts and apolipoprotein B in atherosclerotic lesions of varying severity in WHHL rabbits. Arteriosclerosis 10:336–349

Ross R (1986) The pathogenesis of atherosclerosis: an update. N Engl J Med 314:488–500

Ross R (1992) Endothelial dysfunction and atherosclerosis. In: Simionescu N, Simionescu M (eds) Endothelial cell dysfunctions. Plenum, New York, pp 295–307

Rus HG, Niculescu F, Constantinescu E, Cristea A, Vlaicu R (1986) Immunoelectron-microscopic localization of the terminal C5b-9 complement complex in human atherosclerotic fibrous plaque. Atherosclerosis 61:35–43

Ryan US (1987) Endothelial cell activation responses. In: Ryan US (ed) Pulmonary endothelium in health and disease. Dekker, New York, pp 3–33

Sambandam T, Baker JR, Christner JE, Ekborg SL (1991) Specificity of low density lipoprotein–glycosaminoglycan interaction. Arteriosclerosis Thromb 11:561–568

Schwartz CJ, Valente AJ, Sprague EA, Kelley JL, Nerem RM (1991) The pathogenesis of atherosclerosis: an overview. Clin Cardiol 14:1–16

Schwenke DC, Carew TE (1989) Initiation of atherosclerotic lesions in cholesterol-fed rabbits. I. Focal increases in arterial LDL concentration precede development of fatty streak lesions. Arteriosclerosis 9:895–907

Seifert PS, Hugo F, Hansson GK, Bhakdi S (1989) Prelesional complement activation in experimental atherosclerosis. Lab Invest 60:747–754

Sevanian A, Berliner J, Peterson H (1991) Uptake metabolism, and cytotoxicity of isomeric cholesterol-5,6-epoxides in rabbit aortic endothelial cells. J Lipid Res 32:147–155

Shaikh M, Martini S, Quiney JR, et al. (1988) Modified plasma-derived lipoproteins in human atherosclerotic plaques. Atherosclerosis 69:165–172

Shatos MA, Doherty JM, Hoak JC (1991) Alteration in human vascular endothelial cell function by free radicals. Platelet adherence and prostacyclin release. Arteriosclerosis Thromb 11:594–601

Sima A, Bulla A, Simionescu N (1990) Experimental obstructive coronary atherosclerosis in the hyperlipidemic hamster. J Submicrosc Cytol Pathol 22:1–16

Simionescu D, Iozzo RV, Kefalides NA (1989) Bovine pericardial proteoglycan: biochemical, immunochemical and ultrastructural studies. Matrix 9:301–310

Simionescu N (1988) Prelesional changes of arterial endothelium in hyperlipoproteinemic atherogenesis. In: Simionescu N, Simionescu M (eds) Endothelial cell biology in health and disease. Plenum, New York, pp 385–429

Simionescu M (1992a) Endothelial cell response to normal and abnormal stimuli: modulation, dysfunction, injury-adaptation, repair, death. In: Simionescu N, Simionescu M (eds) Endothelial cell dysfunction. Plenum, New York, pp 3–9

Simionescu N (1992b) Endothelial cell dysfunction and injury in experimental hyperlipidemic atherogenesis. In: Simionescu N, Simionescu M (eds) Endothelial cell dysfunction. Plenum, New York, pp 321–344

Simionescu N, Simionescu M (1985) Interactions of endogenous lipoproteins with capillary endothelium in spontaneously hyperlipoproteinemic rats. Microvasc Res 30:314–332

Simionescu M, Simionescu N (1991a) Endothelial transport of macromolecules: transcytosis and endocytosis. Cell Biol Rev 25:1–78

Simionescu N, Mora R, Vasile E, Lupu F, Filip AD, Simionescu M. (1990) Ann. N.Y. Acad. Sci. 598:1–16

Simionescu N, Simionescu M (1991b) Cellular interactions of lipoproteins with the vascular endothelium: endocytosis and transcytosis. In: Shaw JM (ed) Lipoproteins as carriers of pharmacological agents. Dekker, New York, pp 45–95

Simionescu N, Vasile E, Lupu F, Popescu G, Simionescu M (1986) Prelesional events in atherogenesis: accumulation of extracellular cholesterol-rich liposomes in the intima and cardiac valves of the hyperlipidemic rabbit. Am J Pathol 123:109–125

Sloop CH, Dory L, Roheim PS (1987) Interstitial fluid lipoproteins. J Lipid Res 28:225–237

Small DM, Shipley GG (1974) Physical chemical basis of lipid deposition in atherosclerosis. Science 185:129–177

Smelting-Havinga I, Mommaas M, van Hinsbergh VWM, Daha MR, Daems WT, Vermeer B-J (1989) Immunoelectron microscopic visualization of the transcytosis of low density lipoproteins in perfused rat arteries. Eur J Cell Biol 48:27–36

Smith EB (1986) Plasma macromolecules in interstitial fluid from normal and atherosclerotic human aorta. Monogr Atheroscler 14:179–183

Smith EB (1990) Lipids, lipoproteins and antioxidants in cardiovascular dysfunction. Biochem Soc Trans 19:235–241

Smith EB, Ashall C (1983) Variability of the electrophoretic mobility of low density lipoprotein. Comparison of interstitial fluid from human aortic intima and serum. Atherosclerosis 49:89–98

Smith EB, Staples EM (1980) Distribution of plasma proteins across the human aortic wall. Barrier functions of endothelium and internal elastic lamina. Atherosclerosis 37:579–592

Smith EB, Staples EM (1982) Intimal and medial plasma protein concentrations and endothelial functions. Atherogenesis 41:295–308

Spady DK, Huettinger M, Bilheimer DW, Dietschy JM (1987) Role of receptor-independent low density lipoprotein transport in the maintenance of tissue cholesterol balance in the normal and WHHL rabbit. J Lipid Res 28:32–41

Srinivasan SR, Yost C, Radhakrishnamurthy B, Dalferes ER Jr, Berenson GS (1981) Lipoprotein-elastin interactions in human aorta fibrous plaque lesions. Atherosclerosis 38:137–147

Srinivasan SR, Vijayagopal P, Eberle K, Radhakrishnamurthy B, Berenson GS (1989) Low density lipoprotein binding affinity of arterial wall proteoglycans: characteristics of a chondroitin sulfate proteoglycan subfraction. Biochim Biophys Acta 1006:159–166

Stary HC (1990) The sequence of cell and matrix changes in atherosclerotic lesions of coronary arteries in the first forty years of life. Eur Heart J 11:3–19

Stastny J, Fosslien E, Robertson AL Jr (1986) Human aortic intima protein composition during initial stages of atherogenesis. Atherosclerosis [illegible]

Stein Y, Stein O (1973) Lipid synthesis and degradation and lipoprotein transport in mammalian aorta. In: Atherogenesis: initiating factors. Ciba Foundation, Symposium 12 (new series). Elsevier, Amsterdam, pp 165–183

Stein Y, Stein O, Olivecrona T, Halperin G (1985) Putative role of cholesteryl ester transfer protein in removal of cholesteryl ester from vascular interstitium, studied in a model system in cell culture. Biochim Biophys Acta 834:336–345

Stein O, Halpern G, Stein Y (1986) Cholesteryl ester efflux from extracellular and cellular elements of the arterial wall: model systems in culture with cholesteryl linoleyl ether. Arteriosclerosis 6:70–78

Steinberg D, Pittman RC, Carew TE (1985) Mechanisms involved in the uptake and degradation of low density lipoprotein by the artery wall in vivo. Ann NY Acad Sci 454:195–206

Steinberg D, Parthasarathy S, Carew TE, Khoo JC, Witztum JL (1989) Beyond cholesterol. Modifications of low density lipoprotein that increase its atherogenicity. N Engl J Med 320:915–924

Steinbrecher UP, Parthasarathy S, Leake DS, Witztum, JL, Steinberg D (1984) Modification of low density lipoprotein by endothelial cells involves lipid peroxidation and degradation of low density lipoprotein phospholipids. Proc Natl Acad Sci USA 81:3883–3887

Stemerman MB, Morrel EM, Burke KR, Colton CK, Smith KA, Lees RS (1986) Local variation in artery wall permeability to low density lipoprotein in normal rabbit aorta. Arteriosclerosis 6:64–69

Stender S, Hjelms E (1984) In vivo influx of free and esterified plasma cholesterol into human aortic tissue without atherosclerotic lesions. J Clin Invest 74:1871–1881

Stender S, Hjelms E (1988) In vivo transfer of cholesteryl ester from high and low density lipoproteins into human aortic tissue. Arteriosclerosis 8:252–262

Suits AG, Chait MA, Heinecke JW (1989) Phagocytosis of aggregated lipoprotein by macrophages: low density lipoprotein receptor-dependent foam-cell formation. Proc Natl Acad Sci USA 86:2713–2717

Takano T, Mineo C (1990) Atherosclerosis and molecular pathology: mechanisms of cholesteryl ester-accumulation in foam cells and extracellular space of atherosclerotic lesions. J Pharmacobiodyn 13:385–413

Tanimura N, Asada Y, Hayashi T, Kisanuki A, Sumiyoshi A (1990) Aortic endothelial cell damage induced by β-VLDL and macrophages in vitro. Atherosclerosis 85:161–167

Tedgui A, Chiron B, Curmi P, Juan L (1987) Effect of nicardipine and verapamil on in vitro albumin transport in rabbit thoracic aorta. Arteriosclerosis 7:80–87

Tompkins RG, Yarmush ML, Schnitzer JJ, Colton CK, Smith KA, Stemerman MB (1989) Low-density lipoprotein transport in blood vessel walls of squirrel monkeys. Am J Physiol 257:H452–H464

Trian JE, Meydani SNM, Schaefer EJ (1988) Oxidized low density lipoprotein stimulates prostacyclin production by adult human vascular endothelial cells. Arteriosclerosis 8:810–818

Trillo AA, Prichard RW (1979) Early endothelial changes in experimental primate atherosclerosis. Lab Invest 41:294

van Berkel TJC, De Rijke YB, Kruijt JK (1991) Different fate in vivo of oxidatively modified low density lipoprotein and acetylated low density lipoprotein in rats. Recognition by various scavenger receptors on Kupffer and endothelial liver cells. J Biol Chem 266:2282–2289

van der Wal AC (1989) Atherosclerotic lesions in human. In situ immunophenotypic analysis suggesting an immune mediated response. Lab Invest 61:166–172

Vasile E, Simionescu N (1985) Transcytosis of low density lipoprotein through vascular endothelium. In: Seno E, Copley AL, Ventkatachalam MA, Hamashida Y, Tsujii T (eds) Glomerular dysfunction and Biopathology of vascular wall. Academic New York, pp 87–102

Vasile E, Simionescu M, Simionescu N (1983) Visualization of the binding, endocytosis and transcytosis of low density lipoproteins in the arterial endothelium in situ. J Cell Biol 96:1677–1689

Vasile E, Antohe F, Simionescu M, Simionescu N (1989) Transport pathways of beta-VLDL by aortic endothelium of normal and hypercholesterolemic rabbits. Atherosclerosis 75:195–210

Velican C, Velican D (1986) Atherosclerotic involvement of coronary branch vessels. Atherosclerosis 60:237–250

Vijayagopal P, Srinivasan SR, Radhakrisnamurthy B, Berenson GS (1991) Studies on the mechanism of uptake of low density lipoprotein-proteoglycan complex in macrophages. Biochim Biophys Acta 1092:291–297

Vlaicu R, Niculescu F, Rus HG, Cristea A (1985) Immunochistochemical complex in human aortic fibrous plaque. Atherosclerosis 57:163–170

Volker W, Schmidt A, Oortmann W, Broszey T, Faher V, Buddecke E (1990) Mapping of proteoglycans in atherosclerotic lesions. Eur Hearth J 11 [Suppl E]:29–40

Weis JR, Pitas RE, Wilson BD, Rodgers GM (1991) Oxidized low density lipoprotein increases cultured human endothelial cell tissue factor activity and reduces protein C activation. FASEB J 5:2459–2465

Wiklund O, Carew TE, Steinberg D (1985) Role of the low density lipoprotein receptor in penetration of low density lipoprotein into rabbit aortic wall. Arteriosclerosis 5:135–141

Wilson J, Winter M, Shashy MD (1990) Oxidants, ATP depletion and endothelial permeability to macromolecules. Blood 76:2578–2582

Wissler RW, Vesselinovitch D (1977) Atherosclerosis in nonhuman primates. In: Brandley CA, Cornelius CE, Simpson CF (eds) Advances in veterinary science and comparative medicine, vol 21. Academic, New York, pp 351–420

Witztum JL, Steinberg D (1991) Role of oxidized low density lipoprotein in atherogenesis. J Clin Invest 88:1785–1792

Yla-Herttuala S, Solakivi T, Hirvonen J, et al. (1987) Glycosaminoglycans and apoliproteins B and A-I in human aortas. Chemical and immunological analysis of lesion-free aortas from children and adults. Arteriosclerosis 7:333–340

Yla-Herttuala S, Jaakkola O, Enholm C, Tikkanen MJ, Solaviki T, Sarkioja T, Nikkari T (1988) Characterization of two lipoproteins containing apolipoproteins B and E from lesion-free human aortic intima. J Lipid Res 29:563–572

Yla-Herttuala S, Palinski W, Rosenfeld ME, et al. (1989) Evidence for the presence of oxidatively modified low density lipoprotein in atherosclerotic lesions of rabbit and man. J Clin Invest 84:1086–1095

Yla-Herttuala S, Lipton BA, Rosenfeld ME, et al. (1991) Macrophages express monocyte chemotactic protein (MCP-1) in human and rabbit atherosclerotic lesions. Proc Natl Acad Sci USA 88:5252–5256

Zand T, Nunnari JJ, Hofman AH, Savilonis BJ, MacWilliams B, Majno G, Joris I (1988) Endothelial adaptations in aortic stenosis. Correlation with flow parameters. Am J Pathol 133:407–418

Zhang H, Davis WB, Chen X, Whisler RL, Cornwell DG (1989) Studies on oxidized low density lipoproteins. Controlled oxidation and a prostaglandin artifact. J Lipid Res 30:141–148

Angiogenic Processes in the Pathogenesis of Human Coronary Atherosclerosis

K. SUEISHI, M. KUMAMOTO, H. SAKUDA, and K. TANAKA

1 Introduction

Intimal neovascularization, which represents the newly formed vasa vasorum, has been recognized in atherosclerotic plaques of human coronary arteries for many years (WINTERNITZ et al. 1938; BARGER et al. 1984; KAMAT et al. 1987). Nevertheless, there are still several unresolved questions regarding the origin and pathogenesis of these newly formed blood vessels as well as their pathophysiologic significance in the progression and/or regression of atherosclerosis, and especially the development of its sequelae such as thrombi and intimal hemorrhage. It is well known that neovascularization is a ubiquitous and vital response in various physiologic and pathologic conditions such as embryonic development, the inflammatory–repair process, and the growth of solid cancer (FOLKMAN 1990).

It has been recognized that a critical thickness of the arterial wall is necessary for physiologic and pathologic neovascularization in elastic arteries (WOLINSKY and GLAGOV 1967; LINZBACH 1969). From these observations the hypoxic state has been suggested to induce endothelial ingrowth into the arterial wall from a teleologic perspective. In the arterial wall, however, the interaction between cellular components such as endothelial cells, smooth muscle cells (SMCs), and migrating T lymphocytes and monocyte-macrophages has been thought to be essential in the atherogenic processes. This idea has recently led investigators to refocus their attention on the inflammatory aspects of atherogenesis, including the events of intimal neovascularization. The regulatory mechanisms of neovascularization have recently been studied in close detail from a molecular biologic perspective, but there have been disagreements and controversies

Current Topics in Pathology
Volume 87, Vollmer/Roessner (Eds.)

concerning the pathobiologic role and significance in vivo of many angiogenic factors.

The purpose of this paper is primarily to discuss (a) the three-dimensional distribution of newly formed blood vessels in atherosclerotic plaques of human coronary arteries, (b) the origin of vascular ingrowth into the plaques, with reference to light microscopic observations of serial sections, and (c) the association of intimal neovascularization with intimal hemorrhage and rupture, inflammatory cell infiltrate, and accumulation of atheromatous gruel. An attempt will also be made to clarify the effect of the hypoxic state on SMC modulation of the angiogenic process in vitro.

2 Pathophysiologic Significance of Neovascularization in Human Coronary Atherosclerosis

In cardiovascular lesions, neovascularization occurs ubiquitously as an organization and recanalization of thrombi and aberrant vasa vasora in atherosclerotic intima, and in the reparative stage of angiitis. Several reports have found that newly formed microvessels in atherosclerotic intima of human coronary arteries are generally fragile and tortuous, suggesting that these vessels are related to the occurrence of intimal hemorrhage and rupture of atheroma, and are possibly followed by the formation of occlusive thrombi and vascular spasms with occasionally fatal consequences.

2.1 Coronary Artery Lesions in Acute Myocardial Infarction

Acute myocardial infarction has been shown clinically to be largely caused by coronary thrombosis (DE WOOD et al. 1980). In order to examine the occurrence of coronary thrombosis and histopathologic alterations of thrombotic sites of coronary arteries, a series of 84 autopsies in patients with acute myocardial infarction from Kyushu University Hospital and its affiliates were studied by postmortem angiography with the barium sulfate infusion method and by light microscopic observation of serial sections. Approximately 70% of these patients were observed to have thrombus formation in the epicardial coronary arteries perfusing the infarcted myocardium. Comparison between the types of acute myocardial infarction in respect of the prevalence of coronary thrombosis revealed a higher incidence of thrombi in the massive type of acute myocardial infarction, especially the transmural type (90.2%), than in others (Table 1). The histologic alterations at the sites of coronary thrombosis are shown in Table 2. Almost all thrombi observed in this study were located in the markedly obliterated coronary arteries in more than 75% of the cross-sectional areas, due to atherosclerotic lesions. The main lesions in the target coronary branches

Table 1. Correlation between types of acute myocardial infarction and coronary thrombosis

Type	Case	Thrombosis
Massive	54	46 (85.2%)
Transmural	41	37 (90.2%)
Not transmural	13	9 (69.2%)
Scattered	9	6 (66.7%)
Subendocardial	12	2 (16.7%)
Subtotal	75	54 (72.0%)
Undetermined	9	3 (33.3%)
Total	84	57 (67.9%)

Table 2. Histologic alterations at sites of coronary thrombosis

Histologic changes	Thrombus	Occlusive
Rupture of atheroma	31 (50.0%)	23/31 (74.2%)
Hemorrhage in the intima	14 (22.6%)	8/14 (57.2%)
Marked sclerosis only	17 (27.4%)	5/17 (29.4%)
Total	62 (100%)	36/62 (50.0%)

were the rupture of atheroma and intimal hemorrhage in plaques. These lesions were observed in more than 70% of thrombotic sites and these thrombi were frequently occlusive (Table 2). The frequency and pathophysiologic significance of coronary thrombosis are still the subject of controversy and there have been some discrepancies between pathologic and clinical studies. De Wood et al. (1980), however, supported the significance of coronary thrombosis in acute transmural myocardial infarction on the basis of angiographic findings and demonstrated total coronary occlusion which was consistent with acute occlusive thrombosis in 80% of the patients. Our data obtained in this study confirm the hypothesis that the most drastic and significant coronary lesions in fatal acute myocardial infarctions are occlusive coronary thrombus formations which are frequently associated with rupture of atheroma and hemorrhages in plaques.

A critical event in the process of coronary thrombus formation appears to be the endothelial injuries, not only in the coronary arteries but also in the newly formed vascular channels in atherosclerotic plaques. Such endothelial injury leads to increased permeability, causing intimal hemorrhage and activation of platelets and the coagulation cascade through the initiation of activation of the extrinsic pathway.

The injuries to luminal endothelial cells have been thought to be more critical in the formation of occlusive coronary thrombus, especially in fatal myocardial infarction, than those of newly formed blood vessels originating from both luminal and adventitial endothelial ingrowth. However, the latter vessels are a possible source of intimal hemorrhage. Intimal hemorrhage with luminal thrombus but without a rupture of the fibrous cap overlying the atheromatous lesions is actually not rare (Table 2). This has to be borne in mind when appraising the significance of intimal neovascularization in the pathogenesis of coronary atherosclerosis and the sequelae, including intramural hemorrhage and luminal thrombosis.

2.2 Neovascularization in Human Coronary Arteries

In order to analyze the origins of angiogenic growth from either luminal or adventitial vascular endothelial cells, we investigated 20 patients (average age: 72 years) who died of noncardiac causes such as malignancies, terminal infections,

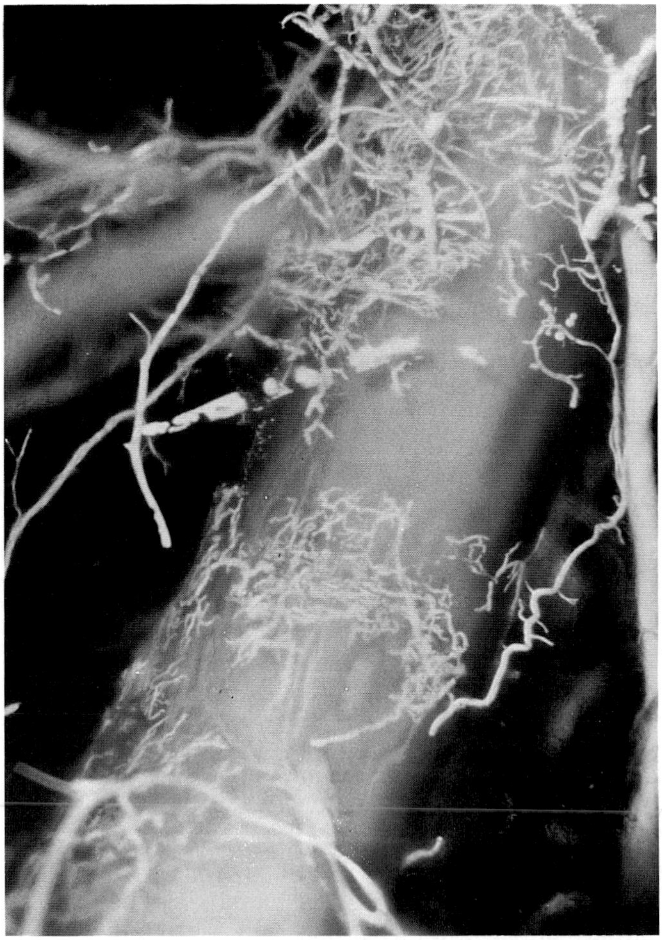

Fig. 1. Neovascularization of coronary artery. The newly formed vascular networks are segmentally documented with silicone polymer infusion; they are located in close vicinity to the lumen of the coronary artery with atherosclerotic narrowing

and cerebrovascular accidents, along with 11 patients (average age: 73 years) who died of cardiac causes. Post-mortem angiography of methyl salicylate-cleared hearts with silicone polymer was utilized (BARGER et al. 1984), while delicate and complicated vascular network or plexuses were segmentally documented in close vicinity to the lumen of coronary arteries and were almost always associated with atherosclerotic narrowing (Fig. 1). These newly formed vessels showed an irregular distribution around the stenotic proper lumen as well as an uneven diameter. Such vascular networks occasionally surrounded the entire circumference of the coronary arteries, and typically were infused from the adventitial blood vessels with silicone polymer under a stereoscopic microscope (Wild, Heerbrugg, FRG) equipped with a fiberoptic light source (Nikon, Tokyo, Japan). Abrupt transition between vascular and avascular portions was occasionally encountered, as reported by BARGER et al. (1984), and this fact seemed to be related to the macro- and microscopic findings that atherosclerotic plaques occurred unevenly and were occasionally well circumscribed.

The light microscopic examinations using serial sections, obtained from about 70 paraffin-embedded blocks approximately 3 mm thick which had been taken from 15 left anterior descending arteries, revealed that newly formed blood vessels in atherosclerotic lesions were derived mainly from adventitial (about 630 arteries in 12 cases) and partly from luminal endothelial growth (about 20 arteries in nine cases) (Fig. 2).

The luminal stenosis of coronary arteries and the intimal vascular density (numbers of blood vessels/intimal area) at 250 sites of 25 left anterior descending branches were morphometrically examined using a Cosmozone-S (Nikon, Tokyo, Japan), and the degree of intimal neovascularization was then compared

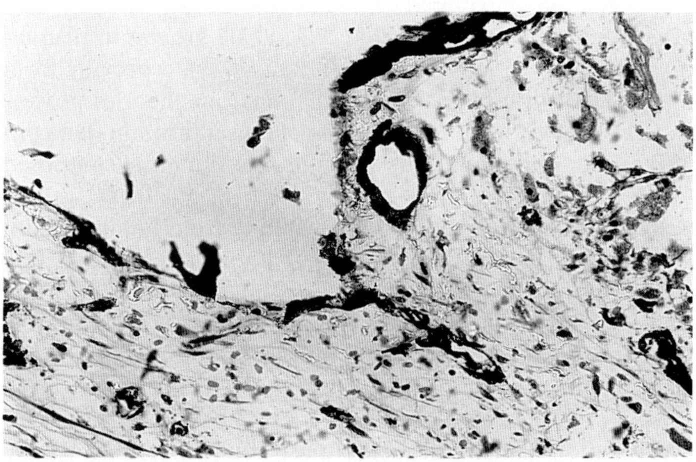

Fig. 2. Light microscopic finding of newly formed vessels in the atherosclerotic intima. A blood vessel connects directly with the lumen of the coronary artery, suggesting that this vessel in the intima is derived from luminal endothelial growth. H&E, × 580

with histopathologic alterations of atherosclerotic plaques. The extent of intimal neovascularization was relatively correlated with the severity of atherosclerosis, especially with luminal narrowing ($r = 0.411$, $P < 0.0001$). This vascular proliferation was frequently associated with inflammatory cell infiltrate, the formation of atheroma and granulation-like tissue, and intimal hemorrhage, but not with calcification or hyalinization.

The distribution of these blood vessels was not simple and varied in each patient; this fact appeared to be fundamentally related to the variety of human atherosclerotic lesions, which may progress and/or regress over a long period. However, newly formed vessels derived from adventitial endothelial growth tended to be localized in the shoulder portion of atherosclerotic plaques as well as in the deeper portion of the atheroma, and the blood vessels from luminal endothelial growth were also distributed not only in the superficial intima but also in the deeper intima, forming vascular plexuses. The intimal vessels ingrowing from the adventitia were frequently associated with the formation of granulation-like tissue and chronic inflammatory infiltrate, but the vessels from the luminal surface rarely showed such histologic alterations. Fresh and old hemorrhages were found in association in about 60% of the intima examined. Fibrinous exudate and accumulation of hemosideraphages were more frequently present around the blood vessels originating from the luminal surface than around those originating from the adventitia.

2.3 Angiogenic Processes in Atherosclerosis

The findings described above support the hypothesis that there are three possible mechanisms of intimal neovascularization, namely, metabolic, thrombogenic, and inflammatory. The metabolic explanation is that the newly formed blood vessels result from the stimulation of endothelial cells which grow into plaques owing to local hypoxia (OSBORN 1963; ZEMPLENYI et al. 1989), especially from adventitial vasa vasora. The thrombogenic and inflammatory theories possess many similarities that exist between the organization of mural thrombi (DUGUID and ROBERTSON 1957) and that inflammatory cell infiltrate is mainly composed of macrophages and T lymphocytes (VAN DER WAL et al. 1989), as well as atherosclerotic processes. The angiogenic process resulting from luminal endothelial ingrowth into plaques has been entirely unclear. Although the organization of mural thrombi seems to be a possible mechanism, intimal neovascularization has not been reported even in the experimental animal models of thrombogenic atherosclerosis. However, the organization of mural thrombi with intimal hemorrhage may leave the intimal sclerosis accompanied by neovascularization as a sequela.

Intimal neovascularization is, therefore, ubiquitously found in human atherosclerotic coronary arteries and is probably a normal response to injury occurring during atherosclerotic processes. These angiogenic processes may involve various factors such as platelet-, macrophage-, fibroblast- and SMC-derived growth factors (PDGF, bFGF, ECDGF, PDECGE, and others) and other modulating factors, including transforming growth factor β (TGF-β) and tumor necrosis factor α (TNF-α). However, the in vivo factors regulating the synthesis, release, and decomposition of angiogenic factors in the context of atherosclerosis are largely unknown.

Intimal neovascularization may be essential as an inflammatory-repair process in both the progression and the regression of coronary atherogenesis and its sequelae, such as intimal hemorrhage, rupture of fibrous plaque, and the formation of occlusive thrombi (possibly leading to acute myocardial infraction). The aforementioned sequelae may be induced by the additional effects of coronary spasm (VINCENT et al. 1983), hypertension (FRYER et al. 1987), or abrupt fluctuations of blood pressure on newly formed blood vessels in the atherosclerotic intima.

3 Angiogenesis In Vitro: Endothelial Cell–Smooth Muscle Cell Interaction

Atherosclerotic lesions are characterized by SMC proliferation, chronic inflammatory cell infiltrate, and extra- and intracellular deposition of lipids. As described above, intimal neovascularization has been shown to correlate with the degree of luminal stenosis in atherosclerotic lesions in vivo; furthermore, it has been speculated that intimal neovascularization is regulated by cell-to-cell interaction in vivo, i.e., by the interaction between endothelial cells and other cells such as SMCs and infiltrating inflammatory cells, especially macrophages and lymphocytes. Therefore, we examined the influence of hypoxia on the modulating effect of SMCs in angiogenesis, using the quantitative assay method of the in vitro angiogenesis model (YASUNAGA et al. 1989).

Bovine capillary endothelial cells (BCEs) were isolated from the bovine adrenal cortex (FOLKMAN et al. 1979) and the eighth to tenth passage of culture was used in the studies. Bovine SMCs were isolated from the bovine aortic media by the explant method (ROSS 1971) and used at the sixth to 13th passage. Confluent SMCs (ca. 9.2×10^4 cells/cm^2) were cultured under conditions of 20%, 5%, or 1% O_2 balanced with N_2 in a humidified 0.5% CO_2 incubator at 37°C (Multigasincubator BL-3200, Astec Co., Fukuoka, Japan). The conditioned media were harvested after 3–48 h. BCEs (6×10^4 cells/well) were seeded on type I collagen gels (0.2%) on Millicell filters (12 mm in diameter, Millipore Co., Bedford, MA) which were inserted onto 12-well plates (Corning Glass Works, Corning, NY). The conditioned media were applied to the outer well, and then BCEs on the Millicell filters were cultured in a conventional CO_2 incubator at an O_2 concentration of 20%. The extent of angiogenesis was assessed by measuring and calculating morphometrically the total length of tubular structures (mm/cm^2) organized by BCEs in type I collagen gels (YASUNAGA et al. 1989).

Table 3. Tube formation by bovine capillary endothelial cells in SMC-conditioned media (SMC-CM)

Culture condition	Total length of tube (mm/mm^2)
Fresh medium	0.343 ± 0.170
SMC-CM	
20% O_2	0.739 ± 0.155*
5% O_2	1.673 ± 0.322**
1% O_2	2.543 ± 0.073***
bFGF (10 ng/ml)	1.580 ± 0.220*

Mean values ($\pm$SD) of three experiments are shown.
*$P < 0.05$; **$P < 0.01$; ***$P < 0.001$ vs control

Table 4. Effects of anti-bFGF or anti-TGF-β_1 polyclonal IgG on tube formation by bovine capillary endothelial cells in SMC-conditioned media (SMC-CM) cultured at an O_2 concentration of 1%

Culture condition	Total length of tube (mm/mm^2)
Fresh medium	0.32 ± 0.08*
SMC-CM	
CM + nonimmune IgG (30 μg/ml)	2.49 ± 0.57
CM + anti-bFGF IgG (30 μg/ml)	2.15 ± 0.54(NS)
CM + anti-TGF-β_1 IgG (30 μg/ml)	0.67 ± 0.19*

Mean values ($\pm$SD) of three experiments are shown.
*$P < 0.01$; NS, not significant vs CM + nonimmune IgG

The effect of SMC-conditioned media on tube formation is shown in Table 3. SMC-conditioned media enhanced the tube formation as compared with the nonconditioned fresh culture medium as a negative control, and bFGF at a concentration of 10 ng/ml as a positive control. These enhancing effects of the SMC-conditioned media on tube formation were apparently dependent on the degree of hypoxia. When anti-bFGF or anti-TGF-β_1 polyclonal IgG was added to SMC-conditioned media cultured at an O_2 concentration of 1%, anti-TGF-β_1 IgG significantly suppressed the effect of the SMC-conditioned media on tube formation while anti-bFGF did not (Table 4). In addition to the in vitro assay of angiogenic reagents, we confirmed the role of possible angiogenic factors in an in vivo assay system. Figure 3 shows the results obtained using the rabbit cornea assay method on the 5th day after application of the stimulant. The polymer mesh containing serum-free SMC-conditioned media at 1% O_2, which was concentrated and dialyzed with phosphate-buffered saline (PBS), was embedded into the cornea. The newly formed blood vessels grew into the embedded portion of the polymer mesh containing SMC-conditioned media from the congested vascular networks at the corneal limbus. No neovascularization was apparent in the negative control using polymer mesh with PBS. Figure 4

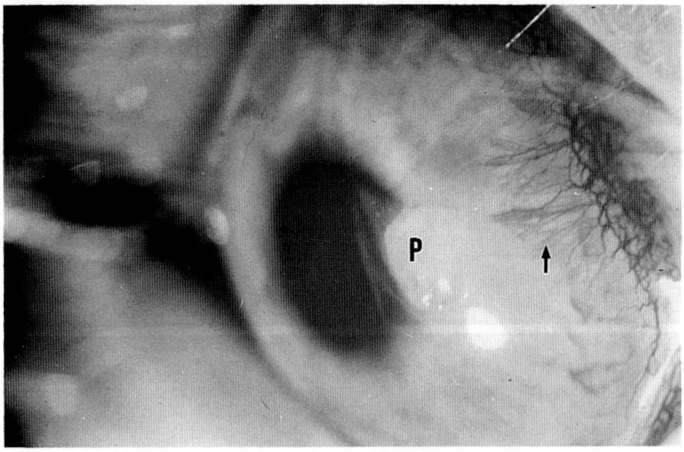

Fig. 3. Angiogenesis in the rabbit cornea effected by SMC-conditioned medium cultured in a hypoxic state. SMCs were cultured in serum-free DMEM at 1% O_2 for 24 h and the conditioned medium was concentrated and dialyzed with PBS. The newly formed blood vessels (*arrow*) are developing toward the intracorneal polymer mesh (*P*), containing SMC-conditioned medium, from the corneal limbus

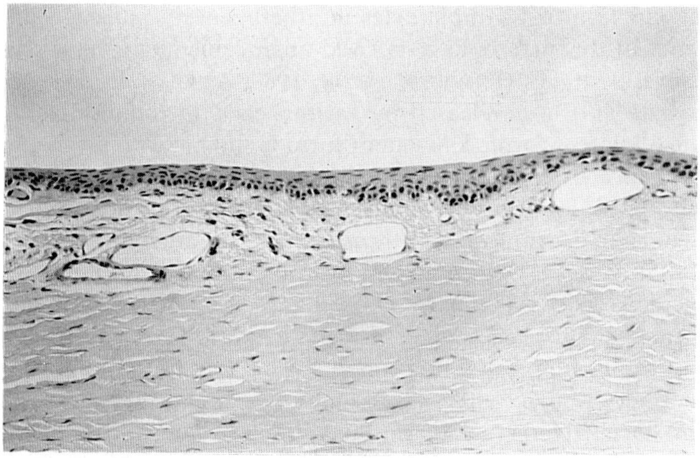

Fig. 4. Light microscopic findings in respect of the rabbit cornea shown in Fig. 3. Newly formed veins and a small muscular artery can be observed in association with minimal inflammatory cell infiltrate composed mainly of macrophages. H&E, × 100

shows the light microscopic findings in respect of the rabbit cornea, which was observed to contain newly formed blood vessels composed of veins and a small muscular artery, and minimal inflammatory cell infiltrate mainly composed of macrophages. The extent of inflammatory cell infiltrate was not substantially different from that found following the application of bFGF.

Thymidine incorporation by BCEs, SMCs and fibroblasts in the two-dimensional and conventional culture system without gel matrix was suppressed by the SMC-conditioned media and this suppression depended on the hypoxic state. The inhibitory effect of the SMC-conditioned media on the growth of these cells was apparently abolished by the simultaneous addition of anti-TGF-β_1 IgG, but not by anti-bFGF or anti-PDGF IgG. These findings suggest that SMCs in a hypoxic state release an active angiogenic factor(s) into the conditioned media and that active TGF-β_1 is closely involved in the expression of the angiogenic effect by SMCs cultured under a hypoxic state.

The relation of tissue hypoxia to angiogenesis has been observed under various conditions and seems to be quite close for vital organs, owing to both the direct influence on endothelial cells and the indirect modulation of angiogenic processes by SMCs and macrophages producing angiogenic factors which may stimulate endothelial cells in a paracrine manner. KNIGHTON et al. (1983) provided evidence that macrophages cultured in a hypoxic environment released angiogenic factor into the conditioned media and speculated that the expression of angiogenic factor by macrophages was influenced by oxygen tension without the necessity for interaction with other cells or biochemical signals. This factor did not accerelate thymidine incorporation by capillary endothelial cells and fibroblasts. Their report is of great interest because our data are quite similar to theirs and macrophages have also been known to play an important role in association with the function of T lymphocytes in atherogenesis, although the biochemical properties of this macrophage-derived angiogenic factor have not yet been clarified. Several studies (LAWRENCE et al. 1984; ASSOIAN et al. 1987) have demonstrated that TGF-β is released by various cells, including macrophages, in a biologically latent form. This latent form is unable to bind to the TGF-β_1 receptor (WAKEFIELD et al. 1987) and the mechanism of activation of the latent form to the active form in vivo still remains unclear. The latent form can be converted to an active form by either transient acid treatment or heating (LAWRENCE et al. 1985) as well as by treatment with proteinases (LYONS et al. 1988, 1990). Angiogenic activity was found to be enhanced in a dose-dependent manner by the addition of Glu-plasminogen to SMC-conditioned media at 1% O_2. Furthermore, aprotinin suppressed this enhancing activity of plasminogen, suggesting that the angiogenic activity expressed by SMCs cultured under a hypoxic state might be partly related to the activation of latent TGF-β by unknown proteases produced by SMCs. Our results suggested that a small amount of active TGF-β was produced in the SMCs cultured in a hypoxic state, although we could not determine the exact amounts of latent and active TGF-β in this study.

We examined the TGF-β_1 gene expression by SMCs cultured under either 20% or 1% O_2. Hypoxic cultivation decreased the amounts of total RNA produced by SMCs. Northern blot analysis of poly(A)$^+$ mRNA demonstrated TGF-β_1-specific 2.5-kb mRNA and the transcripts of the TGF-β_1 gene were not increased by hypoxic cultivation for 24 h. Therefore, the increased production of active TGF-β appeared to be the result of regulation at the posttranscriptional level, or the activation of latent TGF-β by continuous acidic coditions around the cells, or unknown proteinase(s) probably produced by SMCs under hypoxic cultivation.

It is well known that TGF-β_1 is an extremely potent chemotactic agent for macrophages (Wahl et al. 1987). If SMCs were able to produce active TGF-β in vivo in a hypoxic environment, such as atherosclerotic plaques, then neovascularization could also be caused by angiogenic factors derived from macrophages attracted to the TGF-β. Recently, six TGF-β isoforms have been discovered and Merwin et al. (1991) suggested that endothelial cells show different responses to TGF-β_1 and -β_2, depending on the origin of the cells (i.e., from aorta or microvasculature), the experimental conditions (such as two- or three-dimensional cultivation), and the TGF-β concentration.

Although we have proposed various possible mechanisms of intimal neovascularization in atherosclerotic lesions, our findings tend to support the hypothesis that the interaction endothelial cells and vascular SMCs plays a very important role in angiogenic processes even in atherosclerosis, and that active TGF-β participates in the enhancement and regulation of angiogenic processes in a paracrine system. Further studies, however, are necessary to prove the presence of active TGF-β in situ in atherosclerotic lesions and also to clarify the mechanism of activation of latent TGF-β in a hypoxic state.

Acknowledgement. This work was supported in part by Grants-in-Aids for Scientific Research from the Ministry of Education, Science and Culture of Japan (# 63304045, 02219105).

References

Assoian RK, Fleurdelys BE, Stevenson HC et al. (1987) Expression and secretion of type beta transforming growth factor by activated human macrophages. Proc Natl Acad Sci USA 84:6020–6024

Barger AC, Beeuwkes R III, Lainey LL, Silverman KJ (1984) Hypothesis: vasa vasorum and neovascularization of human coronary arteries. N Engl J Med 310:175–177

De Wood MA, Spores J, Notske R et al. (1980) Prevalence of total coronary occlusion during the early hours of transmural myocardial infarction. N Engl J Med 303:897–902

Duguid JB, Robertson WB (1957) Mechanical factors in atherosclerosis. Lancet I:1205–1209

Folkman J (1990) What is the evidence that tumors are angiogenesis dependent? J Natl Cancer Inst 82:4–6

Folkman J, Haudenschild CC, Zetter BR (1979) Long-term culture of capillary endothelial cells. Proc Natl Acad Sci USA 76:5217–5221

Fryer JA, Myers PC, Appleberg M (1987) Carotid intraplaque hemorrhage: the significance of neovascularity. J Vasc Surg 6:341–349

Kamat BR, Galli SJ, Barger AC et al. (1987) Neovascularization and coronary atherosclerotic plaque: cinematographic localization and quantitative histologic analysis. Hum Pathol 18:1036–1042

Knighton DR, Hunt TK, Scheuenstuhl H et al. (1983) Oxygen tension regulates the expression of angiogenesis factor by macrophages. Science 221:1283–1285

Lawrence DA, Pircher R, Kryceve-Martinerie C (1984) Normal embryo fibroblasts release transforming growth factors in a latent form. J Cell Physiol 121:184–188

Lawrence DA, Pircher R, Jullien P (1985) Conversion of a high molecular weight latent β-TGF from chicken embryo fibroblasts into a low molecular weight active β-TGF under acidic conditions. Biochem Biophys Res Commun 133:1026–1034

Linzbach AJ (1969) The anatomy and physiology of the vascular wall. In: Bader H (eds) Handbook of physiology, vol II. American Physiological Society, Williams and Wilkens, Baltimore pp 830–864

Lyons RM, Keski-Oja J, Moses HL (1988) Proteolytic activation of latent transforming growth factor-β from fibroblast-conditioned medium. J Cell Biol 106:1659–1665

Lyons RM, Gentry LE, Purchio AF, Moses HL (1990) Mechanism of activation of latent recombinant transforming growth factor β_1 by plasmin. J Cell Biol 110:1361–1367

Merwin JR, Newman W, Beall LD et al. (1991) Vascular cells respond differentially to transforming growth factors $beta_1$ and $beta_2$ in vitro. Am J Pathol 138:37–51

Osborn GR (1963) The incubation period of coronary thrombosis. Butterworths, London

Ross R (1971) The smooth muscle cell. II. Growth of smooth muscle in culture and formation of elastic fibers. J Cell Biol 50:172–186

van der Wal AC, Das PK, van der Berg DB et al. (1989) Atherosclerotic lesions in humans. In situ immunophenotypic analysis suggesting an immune mediated response. Lab Invest 61:166–170

Vincent GM, Anderson JL, Marshall HW (1983) Coronary spasm producing coronary thrombosis and myocardial infarction. N Engl J Med 309:220–223

Wahl SM, Hunt DA, Wakefield LM et al. (1987) Transforming growth factor type induces monocyte chemotaxis and growth factor production. Proc Natl Acad Sci USA 84:5788–5792

Wakefield LM, Smith DM, Masui C et al. (1987) Distribution and modulation of the cellular receptor for transforming growth factor-beta. J Cell Biol 105:965–975

Winternitz MC, Thomas RM, Le Compte PM (1938) The biology of atherosclerosis. Charles C Thomas, Springfield I11

Wolinsky H, Glagov S (1987) Nature of species differences in the medial distribution of aortic vasa vasorum in animals. Circ Res 20:409–421

Yasunaga C, Nakashima Y, Sueishi K (1989) A role of fibrinolytic activity in angiogenesis: quantitative assay using in vitro method. Lab Invest 61:698–704

Zemplenyi T, Crawford DW, Cole MA (1989) Adaptation to arterial wall hypoxia demonstrated in vivo with oxygen microcathodes. Atherosclerosis 76:173–179

Differentiation and Role of Macrophages in the Early Human Atherosclerotic Plaque

A. ROESSNER, E. VOLLMER, E. JAEGER, J. RAUTERBERG, and W. BÖCKER

1 Introduction

New morphologic investigations on the pathogenesis of atherosclerosis have refocused attention on the role of monocytes and macrophages, especially in the early phases of the disease. The importance of macrophages in the pathogenesis of atherosclerosis had already been pointed out by SCHAEFER and ASSMANN (1980) and SCHAEFER (1981), and current interest in this topic is somewhat in contrast to the former concentration on smooth muscle cells. Various factors have prompted the aforementioned reorientation: Macrophages were found to be essentially involved in the intimal lipoprotein metabolism (BROWN and GOLDSTEIN 1983, 1986; KELLEY 1991; YLÄ-HERTTUALA et al. 1991). They incorporate cholesterol-binding lipoproteins that enter the intima, but if they have taken up more than they can possibly digest, the excess cholesterol will be stored as drop-like cytoplasmic deposits. Recent experimental data have suggested that the majority of foam cells observed in the atherosclerotic plaque must be of this origin. Foam cell transformation of smooth muscle cells was found to be rather less common (WATANABE et al. 1985; SCHWARTZ et al. 1985). Although the functional importance of macrophages in lipoprotein metabolism has been verified in vitro, our knowledge of their behavior, especially in the human atherosclerotic plaque, is still fairly vague, as most of the morphologic studies conducted in this field have been based on experimental models (MASUDA and ROSS 1990a, b).

Monoclonal antibodies revealed a distinct heterogeneity of human aortic intimal cells (OREKHOV et al. 1986). Further phenotypic characterization of macrophages, and their differential identification from other cell types of the

Current Topics in Pathology
Volume 87, Vollmer/Roessner (Eds.)

human atherosclerotic plaque, has been facilitated by application of the monoclonal antibody technique (RADZUN 1985; ZWADLO et al. 1985, 1986). The present study was aimed at a more detailed characterization of the macrophage-derived foam cells in the atherosclerotic plaque. We performed immunohistologic investigations with appropriate antibodies for differentiating the cell types of the mononuclear-phagocyte system.

2 Materials and Methods

Our investigations were performed on samples excised from the ascending aorta of patients undergoing coronary bypass surgery. Since the employed antibodies were also applicable to formol-fixed tissue, the samples were fixed in 4% formol and carefully embedded in paraffin, a procedure that ensures better morphologic preservation than the usual work-up of frozen sections.

Immunohistochemical studies were performed with single and double indirect peroxidase and alkaline phosphatase methods, using the substrate 3,3-diaminobenzidine tetrahydrochloride (DAB) or 3,9-ethylcarbazole (AEC) and naphthol salts as coupling reagent with hexazotic neofuchsin (Sigma, Munich, and Merck, Darmstadt). Endogenous peroxidase was suppressed by $NaNO_3$, and endogenous alkaline phosphatase with levamisole. For secondary and tertiary antibodies we used products of Sigma (Munich), Dakopatts (Hamburg), and Dianova (Hamburg). Nuclear counterstaining was performed with acid hemalum. For negative controls we omitted the primary antibody, or incubated normal serum of the species in question. For positive controls we used the remaining slices of each set.

Light microscopic controls were stained with hematoxylin and eosin. Antibodies for demonstration of monocytes (27-E-10; ZWADLO et al. 1986) and macrophages (25-F-9; ZWADLO et al. 1985) and the antibody against apolipoprotein E were kindly supplied by Prof. Dr. C. Sorg (Institute of Experimental Dermatology, Münster University). The antibody against the inflammatory differentiation antigen (4-D-10) was supplied by Dr. Goerdt from the same institute (GOERDT et al. 1987). The polyclonal antibodies against human apolipoproteins A-I, A-II, and B are commercially available from Boehringer (Mannheim). The monoclonal antibody against muscle-specific α-actin (HHF35; TSUKADA et al. 1987) was purchased from Dakopatts (Hamburg).

3 Demonstration and Differentiation of Macrophages in Fatty Streaks

Conventional light microscopy in H&E staining demonstrated typical foam cells in incipient fatty streaks that are characterized by a lucent cytoplasm and darkly staining nuclei. Their cytologic nature, however, cannot be inferred from the histologic picture alone (Fig. 1). Immunohistologic studies using antibodies against α-1-antichymotrypsin, known to be a marker for cells of the mononuclear-macrophage system, identified the majority of such foam cells as members of the macrophage population. Since antibodies against α-1-antichymotrypsin are known to be nonspecific for demonstrating cells of the mononuclear-phagocyte system (ROESSNER et al. 1987a), we have applied specific monoclonal antibodies to cells of the mononuclear-phagocyte system.

Vessels with incipient fatty streaks showed isolated subendothelial blood monocytes with positive staining with antibody 27-E-10, directed against blood monocytes (Fig. 2). Foam cells would never stain with this antibody. Developing fatty streaks were characterized by a considerable infiltration of macrophages changing to foam cells which displayed negative staining to antibody 27-E-10 against blood monocytes, but strong positive staining to antibody 25-F-9 against mature tissue macrophages. Subendothelial clusters of foamy macrophages were early manifestations. During the progression of lipid streaks we observed extended subendothelial clusters of foam cells thickening the intima. The clusters were identified as mature tissue macrophages by their positive reaction to antibody 25-F-9 (Fig. 3). Only some isolated smooth muscle cells were observed within lipid streaks (Fig. 4). These results permit the conclusion that blood monocytes are able to pervade the endothelial layer, then stay in the intima and be transformed into mature tissue macrophages, from which the majority of foam cells are derived. These foam cells supply the structural characteristics of fatty streaks; the specific antibodies applied in our study allow for appropriate discrimination of infiltrating macrophage populations in the arterial intima (ROESSNER et al. 1987; ROSENFELD and ROSS 1990).

4 Endothelial Pervasion by Macrophages

The next question is how macrophages manage to enter and pervade the vascular endothelium. According to recent investigations, a certain phenotypic modulation of the endothelial cells may be involved in this process (MUNRO and COTRAN 1988). There is increasing experimental evidence for the diversity of endothelial cells, which may be comparable to that of cells belonging to the mononuclear-phagocyte system proper (GOERDT et al. 1987). Is has been possible to raise specific monoclonal antibodies against different subtypes of endothelial cells (GOERDT et al. 1987). We have used an antibody (4-D-19) reacting with a certain differentiation antigen which is expressed exclusively by endothelial cells in tissues undergoing inflammatory changes (GOERDT et al. 1987). The antigen which is recognized by this antibody is known as ELAM (SCHULZE-OSTHOFF et al. 1989).

Investigations performed on endothelial cell cultures have clearly shown that the inflammatory differentiation antigen that reacts with the antibody 4-D-10 can be induced on endothelial cells by various inflammatory stimuli

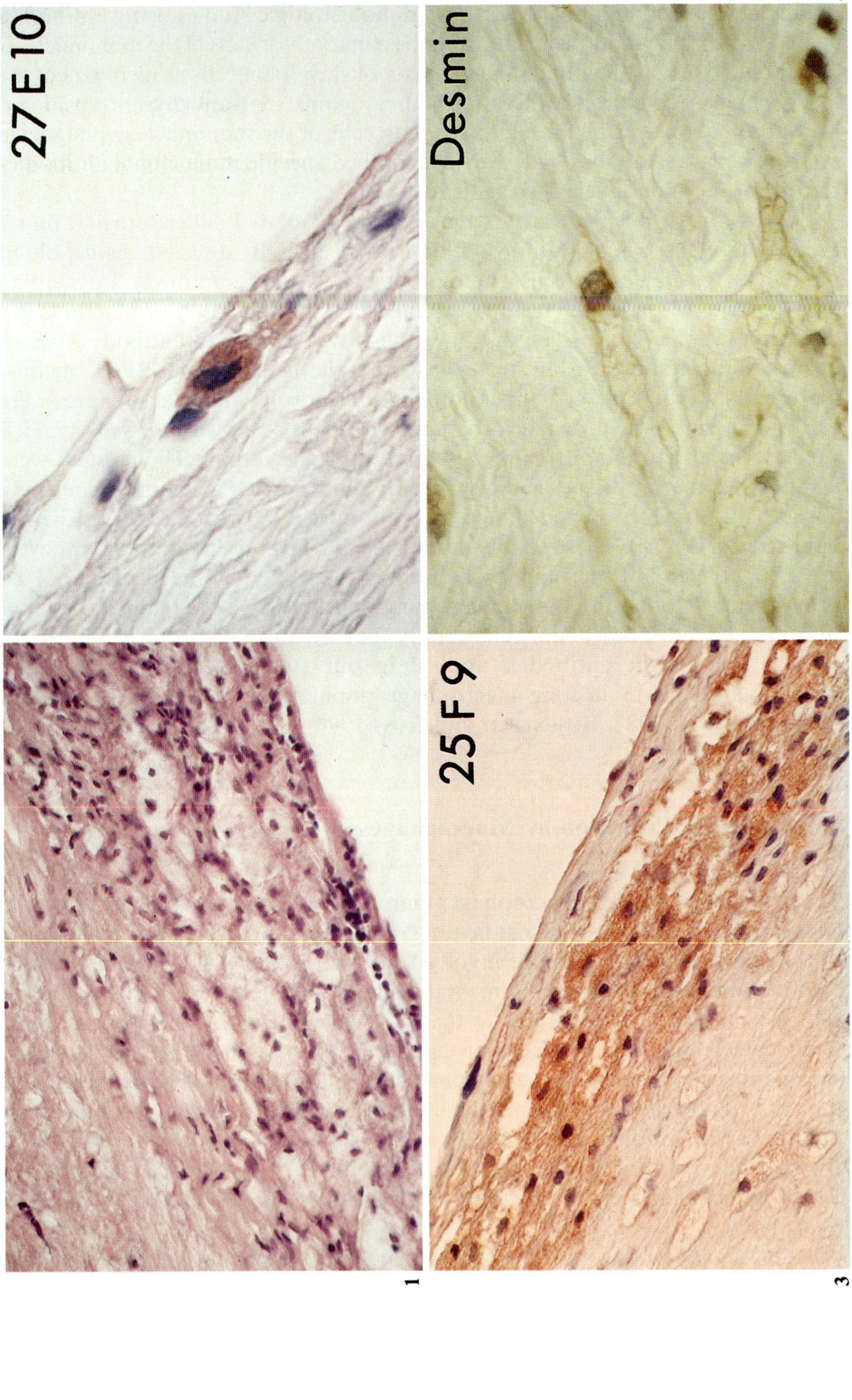

Figs. 1–4

such as endotoxins, phorbol esters, and tumor necrosis factor. If stimulation is discontinued, antigen expression will decrease. Consequently the antibody can be used to discriminate endothelial cells in inflammatory tissue. According to current opinion, there is increasing evidence for the inflammatory basis of atherosclerosis. The similarities between the two processes were recently stressed (MUNRO and COTRAN 1988). We therefore wanted to determine whether expression of the inflammatory differentiation antigen could also be found in the endothelial cells covering early atherosclerotic plaques. Staining of fatty streaks in fibrous/fatty lesions showed distinct positivity for antibody 4-D-10 against the inflamatory differentiation antigen (Fig. 5). In endothelial cells covering unaltered aortic walls the inflammatory differetiation antigen was not detected. These results show that endothelial cells express on their surface selective leukocyte adhesion molecules that can promote local adhesion of different types of leukocytes. CYBULSKY et al. (1990) have recently found that endothelial cells overlying nascent atheromas in experimental atherosclerosis express a surface antigen that appears to function as a monocyte adhesion molecule, called "athero-ELAM." These results correspond well with our findings.

Localization by immunoelectron microscopy reveals expression of the aforementioned antigen in the outer plasma membrane of endothelial cells but not in their cytoplasmic organelles (Fig. 6). Monocytic adherence of endothelial cells is known to increase along with the expression of the inflammatory activation antigen in a highly significant fashion (GOERDT et al. 1987; BEVILACQUA et al. 1985; POBER et al. 1986). Our results have shown that endothelial cells will express inflammatory differentiation antigens on their outer cytoplasmic membrane even above early atherosclerotic plaques, thereby obviously facilitating the entry of blood monocytes through the endothelium into the underlying intima of the vessel.

5 Macrophages and Lipoprotein Metabolism

According to the findings of BROWN and GOLDSTEIN (1983), macrophages function as scavenger cells in lipoprotein metabolism, and their major role in atherogenesis seems to be in the clearance of lipids from the very area where a lesion is forming. Further in vitro studies have shown that macrophages play a major role in lipoprotein metabolism, incorporating various lipoprotein

Fig. 1. Histologic section of typical foam cells in incipient fatty streaks. The cells are characterized by a lucent cytoplasm and densely staining nuclei. × 330

Fig. 2. Incipient fatty streak of human aorta stained with monoclonal antibody 27-E-10 directed exclusively against blood monocytes: single positive monocytes are observed in the subendothelial space. × 550

Fig. 3. Low-power micrograph of fully developed fatty streak in human aorta, stained with 25-F-9 against mature tissue macrophages, and showing abundant clusters of macrophage-derived foam cells. × 136

Fig. 4. Foam cell in the deeper layer of the intima. Staining with antibodies against desmin points to the smooth muscle cell nature of this foam cell. × 330

[low-density lipoproteins (LDL) and β-very low density lipoprotein (β-VLDL)] by receptor-mediated endocytosis (BROWN and GOLDSTEIN 1983; GOLDSTEIN et al. 1980).

The cell surface receptor for modified LDLs, designated the "scavenger" receptor, provides an alternative pathway to the classical LDL receptor for the uptake of lipoproteins by macrophages. Whether this removal of modified lipoproteins is beneficial or detrimental for the development of the atherosclerotic plaque has still to be established (KELLEY 1991). The internalized lipoproteins are transported to lysosomes. Here the cholesterol is hydrolyzed by the enzyme acid cholesteryl ester hydrolase (ACEH). Subsequently the cholesterol is released into the cytoplasm. The cholesterol in the cytoplasm is then re-esterified to form cytoplasmic cholesteryl ester droplets which are hydrolyzed and re-esterified in a continous cycle.

If the surrounding medium contains a cholesterol acceptor such as high-density lipoprotein (HDL), the cholesterol is not re-esterified or stored in cytoplasmic vacuoles but resecreted as unesterified cholesterol. The macrophages are stimulated by cholesterol accumulation to synthesize considerable amounts of apolipoprotein (apo) E. This mechanism is independent of the presence of HDL as cholesterol acceptor (BROWN and GOLDSTEIN 1983; BASU et al. 1981). The current concept of reverse cholesterol transport from the peripheral cells to the liver assumes that HDL absorbs unesterified cholesterol and apo E secreted from macrophages to form the so-called HDLc complex. The HLDc particles target the secreted cholesterol to hepatocytes (MAHLEY 1981), thereby mediating the "reverse cholesterol transport" to the liver. These are, however, so far only the results of in vitro studies. In our morphologic investigations we tried to trace some of the possible steps in this metabolic pathway within the atherosclerotic plaque.

The main lipoprotein component of LDL is apo B. Staining for this substance with antibodies shows distinct and predominantly extracellular deposits in the atherosclerotic plaque (Fig. 7), so we may safely infer that LDL is present in these areas (VOLLMER et al. 1991a). The LDL observed in the arterial intima is most likely incorporated by macrophages. The cholesterol esters are deposited in cytoplasmic lipid vacuoles which ultimately appear as foam cells, and can be demonstrated by conventional electron microscopy. According to ultrastructural findings, the number of lipid vacuoles increases, and the typical foam cells develop, forming the cytologic basis of fatty streaks. Eventually, these macrophage-

Fig. 5. Fibrous/fatty plaque of the human aorta, stained with antibody 4-D-10 against an inflammatory differentiation antigen, revealing strong positivity in the endothelial cells. × 136

Fig. 6. Immunoelectron microscopic demonstration of the inflammatory differentiation antigen using the monoclonal antibody 4-D-10 in the immunoperoxidase technique. The reaction product is revealed exclusively on the outer cytoplasmic membrane, where the antigen is obviously present. × 9300

Fig. 7. Staining of a fibrous/fatty plaque with antibodies against apo B reveals considerable deposits which are localized mostly in the extracellular spaces. × 330

Fig. 8. Fatty streak stained with a monoclonal antibody against apo E. A strongly positive reaction is observed in the cytoplasm of foam cells. × 550

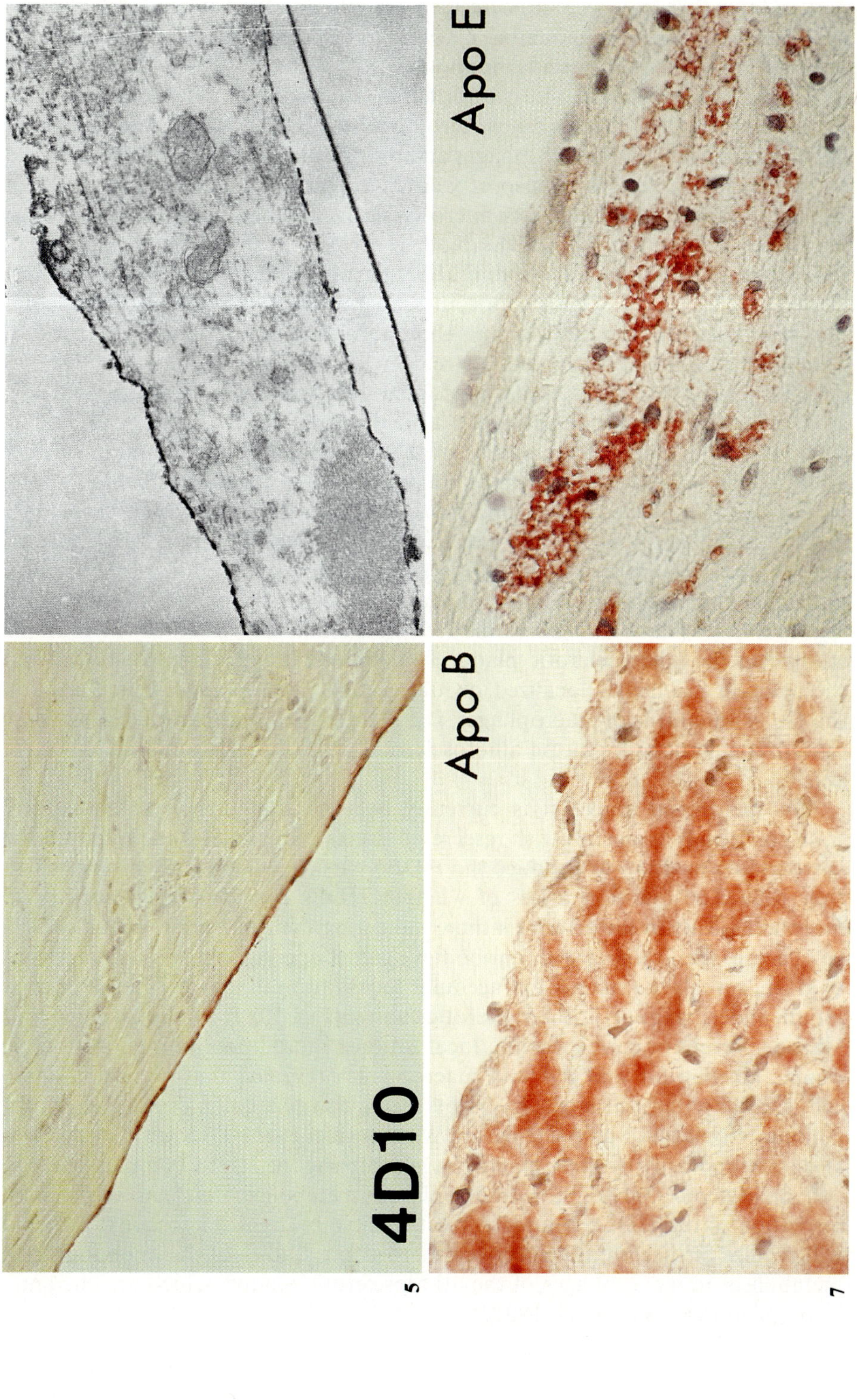

Figs. 5–8

derived foam cells may become necrotic to form the so-called atheroma (FAGIOTTO et al. 1984). It was also suggested by FAGIOTTO et al. that lipid-laden macrophages may again re-enter the vascular lumina.

As has been pointed out, macrophages are also able in vitro to resecrete cholesterol via the reverse cholesterol transport. The exact mechanism of cholesterol secretion by macrophages and the origin of plasma HDL with regard to the reverse cholesterol transport were investigated by SCHMITZ et al. (1985) using biochemical and electron microscopic techniques. These investigations led to the assumption that HDLs bind to specific receptors on the surface of macrophages. Subsequently, bound HDL particles are internalized and transported in endosomes. These endosomes do not fuse with the lysosome compartment, but take up cytoplasmic cholesterol and are ultimately resecreted. Staining histologic sections of fatty streaks with antibodies against apo E shows distinct positivity in the cytoplasm of foam cells which obviously contain apo E (Fig. 8). Comparable results were also observed by MURASE et al. (1986). To confirm the macrophage nature of these foam cells which contain or probably secrete apo E, we performed immunohistologic double labeling: apo E was stained red using the alkaline phosphatase method, while the peroxidase method using antibody 25-F-9 identified these cells as mature tissue macrophages. The cytoplasm of foam cells appeared in a mixed, reddish-brown color, indicating these cells to be macrophages carrying or probably actively secreting apo E (Fig. 9; VOLLMER et al. 1991b). Preliminary electron microscopic studies on the atherosclerotic plaque to demonstrate apo E have shown that the reaction product is localized on the granular endoplasmic reticulum and the Golgi apparatus of macrophages, i.e., their secretory apparatus. So we may infer that macrophages in the atherosclerotic plaque are indeed able to secrete apo E.

As mentioned above, it is currently believed that in reverse cholesterol transport apo E associates with resecreted cholesterol and HDLs present in the surrounding medium to produce the HDLc particle, which is then targeted to liver cells. The question arises of whether HDLs can also be demonstrated morphologically in the arterial intima, indicating their potential role as cholesterol acceptors. Staining with antibodies against apo A-I, the main component of HDL, reveals the mainly extracellular localization of apo A-I in the arterial intima undergoing early atherosclerotic change (Fig. 10). It can be assumed that HDL is present in corresponding localizations. In addition, immunohistologic double labeling for apo A-I and macrophages revealed that numerous foam cells characterized as macrophages by their brownish color using 25-F-9 also contain cytoplasmic apo A-I (Fig. 11). We may infer that HDLs are incorporated at least temporarily by these macrophages, forming the HDLc complexes. However, an in-depth study of the intracytoplasmic metabolism that leads to potential formation of the HDLc complex is not feasible by light microscopy; rather it will require further immunoelectron microscopic studies of the apolipoprotein metabolism in macrophages of the atherosclerotic plaque, which are currently in progress (VOLLMER et al. 1991a).

9

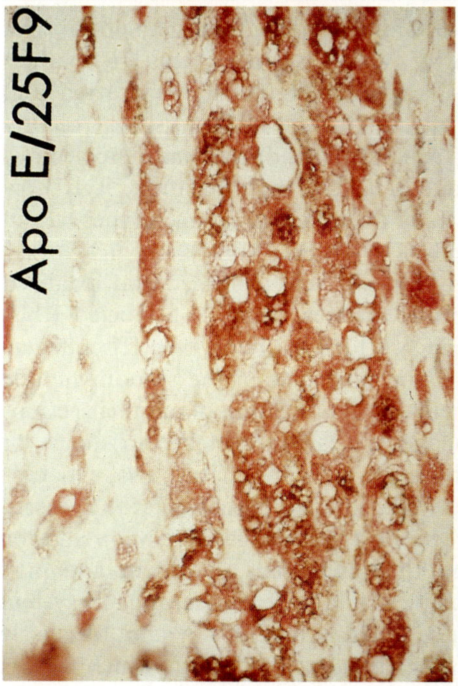

10

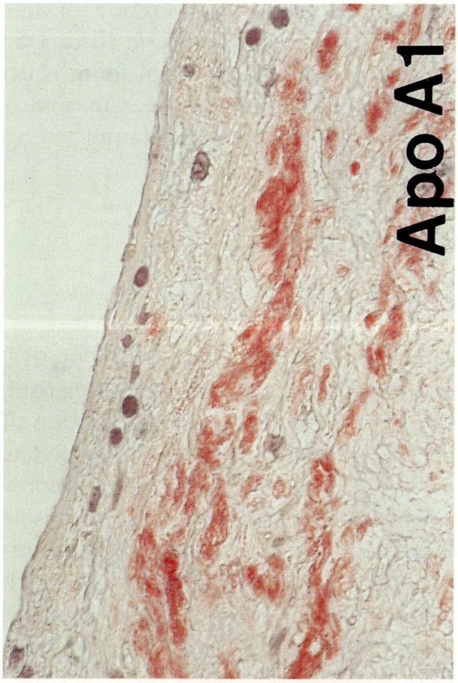

11

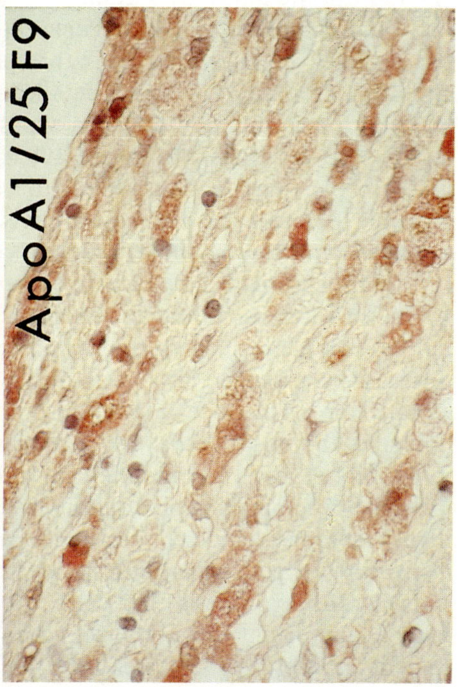

Fig. 9. Double labeling of a fatty streak with an antibody against mature tissue macrophages (25 F 9, brown) and apo E (red) reveals a mixed brown-reddish color of the foam cells, pointing to the macrophage nature of the E-secreting cells. × 330

Fig. 10. Fibrous/fatty plaques stained with an antibody against apo A-I. Deposits are mainly localized in the extracellular spaces. × 330

Fig. 11. Double labeling of a fibrous/fatty plaque with a monoclonal antibody against mature tissue macrophages (25 F 9) and apo A-I reveals a brownish red-mixed color. These results show that macrophages contain cytoplasmic apo A-I. × 330

In conclusion, our morphologic data demonstrating the secretion of apo E by macrophage-derived foam cells, and the occurrence of HDL in the extracellular spaces of the arterial intima and also in the cytoplasm of foam cells, suggest that the so-called reverse cholesterol transport to the liver may also play a significant role in the development of the atherosclerotic plaque.

6 The Role of Macrophages in the Synthesis of Collagen by Smooth Muscle Cells

Increased biosynthesis and deposition of proteins in the extracellular matrix, especially of collagens, makes an essential contribution to the atherosclerotic transformation of the arterial wall. In the course of the disease, modification of smooth muscle cells from a contractile phenotype to a synthetic phenotype has been observed (CAMPBELL and CAMPBELL 1985). The potential role of macrophages in the synthesis of collagen types principally effected by smooth muscle cells is still insufficiently explained. These smooth muscle cells are readily identified in the proliferating fibrous plaque by immunohistology after staining with antibodies against muscle-specific α-actin (TSUKADA et al. 1987). The substances synthesized by smooth muscle cells can also be detected on histologic sections by appropriate antibody staining.

Studies of VOSS and RAUTERBERG (1986) have shown that incipient fibrous plaques will manifest collagens (primarily type I, but also type III) in their intercellular matrix. A more detailed description of the demonstration and distribution of different collagen types in human atherosclerosis has recently been given by KATSUDA et al. (1992), who also conducted immunoelectron microscopic investigations. With the aid of in situ hybridization, it is now possible to detect and distinguish mRNAs of the different collagen types within collagen-synthesizing smooth muscle cells (JAEGER et al. 1991).

Thus, cells with active collagen biosynthesis were identified and localized in frozen sections of human atherosclerotic arteries, using 25-S-labeled RNA probes complementary to the messenger RNA for type I and type III collagen. Increased messenger RNA was observed in particular in the smooth muscle cells of fibrous plaques. Immunohistochemical identification of parallel sections for smooth muscle cells and macrophages revealed regular coexistence or proximity of mRNA-containing smooth muscle cells and mature tissue macrophages or immigrating blood monocytes in the intima of atherosclerotic vessels. From these results the connection between the macrophage infiltration and the activation of collagen synthesis in smooth muscle cells is evident and may support the hypothesis that cells from the mononuclear-macrophage system play an important role in the activation of collagen synthesis in smooth muscle cells of atherosclerotic vessels. On the other hand it is not clear which factors might be responsible for induction of the collagen synthesis at the transcriptional level. As regards the macrophage-derived cytokines, mainly transforming growth factor-β has been described to stimulate synthesis of extracellular matrix proteins in a number of mesenchymal cells (ROBERTS et al. 1988).

Furthermore, interleukin-1 is also thought to be of great importance in the activation of connective tissue (WAHL 1986; DAYER and DAMCZUK 1984). On the other hand, reports on the effect of interleukin-1 on collagen synthesis are contradictory, and interleukin-1 has also been considered inhibitory (MAUVIEL et al. 1988). Further studies focusing on the proteins which play a role in macrophage-dependent induction of collagen synthesis by fibroblasts in atherosclerotic vessels will probably eludicate the mechanisms of this stimulatory effect.

7 Conclusion

In its early stages, atherosclerosis is in fact an intimal disease. Monocytes migrate from the vascular lumen through the endothelium into the arterial intima. Obviously, a certain phenotypic modulation of endothelial intimal cells, expressing an inflammatory differentiation antigen with increased monocytic adherence, plays an important role in this process. According to immunohistologic observations with differentiating antibodies, the immigrating monocytes undergo transformation to tissue macrophages in the arterial intima. These macrophages are actively involved in lipoprotein metabolism, ingesting cholesterol-carrying lipoproteins that have penetrated into the intima through the endothelium and thereby acting as scavenger cells. If they have incorporated more cholesterol than they are able to excrete under the conditions prevailing in the atherosclerotic plaque, macrophages are transformed to foam cells. So far, little is known about the fate of the intimal macrophages. One theory suggests that some of them may pass through the endothelium and begin to recirculate after transformation into foam cells. However, our immunohistologic results have shown that macrophages secrete apo E, and that in the presence of HDL in the arterial intima, the so-called reverse cholesterol transport towards the liver may play a significant role in the pathogenesis of the atherosclerotic plaque. This ability of macrophages to secrete apo E after loading with cholesterol could be interpreted as a potentially antiatherogenic property. On the other hand, the function of macrophages may also be a negative one. In the progression of an atherosclerotic lesion, the metabolically transforming macrophage seems to be able, by activating the collagen synthesis of smooth muscle cells, to enhance and advance the atherosclerotic process itself.

References

Basu SK, Brown MS, Ho YK, Havel RJ, Goldstein JL (1981) Mouse macrophages synthesize and secrete a protein resembling apolipoprotein E. Proc Natl Acad Sci USA 78:7545–7549

Bevilacqua MP, Pober JS, Wheeler ME, Cotran RS, Gimbrone MA Jr (1981) Interleukin-1 activation of vascular endothelium: effects on procoagulant activity and leukocyte adhesion. Am J Pathol 121:394–400

Brown MS, Goldstein JL (1983) Lipoprotein metabolism in the macrophage: implications for cholesterol deposition in atherosclerosis. Annu Rev Biochem 52:223–261

Brown MS, Goldstein JL (1986) A receptor-mediated pathway for cholesterol homeostasis. Science 232:34–47

Campbell GR, Campbell JH (1985) Smooth muscle phenotypic changes in arterial wall homeostasis: implications for the pathogenesis of atherosclerosis. Exp Mol Pathol 42:139

Cybulsky MI, Gimbrone MAJ (1990) Endothelial cells express a monocyte adhesion molecule during atherosclerosis. FASEB J 4:A 1135

Dayer JM, Damczuk S (1984) Cytokines and other mediators in rheumatoid arthritis. Springer Semin Immunopathol 7:387

Fagiotto A, Ross R (1984) Studies of hypercholesterolemia in the non-human primate. II. Fatty streak conversion to fibrous plaque. Arteriosclerosis 4:341–356

Fagiotto A, Ross R, Harker L (1984) Studies of hypercholesterolemia in the non-human primate. I. Changes that lead to fatty streak formation. Arteriosclerosis 4:323–340

Goerdt S, Zwadlo G, Schlegel R, Hagemeier HH, Sorg C (1987) Characterization and expression kinetics of an endothelial cell activation antigen present in vivo only in acute inflammatory tissue. Exp Cell Biol 55:117–126

Goldstein JL, Ho YK, Brown MS, Innerartiy TL, Mahley RW (1980) Cholesteryl ester accumulation in macrophages resulting from receptor-mediated uptake and degradation of hypercholesterolemic canine β-very low density lipoproteins. J Biol Chem 255:1839–1848

Jaeger E, Rust S, Roessner A, Kleinhans G, Buchholz B, Althaus M, Rauterberg J, Gerlach U (1991) Joint occurrence of collagen mRNA containing cells and macrophages in human atherosclerotic vessels. Atherosclerosis 31:55–68

Katsuda S, Okada Y, Minamoto T, Oda Y, Matsui Y, Nakanishi I (1992) Collagens in human atherosclerosis. Immunohistochemical analysis using collagen type-specific antibodies. Arteriosclerosis Thromb 12:494–502

Kelley JL (1991) Macrophages Scavenger receptor(s) for modified low density lipoproteins. Prog Lipid Res 30:231–235

Mahley RM (1981) Cellular and molecular lipoprotein metabolism in atherosclerosis. Hum Pathol 16:3–5

Masuda J, Ross R (1990a) Atherogenesis during low level hypercholesterolemia in the nonhuman primate. I. Fatty streak formation. Arteriosclerosis 10:164–177

Masuda J, Ross R (1990b) Atherogenesis during low level hypercholesterolemia in the nonhuman primate. II. Fatty streak conversion to fibrous plaque. Arteriosclerosis 10:178–187

Mauviel A, Teyton L, Bhatnagar R, et al. (1988) Interleukin -1α modulates collagen gene expression in cultured synovial cells. Biochem J 252:247

Munro JM, Cotran RS (1988) The pathogenesis of atherosclerosis: atherogenesis and inflammation. Lab Invest 58:249–261

Murase T, Oka T, Yamada N, Mori N, Ishibashi S, Takaku F, Mori W (1986) Immunohistochemical localization of apolipoprotein E in atherosclerotic lesions of the aorta and coronary arteries. Atherosclerosis 60:1–6

Orekhov AN, Kalantarov GF, Andreeva ER, Prokazova NV, Prakht JN, Bergelson LD, Smirnov VN (1986) Monoclonal antibody reveals heterogeneity in human aortic intima: detection of ganglioside antigen associated with subpopulation of intimal cells. Am J Pathol 122:279–385

Pober JS, Bevilacqua MP, Mendrick DL, Lapierre LA, Fiers W, Gimbrone MA Jr (1986) Two distinct monokines, IL-1 and TNF, each independently induce biosynthesis and transient expression of the same antigen on the surface of cultured vascular endothelial cells. J Immunol 136:1680–1687

Radzun HJ (1985) Immunhistochemie des menschlichen mononukleärphagozytischen Systems. Gustav Fischer, Stuttgart

Roberts AB, Flanders KC, Kondaiah P, et al. (1988) Transforming growth factor β: biochemistry

and roles in embryogenesis, tissue repair and remodelling, and carcinogenesis. Recent Prog Horm Res 44:157
Roessner A, Zwadlo G, Vollmer E, Sorg C, Grundmann E (1987a) Biologic characterization of human bone tumors. IX. Occurrence of macrophages. Pathol Res Pract 182:336–343
Roessner A, Herrera A, Höning HJ, et al. (1987b) Identification of macrophages and smooth muscle cells with monoclonal antibodies in the human atherosclerotic plaque. Virchows Arch [A] 412:169–174
Rosenfeld ME, Ross R (1990) Macrophage and smooth muscle cell proliferation in atherosclerotic lesions of WHHL and comparably hypercholesterolemic fat-fed rabbits. Arteriosclerosis 10:680–687
Schaefer HE (1981) The role of macrophages in atherosclerosis. In: Schmalzl F, Huhn D, Schaefer HE (eds) Haematology and blood transfusion, vol 27. Springer, Berlin Heidelberg New York, pp 137–142
Schaefer HE, Assmann G (1980) Bedeutung der Makrophagen für die Genese der Arteriosklerose. MMW 122:S228–238
Schmitz G, Robenek H, Lohmann U, Assmann G (1985) Interaction of high density lipoproteins with cholesteryl ester-laden macrophages: biochemical and morphological characterization of cell surface receptor binding, endocytosis and resecretion of high density lipoproteins by macrophages. EMBO J 4:613–622
Schulze-Osthoff K, Meinardus-Hager G, Sorg C (1989) Das Endothel und seine Schlüsselrolle in der Entzündung. Jahrb Dermatol: 41–52
Schwartz CJ, Sprague EA, Kelley JL, Valente AJ, Suenram CA (1985) Aortic intimal monocyte recruitment in the normo- and hypercholesterolemic baboon (*Papio cynocephalus*). Virchows Arch [A] 405:175–191
Tsukada T, Tippens D, Gordon D, Ross R, Gown AM (1987) HH F 35, a muscle-actin specific monoclonal antibody. I. Immunocytochemical and biochemical characterization. Am J Pathol 126:51–60
Vollmer E, Brust J, Roessner A, et al. (1991a) Distribution patterns of apolipoproteins A_1, A_2, and B in the wall of atherosclerotic vessels. Virchows Arch [A] 419:79–88
Vollmer E, Roessner A, Bosse A, et al. (1991b) Immunohistochemical double labelling of macrophages, smooth muscle cells and apolipoprotein E in the atherosclerotic plaque. Pathol Res Pract 187:184–188
Voss B, Rauterberg J (1986) Localization of collagen types I, III, IV and V, fibronectin, and laminin in human arteries by the indirect immunofluorescence method. Pathol Res Pract 181:568–575
Wahl SM (1986) The role of lymphokines and monokines in fibrosis. Ann NY Acad Sci 460:224
Watanabe T, Hirata M, Yoshikawa Y, Nagafuchi Y, Toyoshima H, Watanabe T (1985) Role of macrophages in atherosclerosis. Sequential observations of cholesterol-induced rabbit aortic lesion by the immunoperoxidase technique using monoclonal antimacrophage antibody. Lab Invest 53:80–90
Ylä-Herttuala S (1991) Macrophages and oxidized low density lipoproteins in the pathogenesis of atherosclerosis. Ann Med 23:561–567
Zwadlo G, Bröcker EB, von Bassewitz DB, Feige U, Sorg C (1985) A monoclonal antibody to a differentiation antigen present on mature human macrophages and absent from monocytes. J Immunol 134:1487–1492
Zwadlo G, Schlegel R, Sorg C (1986) A monoclonal antibody to a subset of human monocytes found only in the peripheral blood and inflammatory tissues. J Immunol 137:512–518

Lipoprotein Receptors on Macrophages and Smooth Muscle Cells

H. ROBENEK and N. J. SEVERS

1 Introduction

Atherosclerosis is now recognised as a multifactorial disease process in which a number of distinct but overlapping pathways of pathogenesis are involved. The major current hypotheses of atherogenesis focus on (a) response of the arterial wall to injury, (b) lipid infiltration into the intima, (c) smooth muscle cell transformation, (d) thrombosis, (e) immune mechanisms and (f) viruses as aetiological agents (ROSS 1986; Steinberg et al. 1989; SCOTT 1989; PENN et al. 1986; LIBBY

Current Topics in Pathology
Volume 87, Vollmer/Roessner (Eds.)

and Hansson 1991; Hajjar 1991). These hypotheses are not mutually exclusive, but reflect different aspects of an interactive disease process in which various factors may assume different degrees of importance in different stages and instances of the disease. Underlying all these processes is a complex web of interactions between the cellular constituents of the arterial wall, their secreted products and lipoproteins.

The principal cell types of the artery wall—the endothelial cell, the smooth muscle cell and the monocyte/macrophage—are major players in the events involved in initiation and evolution of the atherosclerotic plaque. Other important participants are platelets and lymphocytes, which have modulating influences on smooth muscle cell and macrophage behaviour. The interaction of macrophages with and their handling of lipoproteins are generally recognised as particularly crucial in disease initiation and progression. How cells interact with lipoproteins is determined by the nature of the specific cell surface lipoprotein receptors that they express. Much has been learned in recent years about the properties of lipoprotein receptors, and recent developments in electron microscopy and cytochemistry make it possible to detect, visualise and track these receptors through their cycles of display, ligand binding, internalisation and subsequent passage through intracellular compartments. In this chapter, we set out to examine the properties of the lipoprotein receptor systems of macrophages and smooth muscle cells, as explored in cultured cells, by applying these and related techniques. To put these studies in perspective, we start by introducing, in the context of atherosclerosis, the structure and function of the cell types on which our studies are focussed.

2 Cellular Constituents of the Normal Artery and Atherosclerotic Plaque

2.1 The Endothelial Cell

Although the smooth muscle cell and the macrophage are the dominant cell types of the normal and diseased artery, and the principal subjects of this chapter, no discussion of atherosclerosis can ignore the importance of the endothelial cell. Endothelial cells form the squamous epithelium that lines the entire inner surface of the cardiovascular system. The organisation of the endothelium and smooth muscle in a typical muscular artery, the rabbit coronary artery, is illustrated in Fig. 1. Major functions of the endothelial lining are to provide a non-thrombogenic surface and a selective permeability barrier between the blood and tissue fluid. Endothelial cells synthesise a complex range of substances that control growth, differentiation and function of smooth muscle cells and macrophages. Blood-borne lipoproteins have to cross the endothelial barrier before they can interact with smooth muscle cells and macrophages in vivo. Similarly,

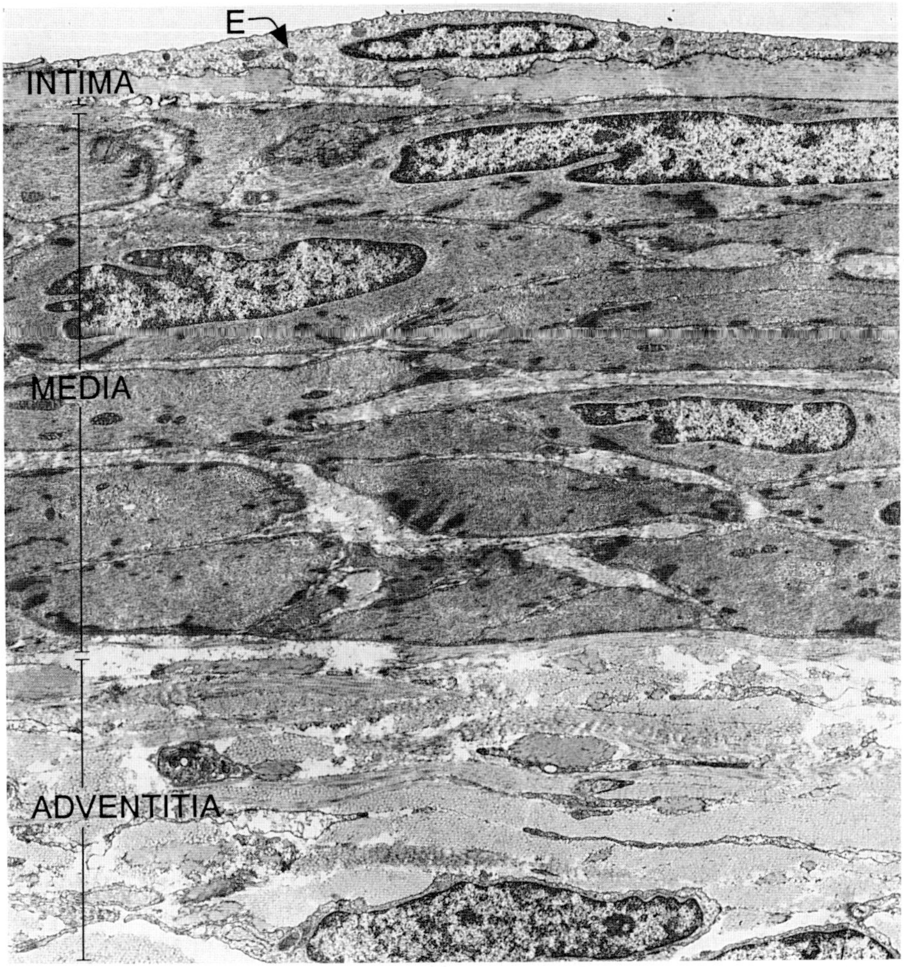

Fig. 1. Cellular structure of the wall of a typical muscular artery, the rabbit coronary artery. The intima consists of a single layer of endothelial cells (*E*), resting on the internal elastic lamina. The media consists of smooth muscle cells showing the typical feature of the contractile phenotype, embedded in the matrix they secrete. The adventitia is rich in connective tissue and contains scattered fibroblasts. × 6000

monocytes, the precursors to macrophages, migrate between the boundaries of adjacent endothelial cells in order to gain access to the intima. Endothelial cells thus have multiple roles in the pathogenesis of atherosclerosis, as recognised by their prime of place in the "response to injury hypothesis" refined by Ross (1986). Our subject here, however—the interactions of lipoproteins with macrophages and smooth muscle cells—, concerns events that, in the in vivo situation, occur after the endothelial barrier has been breached.

2.2 The Smooth Muscle Cell

Vascular smooth muscle cells are the sole cell type of the arterial media (Fig. 1), and are also a normal constituent of the intima of the human coronary artery (STARY 1989). Normal medial smooth muscle cells are elongated, flattened contractile cells of irregular shape. Through periodic contacts, they are organised together with their long axes in parallel, forming layers surrounded by extracellular matrix. Contractile smooth muscle cells have the capacity to undergo remarkable changes in length. They contract slowly and are capable of sustaining tension for longer periods than other muscle cells. These properties enable them to control blood vessel calibre, and so regulate blood distribution and flow.

Normal medial smooth muscle cells are characteristically packed with bundles of myofilaments and intermediate filaments, reflecting their specialised contractile function (Fig. 1). A filament-free zone of cytoplasm on either side of the nucleus accommodates most of the mitochondria and other organelles. Elements of sarcoplasmic reticulum, and some mitochondria, are distributed widely throughout the cell. Densely staining amorphous structures, the dense bodies, act as insertion sites for the contractile filaments and intermediate filaments (TRAVO et al. 1982), thereby mechanically coupling the cytoskeleton and contractile systems (KARGACIN et al. 1989; DRAEGER et al. 1990). Most of the dense bodies are wedge-shaped and attached to the plasma membrane, but some occur as free-floating structures in the cell interior. The plasma membrane between the membrane-associated dense bodies contains caveolae organised in rows and bands parallel with the long axis of the cell. An external lamina ("basement membrane") covers the cell, to which matrix components attach. Smooth muscle cells are anchored to one another by adherens junctions and are electrically coupled by gap junctions (MOORE et al. 1991). Their plasma membrane houses a variety of receptors, notably to neurotransmitters, and, of particular importance in the context of atherosclerosis, to platelet-derived growth factor (PDGF) and to low density lipoprotein (LDL), the principal carrier of cholesterol in the plasma.

Although in the normal vessel of the mature animal, smooth muscle cells are differentiated as specialised contractile cells, they nevertheless have an important synthetic function, manufacturing the spectrum of extracellular matrix components, including collagen, elastin, proteoglycans, fibronectin and laminin, in which they are embedded. An important property of the smooth muscle cell is its ability, under the influence of PDGF and other growth factors and mediators released by macrophages, endothelial cells or platelets, to undergo phenotypic modulation to a synthetic form in which contractile features are lost, and migration and proliferation occur (CAMPBELL and CAMPBELL 1990; CAMPBELL et al. 1989). In the synthetic phenotype, the contractile apparatus becomes rudimentary, the Golgi apparatus and rough endoplasmic reticulum hypertrophy, and enhanced matrix production occurs (Fig. 2). These changes resemble the phenotype expressed during development, and can be simulated in culture. Modulation to the synthetic phenotype occurs as part of the natural repair response to arterial

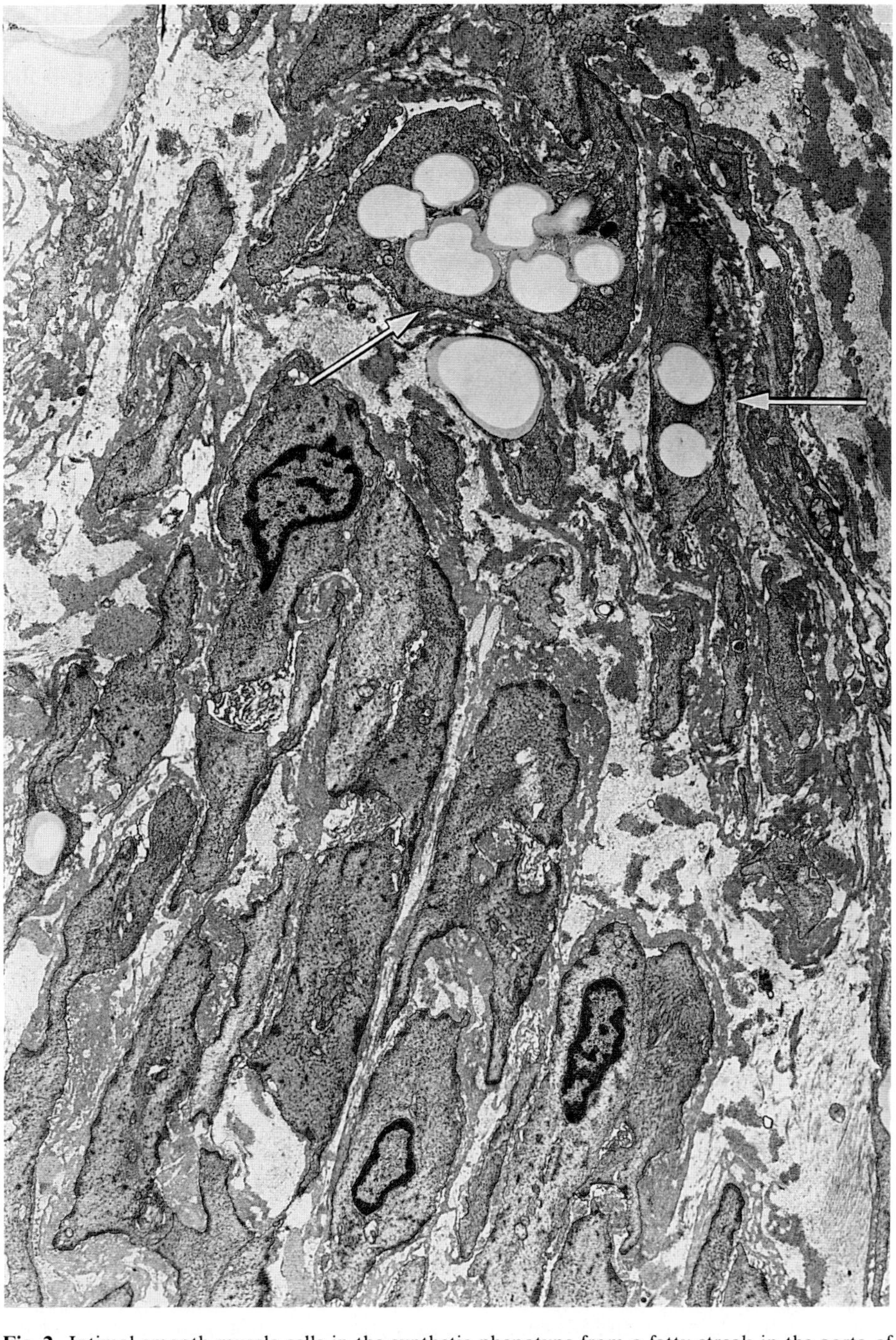

Fig. 2. Intimal smooth muscle cells in the synthetic phenotype from a fatty streak in the aorta of a 55-year-old male. Uptake of lipid has occurred in some of the smooth muscle cells to the top of the field (*arrows*), giving the cells a foamy appearance. × 9000

injury and is an indispensable step for participation of smooth muscle cells in the formation of the atherosclerotic lesion.

Not all contractile smooth muscle cells appear to be equally sensitive to the effects of chemoattractants and mitogens, and variable expression of properties over a continuum between the archetypal contractile and synthetic forms may occur. Thus, the description of smooth muscle cells as being of either a contractile or a synthetic phenotype is oversimplistic. However, the fact that smooth muscle cells can be readily induced to abandon their normal contractile function to migrate, divide and engage in augmented synthesis of matrix components is identified in all hypotheses of atherosclerosis as the basis for the bulk growth of fibromuscular material in the raised atherosclerotic lesion.

2.3 The Macrophage

Macrophages are mobile, phagocytotic cells, specialised in clearing unwanted cellular material and foreign matter. They are widely distributed in the body, occurring in the loose connective tissue of most organs, and are rapidly recruited in inflammatory responses. Macrophages are normal, isolated residents of the arterial wall (Massmann 1979; Stary 1989), but their accumulation in the intima in fatty streaks and advanced lesions has increasingly focussed attention on their role in atherosclerosis (Watanabe et al. 1985; Brown and Goldstein 1983; Gerrity 1981a, b; Fan et al. 1991; Watanabe et al. 1989).

Macrophages originate from blood-borne monocytes, which adhere to the luminal surface of the endothelium before crawling in between adjacent endothelial cells, which temporarily part to admit them (Gerrity 1981a). Once within the intima, monocytes undergo transformation into macrophages, a process involving enlargement, onset of endocytotic activity, and appearance of lysosomes. The shape and appearance of the macrophage are variable; active cells typically have an irregular profile with abundant pseudopodia, while resident cells have a smoother, drawn out profile. The cytoplasm is filled with polymorphic vacuoles, vesicles, lysosomes and residual bodies, representing various stages in the uptake and digestion of engulfed products. The endoplasmic reticulum and Golgi apparatus are particularly well developed, reflecting intense synthetic and secretory activities. Macrophages have no external lamina. Apart from developing from monocytes, fully formed macrophages may themselves divide on occasion to give rise to new macrophages.

The hallmark of the macrophage is its avid capacity for phagocytosis and other forms of endocytosis. These processes are mediated by various plasma membrane receptors, notably the Fc receptor and complement receptors (CR3 and CR1) (Mellman et al. 1988; Law 1988; Ravetch and Kinet 1991). Other receptors, for example those that recognise components of the extracellular matrix such as laminin and fibronectin and which affect migratory and secretory activities, also appear to influence phagocytotic activity. Cell movement and shape changes triggered by ligand–receptor interactions are mediated via dynamic changes in the cytoskeleton, a three-dimensional network of actin filaments cross-linked by filamin. Upon stimulation of receptors, the cytoskeleton is rapidly assembled at the cell cortex to initiate cell movement (YIN and HARTWIG 1988).

The Fc and complement component receptors are but few of an unusually diverse and abundant population of cell surface receptors (GORDON et al. 1988; GORDON 1988). More than 60 ligands have been reported to bind to macrophage receptors, but as some ligands bind to more than one receptor, and some of the receptors recognise more than one ligand, the precise number of macrophage receptors is difficult to define. Three main superfamilies of macrophage receptors are generally recognised, the immunoglobulin-interacting receptors, complement component (C3b/C4b)-interacting receptors and integrins. In addition, there are various lectin-like receptors. These receptors enable the macrophage to respond sensitively to its environment, allowing versatile differentiation suited to the particular purpose required.

This versatility is reflected in the multitude of immunoregulatory molecules, chemoattractants, growth factors and cytokines that macrophages are capable of synthesising and releasing. Among these products are prostaglandins, leukotriene B_4 (a potent chemoattractant), monocyte chemoattractant protein (WOLPE and CERAMI 1989), PDGF (ROSS et al. 1990), transforming growth factor (MASSAGUÉ 1990), tumour necrosis factor (JONES and STUART 1990) and interleukin-1. These substances all exercise potent effects on the activities of smooth muscle cells, endothelial cells and macrophages themselves. In particular, they form a major source of the stimuli that entice smooth muscle cells to migrate to the intima, proliferate and adopt the synthetic phenotype. Macrophages do not express simultaneously the full range of their synthetic potential. Signalling molecules released by other cells, and the precise nature of the extracellular matrix environment, both of which are sensed by the macrophage's receptors, determine expression of the appropriate response. T-lymphocytes may contribute to this process by releasing various lymphokines that modulate macrophage differentiation.

Macrophage receptors of critical importance in the context of atherosclerosis are those concerned with lipoprotein binding and uptake (BROWN an GOLDSTEIN 1983; FOGELMAN et al. 1988). Although, like smooth muscle cells, macrophages possess LDL receptors, these receptors are not abundant. However, activated macrophages express additional types of lipoprotein receptor, notably one that recognises β-migrating very low-density lipoprotein (β-VLDL) and one referred to as the scavenger receptor (HERZ et al. 1988; FOGELMAN et al. 1988). These receptors profoundly influence the fate of lipoproteins in the artery wall, and will be examined in more detail in Sects. 3.2 and 5.2.

2.4 The Foam Cell

Foam cells are a characteristic and major cellular constituent of the fatty streak and atherosclerotic plaque. They are characterised by a cytoplasm packed full of lipid droplets, which gives them the "foamy" appearance from which their name derives. Some lipid-laden foam cells are thought to be able to migrate to the bloodsteam, thereby removing lipid from the lesion (GERRITY 1981b; GERRITY and NAITO 1980). Others, however, remain trapped in the arterial wall, forming the major source of chemoattractants and mitogens that act on smooth muscle cells and cause them to migrate, divide and modulate to the synthetic phenotype. Foam cells that remain immobilised with their lipid overload eventually perish, contributing to the accumulation of necrotic material and lipid in the core of the plaque. Foam cells are now known to originate mainly but not exclusively from macrophages (ROSS 1986; GERRITY 1981a; JORIS et al. 1983; KLURFELD 1985). Smooth muscle cells are the alternative cell type of origin. Examples of foam cells derived from these two cells types are illustrated in Figs. 3 and 4. Foam cell formation occurs by processes that involve the interaction of macrophages and smooth muscle cells with cholesterol-rich lipoproteins, and these processes are thus fundamental to our understanding of the link between cholesterol and atherosclerosis (STARY 1987; AQUEL et al. 1985; WATANABE et al. 1985; HABERLAND et al. 1988).

One of our principal interests has been to investigate, at the ultrastructural level, the mechanisms underlying cholesterol influx and accumulation in macrophages, in order to understand the mechanisms underlying foam cell formation (ROBENEK et al. 1984; ROBENEK and 1985; SCHMITZ 1985; SCHMITZ et al. 1990c). We have examined the receptor-mediated pathways by which cultured macrophages take up lipoprotein-bound cholesterol in the form of β-VLDL (ROBENEK et al. 1987) and chemically modified low-density lipoproteins (LDL) (SCHMITZ et al. 1988, 1990a; ROBENEK and SCHMITZ 1988, 1991). Both these lipoproteins are potent effectors of macrophage–foam cell conversion in vitro (PARTHASARATHY et al. 1986; POLACEK et al. 1989; ELLSWORTH et al. 1990; HENSON et al. 1989; JAAKKOLA et al. 1989; HEINECKE et al. 1991; HUFF et al. 1991). The receptor processes responsible for uptake of these lipoproteins are not strictly regulated, i.e. the expression of the lipoprotein receptors involved cannot be down-regulated, however high the external concentration of lipoproteins (GOLDSTEIN et al. 1979b, 1980; BROWN et al. 1979 STEINBERG et al. 1989; SPARROW et al. 1989; FOGELMAN et al. 1980; INNERARITY et al. 1986). In this situation, the only way accumulation of cholesterol can be avoided is by interaction of the cell with cholesterol accepters. High-density lipoproteins (HDL) are thought to fulfil this function. We have therefore examined the ability of HDL to remove cholesterol from macrophages in culture, an important step in the proposed process by which cholesterol is transported from peripheral tissues back to the liver in vivo (SCHMITZ et al. 1985a,c; GLOMSET 1968; BADIMORE et al. 1989; HO et al. 1980). Additional processes that may contribute to this process of "reverse cholesterol transport" include: (a) an HDL-independent mechanism by which macrophages release excess cholesterol, and (b) resumption of motility in appropriately stimulated foam cells. We will present evidence for both these processes later in this chapter.

Although in vivo a proportion of foam cells in lesions are demonstrated by immunohistochemical marking to be of smooth muscle cell origin, feeding

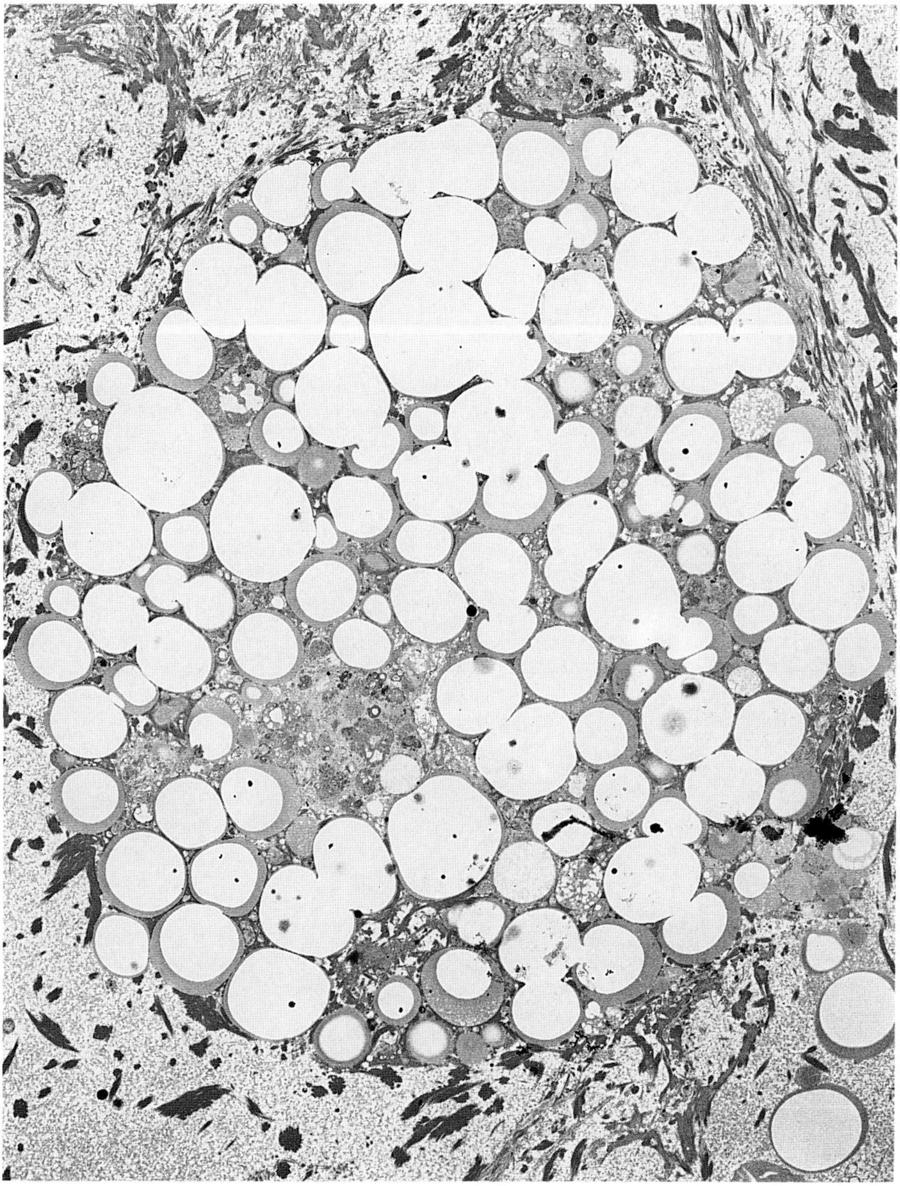

Fig. 3. Typical morphology of a macrophage-derived foam cell. This example comes from an atherosclerotic lesion from human femoral artery. × 3300

smooth muscle cells in vitro with β-VLDL or chemically modified LDL does not, in contrast to the case with macrophages, lead to foam cell formation (HOFF et al. 1991; HUFF et al. 1991; HEINECKE et al. 1991). The reason for this difference in response relates to differences in the types and properties of the lipoprotein receptors expressed in cultured macrophages and cultured smooth muscle cells.

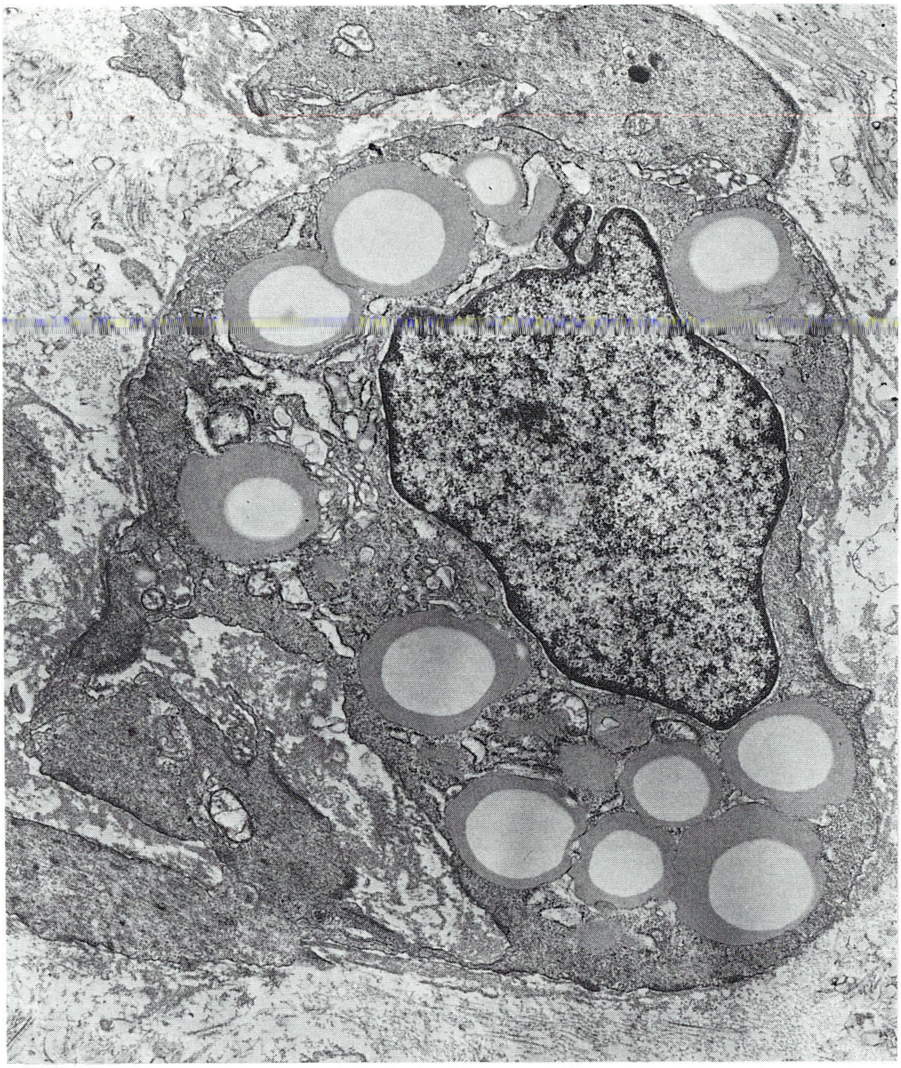

Fig. 4. Example of a smooth muscle cell-derived foam cell from the same fatty streak as that in Fig. 2. Contractile features are reduced in prominence, abundant endoplasmic reticulum is present, and the cell is packed with large lipid droplets. X 11000

Smooth muscle cells, like fibroblasts (the cell type on which the classical studies were conducted), are typical LDL receptor cells (GOLDSTEIN and BROWN 1977a). In these cells, the numbers of receptors displayed, and the rate-limiting step of intracellular cholesterol synthesis, are strictly regulated, in tune with cellular needs. LDL receptor cells are consequently protected from excessive accumulation of cholesterol or cholesteryl esters; in the presence of a high external concentration of LDL, uptake of the lipoprotein ceases because the number of cell surface receptors is greatly reduced. As a result, conversion to foam cells does not occur (GOLDSTEIN and BROWN 1977b; MAHLEY and INNERARITY 1983; GOLDSTEIN et al. 1985; BRADLEY and GIANTURCO 1988; HOBBS et al. 1990).

Given this situation, how can smooth muscle cells in vivo become transformed to foam cells within the plaque? Clues to this process have been provided by studies on the effects of incorporating artificially generated fragments of macrophages into smooth muscle cells in culture (WOLFBAUER et al. 1986; MINOR et al. 1986). Under defined conditions, cholesteryl ester-rich lipid droplets extracted from macrophages can be incorporated into smooth muscle cells in vitro, and a foam cell-like transformation occurs. These experiments raise the possibility that in vivo conversion of smooth muscle cells to foam cells occurs via interactions between the smooth muscle cell and the macrophage/foam cell or its components. Such an explanation is consistent with the observation that macrophages and macrophage-derived foam cells apparently precede smooth muscle cell-derived foam cells in the natural history of lesion progression.

In our current work, we are extending investigation of this possibility by establishing methods for fusing macrophages and their components with smooth muscle cells, and investigating the altered properties of lipoprotein handling in the resulting hybrids. Our working hypothesis is that analogous processes occurring in vivo could lead to acquisition of the macrophage scavenger receptor by smooth muscle cells, thus endowing the altered smooth muscle cell with the potential for foam cell transformation.

Before proceeding to discuss these studies in detail, we will first provide some basic background to the subject of lipoproteins and lipoprotein receptors, and then explain the ultrastructural techniques we have applied to visualise lipoprotein receptor pathways in action.

3 Plasma Lipoproteins and Lipoprotein Receptors

3.1 Plasma Lipoproteins

Lipoproteins are spheroid macromolecules consisting of complexes between lipids (triglycerides, cholesterol and phospholipids) and one or more apolipoproteins (for reviews see GOLDSTEIN and BROWN 1977b; MAHLEY and INNERARITY 1983; GOLDSTEIN et al. 1985; BRADLEY and GIANTURCO 1988; ASSMANN 1982). There are four major classes of lipoproteins, defined by differences in density: (a) chylomicrons, (b) VLDL, (c) LDL and (d) HDL. Various subtypes of these lipoproteins are recognised, and several less abundant lipoproteins are also present in normal plasma. These include intermediate-density lipoprotein (IDL), which has physical and chemical properties intermediate between those of VLDL and LDL, and Lp(a), highly atherogenic variant of LDL.

Apolipoproteins are divided into five groups, designed A, B, C, D and E. These proteins have a number of important functions: they bind and solubilise lipids, allowing them to be transported as stable lipoprotein complexes in the plasma, they act as ligands for the specific binding of lipoproteins to their receptors, and in some cases they regulate the activities of enzymes involved in lipoprotein metabolism. With the exception of LDL, each class of lipoprotein contains a variety of dffferent apolipoproteins. Apolipoprotein (apo) A, which occurs in three main forms (A-I, A-II and A-IV), is the major protein of HDL. Two forms of apo B exist, apo B-100 and apo B-48. LDL contains only one apolipoprotein, apo B-100; this apolipoprotein is also an obligate constituent of VLDL and IDL. Apo B-48 occurs in chylomicrons and chylomicron remnants. Apo C and apo E are present in various proportions in all lipoproteins except LDL. It is useful to distinguish two forms of HDL, according to the presence or absence of apo E; HDL with apo E are cholesterol-rich, and HDL without apo E are cholesterol-poor.

In addition to these lipoproteins, a number of abnormal lipoproteins and apolipoproteins occur in the plasma in human disease and in experimental animals fed diets high in fat and cholesterol. LpX is found in obstructive liver disease and in familial lecithin: cholesterol acyl transferase (LCAT) deficiency. Patients with the genetic disorder type III hyperlipoproteinemia have only the E2 isoform of apo E, and high levels of β-VLDL (Mahley and Innerarity 1983; Robenek et al. 1987). β-VLDL are cholesterol-enriched lipoproteins that contain apo B and apo E as their major protein constituents. Animals fed diets rich in fat and cholesterol also produce β-VLDL; they also show an increase in HDL with apo E and a reduction of the usual form of HDL without apo E (Mahley and Innerarity 1983).

Lipoprotein variants of particular importance are those that have undergone chemical modification. Oxidative change to LDL, a process which may occur in vivo, either during circulation in the plasma, perfusion through the arterial wall or in the microenvironment of the subintimal matrix, is pivotal to the lipid hypothesis of atherosclerosis in its current form (Parthasarathy 1987; Steinberg et al. 1989; Palinski et al. 1989; Luc and Fruchart 1991). Apart from oxidation, the effects of other chemically modified forms of LDL have been studied in in vitro experiments on cultured cells. The modified forms studied include acetylated LDL (Goldstein et al. 1979b; Brown et al. 1979), acetoacetylated LDL (Mahley and Innerarity 1983), malondialdehyde-treated LDL (Fogelman et al. 1980) and LDL–proteoglycan complexes (Hurt and Camejo 1987; Vijayagopal et al. 1985).

3.2 Lipoprotein Receptors

The LDL receptor, which recognises apo B-100 and apo E as ligands, is the most extensively characterised of all the lipoprotein receptors, largely through pioneering studies (Goldstein and Brown 1977a; Goldstein et al. 1979a;

SCHNEIDER et al. 1982) on cultured fibroblasts. Further lipoprotein receptor systems have been identified, some of which are well characterised, while others remain to be elucidated in detail. Most lipoprotein receptors function to provide a mechanism for receptor-mediated endocytosis and subsequent catabolism of specific plasma lipoproteins, but some receptors appear to have additional functions.

Lipoprotein receptors other than the LDL receptor have been documented in a number of cell types and tissues. In macrophages, receptors or binding sites for at least four different types of lipoproteins have been described: (a) normal LDL, i.e. the LDL receptor, (b) β-VLDL (from patients with type III hypercholesterolaemia and from animals fed high cholesterol diets), i.e. the "β-VLDL receptor" (MAHLEY and INNERARITY 1983), (c) negatively changed or oxidised LDL, i.e. the "scavenger receptor" (KODAMA et al. 1990; ROHRER et al. 1990) and (d) HDL, the A-I or HDL receptor (SCHMITZ et al. 1985c).

The HDL receptor is poorly characterised, although candidate proteins for this receptor have been identified. The "β-VLDL receptor" is immunologically related to the LDL receptor (FOGELMAN et al. 1988) but it has only a low affinity for LDL, binding avidly to β-VLDL and chylomicron remnants, i.e. lipoproteins that contain apo E. A specific receptor for apolipoprotein E-containing lipoproteins, the LDL-related protein (LRP), has recently been identified in liver (HERZ et al. 1988, 1990). LRP is responsible for the clearance by the liver of chylomicrons and chylomicron remnants, and from current evidence the "β-VLDL receptor" appears to be equivalent to this receptor.

The scavenger receptor mediates the uptake of oxidatively or chemically modified LDL, which no longer binds with high affinity to the LDL receptor. Two types of macrophage scavenger receptor have been identified by complementary DNA cloning; both have an unusual α-helical coiled coil domain joined to a collagen-like triple helix exposed on the external surface of the membrane; one or both of these regions may be the recognition sites for the ligand (KODAMA et al. 1990; ROHRER et al. 1990). It is because both the scavenger receptor-mediated and the β-VLDL uptake processes are not down-regulated that the macrophage takes up as much oxidatively modified LDL (oxLDL) and β-VLDL and transforms into a foam cell.

4 Ultrastructural Localisation of Lipoproteins and Lipoprotein Receptors: Methodology

4.1 Advantages of Colloidal Gold as a Marker

Major improvements in methods for localising receptors at the electron microscopic level have been taken place over the last decade. The most important of these has been the development of colloidal gold labelling (HANDLEY 1989b).

Colloidal gold particles can be prepared in a range of sizes, suitable for high, intermediate or "low" resolution work (Frens 1973; Mühlpfordt 1982; Doerr-Schott 1989; Handley 1989a). The high electron density of the marker particles ensures that they stand out clearly against background detail, whether in sectioned specimens or in platinum-carbon replicas of cell surfaces and membrane faces. Apart from facilitating precision of localisation, these properties offer opportunities for comparative quantification of results.

4.2 Colloidal Gold Labelling of Cell Surface Receptors

The combination of gold labelling with platinum/carbon (Pt/C) replication techniques, which we played a part in developing and exploiting (Severs and Robenek 1983), has revolutionised the study of the surface distribution of lipoprotein receptors. The essence of the approach is first to carry out gold labelling of the target receptors, and follow this with platinum-carbon replication in such a way that the gold remains attached to the replica, marking the positions of the receptors or bound lipoproteins. Gold-labelled replicas provide "non-averaged" information on the distribution and numbers of receptors as viewed from above the cell—information that cannot easily be obtained by other structural or biochemical analytical techniques (Severs and Robenek 1983; Robenek et al. 1982, 1991; Robenek 1989a, b). The dense, particulate nature of the gold marker facilitates accurate identification of the labelled structure at high magnifications, and is equally useful at lower magnifications for rapid sampling and preliminary screening of experimental interventions. Moreover, by combining this approach with experiments designed to follow ligand—receptor interactions and receptor expression over time, a dynamic aspect to experimental investigations becomes possible.

A number of different cytochemical methods are available for carrying out the labelling step. We use two main methods, which give different but overlapping types of information. In the first, lipoprotein–gold complexes are prepared and presented to the cultured cells; this permits identification of the sites to which the lipoprotein–gold binds on the plasma membrane surface. The complexes are added to the culture medium of living cells, and the cells incubated at 4°C for various periods of time, before termination of the experiment by thorough washing with ice-cold buffer. The samples are aldehyde fixed and platinum–carbon replicas prepared. As an alternative, labelling can be carried out after the aldehyde fixation step.

In the second method, the approach involves indirect (two-step) immunocytochemical labelling of receptors or receptor-bound lipoproteins. Here, the cells are exposed to specific antibodies directed either against the receptor or against the lipoprotein which has been prebound to the cells. This step is followed by incubation with protein A–gold complexes or peroxidase-/gold-labelled secondary antibodies at 4°C. As before, washing with ice-cold buffer, fixation and processing for replication completes the procedure.

In both the above procedures, standard thin-section electron microscopy can be carried out in parallel for comparison with the replica results. An additional cytochemical method, allowing immunocytochemical labelling of receptor-bound lipoproteins in sectioned material, has proved useful in our studies. This involves incubating living cells with unlabelled lipoproteins and after fixation, processing for cryo-ultrathin sectioning or embedding in Lowicryl resin. Sections are then prepared and treated sequentially with specific antibodies directed against apolipoproteins followed by protein A–gold or secondary antibody–gold complexes.

All three procedure conducted at 4°C give information on the distribution of surface receptors captured in a state of "arrest" by the low temperature. Warming the cells to 37°C initiates dynamic changes that, with the aid of these detection systems, allow the dynamic surface changes and subsequent intracellular pathways of the lipoprotein receptor systems to be traced.

4.3 Surface Replication Techniques

The preparation of surface replicas of dried cultured cells is a simple and versatile technique for visualising receptors at the cell surface. The essential steps in the procedure are as follows:

$$\text{Label} \rightarrow \text{Fix} \rightarrow \text{Dry} \rightarrow \text{Pt/C replication} \rightarrow \text{Replica cleaning}$$

Cultured cells are gold-labelled using either the first or the second method detailed above. They are then fixed, dried and replicated with platinum–carbon in a standard vacuum evaporator or a freeze-etch machine (using without freeze-fracture-etch). The drying step can be accomplished quickly by air drying after ethanol dehydration, or if improved preservation of surface structural detail is required, by critical point drying or freeze-drying. Upon platinum–carbon evaporation, the gold particles become partially embedded within the replica. Gentle cleaning conditions are used to remove the biological material from the replica, leaving the gold particles attached to it. Upon examination in the electron microscope, the gold particles marking the positions of the receptors are clearly viewed from above the cell, over extensive replica views of the external surface of the plasma membrane. Standard surface replicas are quick and easy to make, and extensive areas of the cell surfaces of multiple cells are viewed, enabling rapid sampling and assessment of results. This approach is especially useful for analysing the distribution of receptors, and the dynamic changes that occur upon ligand binding.

Apart from the standard surface replica technique, a number of more sophisticated label-replica approaches are now available, and these are useful for more specialised applications (Severs 1989). The label-fracture technique, developed by Pinto da Silva and Kan (1984), is one that we have found useful. This technique allows label on the external surface of the plasma membrane to be viewed superimposed upon a freeze-fracture replica view of the E-face of the plasma membrane. The strategy is summarised as follows:

Label → Fix → Cryoprotect → Freeze-fracture → Pt/C replication → Replica rinsed in water (no cleaning in bleach or acid)

The cells are first labelled, and then the routine freeze-fracture sequence is followed up to and including the stage of platinum–carbon replication. Instead of cleaning the replicas in bleach or acids, however, they are washed extensively in distilled water, mounted and viewed in the electron microscope with portions of the fractured cells still attached (Pinto da Silva and Kan 1984). Where cells are fractured to reveal the E-face of the plasma membrane, the external half-membrane leaflet with still attached label remains stuck to the replica, allowing simultaneous visualisation of surface label and E-face structural detail. To facilitate generation of the right type of fracture through the cultured cells, we invert cells grown on coverslips on drops of polyvinyl alcohol on specimen holders. The specimens thus prepared and frozen, and then fractured by seperating the coverslip from the frozen medium under high vacuum (Brown 1981).

The standard surface replication technique thus allows visualisation of the external surface of the "dorsal" (i.e. uppermost) plasma membrane with attached label, and the label-fracture technique combines the viewing of label on this same surface with a replica view of the membrane interior (E-face). To gain access to the protoplasmic aspects of the plasma membranes of cultured cells, as is required for the investigation of the role of cytochemically identified cytoskeletal elements in receptor dynamics, different procedures are required. These involve "lysis-squirting" or "sandwich mounting/breaking" techniques (Nicol et al. 1987; Semich et al. 1989; Semich and Robenek 1990; Nermut 1989). The "lysis-squirting" technique involves the following steps:

Lysis → Squirting → Label → Fix → Dry → Pt/C replication → Replica cleaning

Cells attached to coverslips are incubated in hypotonic buffer, and then the bulk of the cells and their contents are sheared away using a stream of buffer from a syringe or Pasteur pipette. The protoplasmic surface of the "ventral" plasma membrane is thus exposed for immunolabelling. Gold labelling is carried out, the sample dried (freeze-drying, critical point drying, or air-drying following partial dehydration in ethanol) and platinum–carbon surface replicas prepared.

The "sandwich mounting/breaking" technique is designed to reveal, in similar manner, the protoplasmic aspect of the "dorsal" plasma membrane. Here, a monolayer of cells is sandwiched between polylysine-coated coverslips, and the coverslips are separated to break the cells apart. Once the sample has been labelled, drying is again done by either freeze-drying, critical point drying, or simple air-drying after ethanol dehydration, and replication carried out.

All these labelling/replica techniques are limited to investigations of receptors on the surfaces of membranes, and their application is restricted to cultured cell monolayers, cell suspensions and the luminal membranes of surface epithelia.

A standard approach we have used to follow the fate of internalised lipoproteins is to examine, by standard thin-section electron microscopy, cell cultures that had been fixed at intervals after exposure to lipoprotein–gold complexes at 37°C. The disadvantage of this approach is that the intracellular pathway of the lipoprotein can normally only be followed for a limited period owing to dissociation of lipoprotein and marker (e.g. upon lysosomal degradation of lipoprotein). Such aspects as receptor recycling, and the initial synthesis and trafficking of receptors and lipoproteins, cannot be investigated with this approach. To overcome these problems in the localisation of lipoproteins and lipoprotein receptors within tissues or cells, rather different approaches have to be adopted. The most successful of these are pre-embedding and post-embedding immunocytochemical methodologies combined with sectioning.

4.4 Pre-embedding Immunocytochemistry

The principle of pre-embedding immunocytochemistry is to permeabilise the cells to allow penetration of cytochemical reagents before processing for thin-section electron microscopy. We do this by fixing cells in McLean and Nakane's fixative (McLean and Nakane 1974) for 2–4 h at room temperature, and after washing, permeabilising using 0.05/ (w/v) saponin in phosphate-buffered saline (PBS) containing 0.2% gelatin (incubation buffer). The cells are then incubated with an appropriate dilution of primary antibodies against lipoproteins or lipoprotein receptors, and thoroughly washed. Incubation with secondary peroxidase-conjugated antibodies follows for 1 h at room temperature. Cells are washed with PBS, and fixed for 1 h at 4°C in 2.5% glutaraldehyde, 5% sucrose, 0.1 *M* sodium cacodylate buffer (pH 7.4). After intensive washing in 0.05 *M* Tris-HCl (pH 7.6), 5% sucrose, peroxidase activity is revealed by incubation with 0.05% (w/v) 3,3-diaminobenzidine tetrahydrochloride (DAB) in 0.05 *M* Tris-HCl (pH 7.6) for 10 min and 0.01% H_2O_2, 0.05% DAB in 0.05% *M* Tris-HCl for 3–6 min. Cells are postfixed with 1.3% OsO_4 in 0.1 *M* collidine buffer, dehydrated and embedded in Epon 812. Thin sections are examined without further staining.

4.5 Post-embedding Immunocytochemistry

The two low denaturing preparation procedures most widely used for intracellular localisation of proteins are cryofixation followed by cryoultramicrotomy, and low temperature embedding in hydrophilic acrylic resins such as Lowicryl followed by conventional sectioning (Brown 1989; Hobot 1989; Van Bergen en Honegouwen 1989). In both procedures, the strategy is to carry out immunogold labelling of thin sections after they have been cut, rather than labelling specimens before embedding, as in the method described above in Sect. 4.4 (Roth 1982; Bendayan 1984; Van Bergen et Honegouwen 1989). Components in the cell interior are thus exposed by the sectioning process itself; hence prior permeabilisation of the cells is not required for reagent access.

These post-embedding techniques have, in our hands, proved to be highly effective approaches for the detection of intracellular lipoproteins. For ultracryomicrotomy, we process cells or tissues according to the method of TOKUYASU (1980). Tissue blocks or cultured cells are fixed with 5% formaldehyde in 0.2 *M* piperazine-1,4-bis(2-ethanesulfonic acid) (PIPES), pH 7.0, for 2 h at room temperature. After washing in PIPES buffer, the fixed cells are infused with a mixture containing 1.6 *M* sucrose and 25% (w/v) polyvinylpyrrolidone (M_r = 10000), and frozen and mounted on silver pins. Ultrathin frozen sections are cut at −100°C (chamber) and −90°C (knife) using a Reichert-Jung FC 4 E equipped with a diamond knife. Sections are picked up on Formvar-coated copper grids and immunolabelled at room temperature. Immunocytochemical labelling is routinely done by floating grids serially, section side down, on 10- to 20-μl droplets of the following solutions: (a) PBS containing 0.2% glycine and/or 1% bovine serum albumin, (b) an appropriate dilution of specific primary antibodies, (c) PBS wash and (d) protein A–gold or secondary antibody–gold complexes. After the labelling procedure, sections are washed thoroughly with distilled water. The subsequent staining procedure includes a 10-min uranyl acetate oxalate (pH 7.4) stain, three 1-min rinses in distilled water, and a 10-min 2% uranyl acetate stain in distilled water. The grids are then floated on drops of 1% tylose in 0.5% uranyl acetate three times for 1 min each at 0°C.

For embedding in Lowicryl, the cells are fixed in 4% formaldehyde or in a mixture of 0.5%–3% glutaraldehyde and 4% formaldehyde in 0.1 *M* sodium cacodylate buffer, pH 7.2, for 1 h at room temperature, and subsequently washed in the same buffer. After dehydration in an ascending series of dimethylformamide, low temperature embedding in Lowicryl K4M is carried out according to VÖLKER et al. (1985). Sections are immunolabelled as described for cryosections above, and stained with uranyl acetate for 10 min.

In the two-step indirect cytochemical procedures used for pre-embedding and post-embedding immunocytochemistry, optimal retention of antigenicity combined with antibodies of high specificity and affinity is required if adequate labelling is to be obtained (NEWMAN and HOBOT 1989). Where chemical fixation is necessary, "mild" fixation in formaldehyde is the standard, as this is associated with less reduction in antigenicity than are the other eldehydes. The retention of antigenicity in cryosections is generally superior to that of other techniques because fewer tissue processing steps are involved; although the cells are fixed before freezing, there is no subsequent exposure to alcohols or embedding resins.

4.6 Antibodies

Successful intracellular localisation of lipoproteins and lipoprotein receptors requires antibodies of appropriate specificity and high affinity against the various lipoproteins and apolipoproteins. Despite the range of polyclonal and monoclonal antibodies available, however, electron microscopic localisation studies have remained limited. One reason for this relates to the preparation procedures used for electron microscopy. Even the standard "mild" formaldehyde fixation may adversely influence the antigenicity of lipoproteins, resulting in a much reduced labelling intensity. Formaldehyde is known to react with the amino groups of proteins and to cross-link polypeptide chains, and so may impair or even abolish immunological reactions (HOLUND et al. 1981; MELOAN et al. 1984). As some form of chemical fixation is required to preserve cell structure, such fixation-induced changes of antigenicity cannot always be avoided by using fixation-independent preparation procedures.

We have approached the problem of improving recognition of target lipoproteins in fixed cells by raising polyclonal antibodies to lipoproteins or apolipoproteins that had been chemically modified by formaldehyde fixation before immunisation of rabbits (HARRACH and ROBENEK 1990). In this way, we reasoned that the resulting antibodies might be directed against the antigenic determinants that are normally altered by fixation. Antibodies to prefixed apo A-I (anti-fix. apo A-I) and LDL (anti-fix. LDL) were produced in this way. Characterisation of these antibodies and practical experience have confirmed our prediction that this approach can improve labelling efficiency in intracellular immunolocalisation studies of fixed material.

Compared with lipoproteins and apolipoproteins, comparatively few immunolocalisation studies have used antibodies raised directly against lipoprotein receptors; indeed, only one receptor type, the LDL receptor, has been studied in this way (ANDERSON et al. 1982). Monoclonal anti-LDL receptor antibodies have been successfully used to localise LDL receptors in the plasma membrane of cultured fibroblasts (ROBENEK 1989a,b; ROBENEK et al. 1991; ANDERSON et al. 1982). The intracellular distribution of LDL receptors studied by pre-embedding and post-embedding immunolabelling techniques has so far been the subject of just two reports (PATHAK et al. 1988, 1990).

5 Receptor-Mediated Uptake of Cholesterol-Rich Lipoproteins

Cells organize and display their various classes of receptor in different ways, according to the functions they are required to perform. Here, we present a survey of our recent findings obtained using the techniques described above on the LDL receptor, binding sites for β-VLDL and the macrophage scavenger receptor. HDL receptors will be considered later, in the context of cholesterol removal from cells (Sect. 7.1).

5.1 LDL Receptor and Cholesterol Homeostasis in the Fibroblast and Smooth Muscle Cell

Initially, LDL receptors were thought to be displayed in a dispersed fashion on the plasma membrane, with clustering involving long-distance lateral migration, occurring after the binding of LDL (ANDERSON et al. 1977). Aggregation of receptor–LDL complexes into clusters was envisaged as the prelude to the classical events of receptor-mediated endocytosis. The original view that LDL receptors start their sojourn at the cell surface as individual widely dispersed units came from experiments on fibroblasts using ferritin–LDL conjugates and thin-section electron microscopy (ANDERSON et al. 1977). Later work with ferritin–anti-receptor antibody labelling, also examined by thin sectioning, did not lead to revision of this view (ANDERSON et al. 1982). However, the true surface distributions as viewed from above the cell are difficult to deduce from the

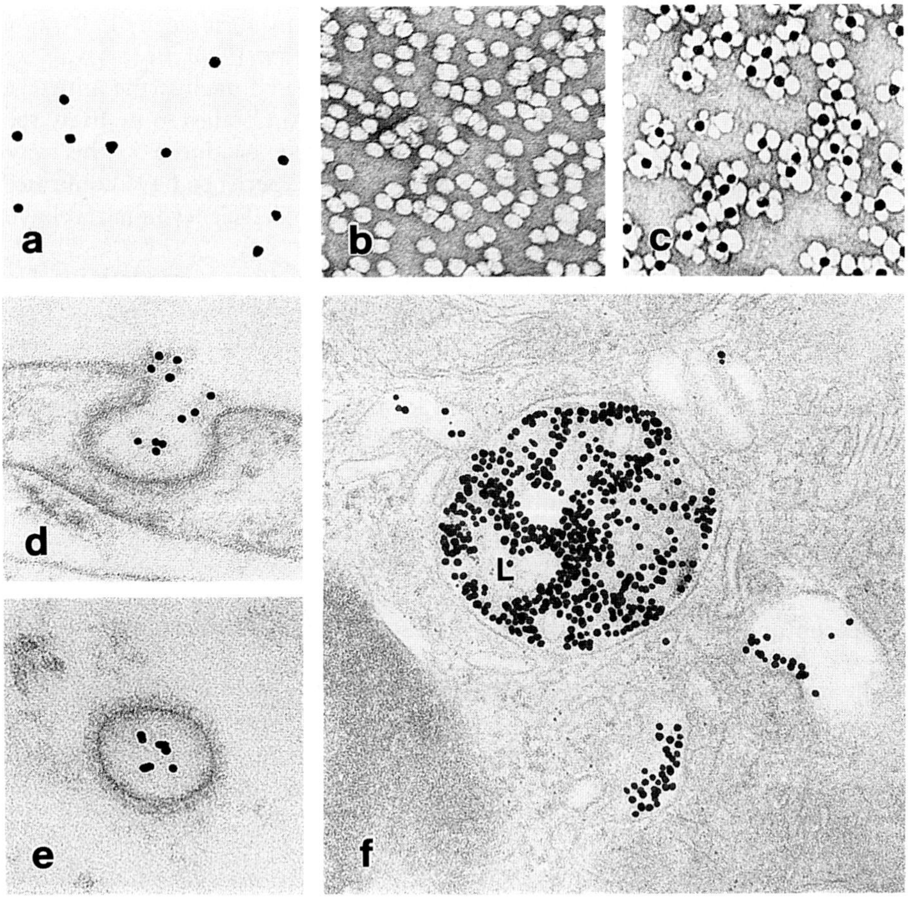

Fig. 5a–f. Gold markers, native lipoproteins, lipoprotein–gold complexes, and the labelling of LDL receptors as viewed by thin-section transmission electron microscopy. **a** Example of a preparation of colloidal gold particles (average diameter 15 nm). **b** Unconjugated (native) LDL molecules. **c** LDL–gold conjugate. **d–f** The major events of receptor-mediated endocytosis of LDL. Bound LDL–gold conjugates are concentrated in clathrin-coated invaginations (**d**). These detach into the cytoplasm as coated vesicles, internalising the bound LDL (**e**). The LDL is ultimately directed to the lysosomes for degradation (**f**). *L*, lysosome. **a–c** × 100 000; **d, e** × 90 000; **f** × 75 000

limited perpendicular views provided by thin sections. Our experiments, exploiting the technical advantages afforded by gold labelling (Fig. 5a–b) and surface replicas (Figs. 6, 7), suggested a rather different picture of LDL receptor display. These experiments have been conducted both on fibroblasts (the cell type on which the LDL receptor system was first analysed in detail) and on smooth muscle cells.

When fibroblasts or smooth muscle cells, previously maintained in lipoprotein-deficient medium, are incubated at or just below 4°C for 1 h in the presence of LDL–gold complexes, standard surface replica and label-fracture preparations show the label to be distributed as aggregates consisting of loosely organised clusters on the cell surfaces, with virtually no solitary gold particles in the intervening areas (Figs. 6, 7). Typically, the individual gold particles within the clusters are separated by distances of the order of 20–100 nm, indicating binding of individual complexes to individual receptors, rather than artefactual complex–complex binding (where closely packed gold particles would be the outcome). By using thin sectioning, and the technique of filipin treatment after LDL–gold

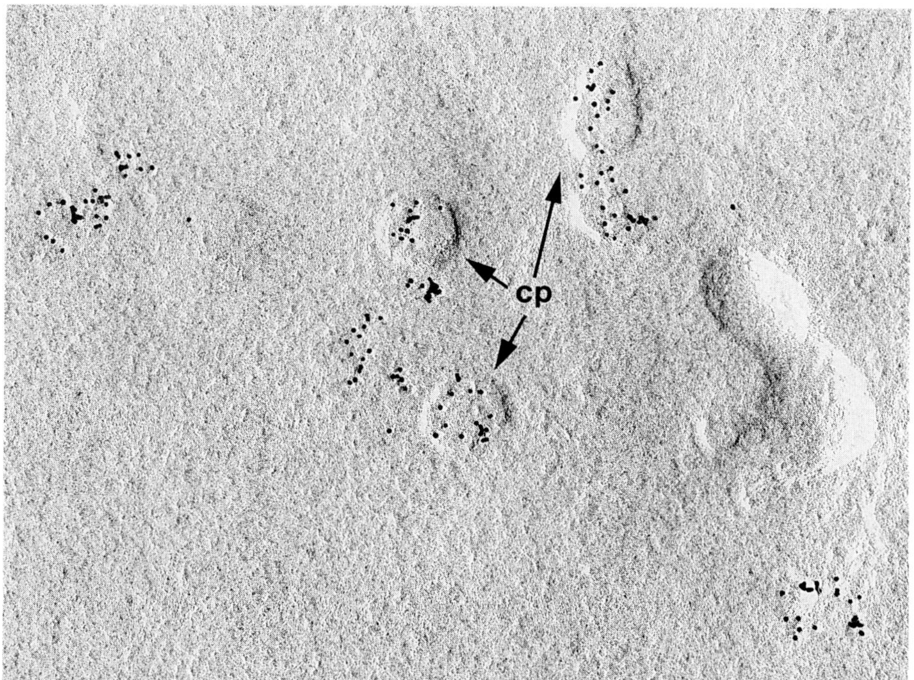

Fig. 6. Surface replica of a cultured smooth muscle cell after exposure to LDL–gold conjugates for 1 h at 4°C. The gold particles, marking positions of LDL receptors, are organised in clusters over flat and indented areas of the plasma membrane. The indented areas probably represent coated pits (*cp*). × 55 000

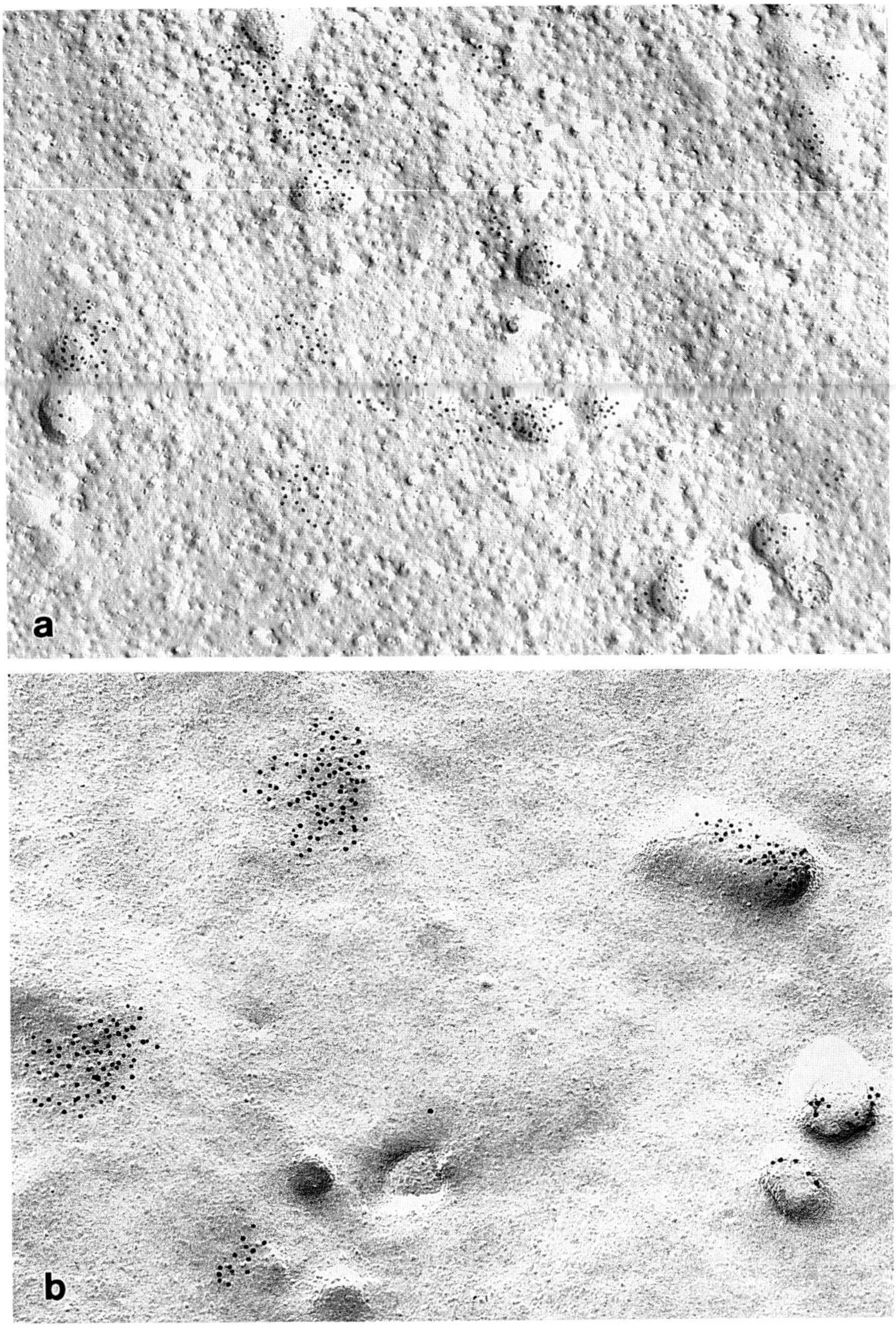

Fig. 7a, b. Label-fracture preparation from a fibroblast (**a**) and smooth muscle cell (**b**) treated with LDL–gold conjugates like those in Fig. 6 for 1 h at 4°C. Note that all the gold particles occur in clusters. Almost no single gold particles are present. The fibroblast (**a**) was treated with filipin (in glutaraldehyde) after the LDL–gold to discriminate between clathrin-coated and uncoated regions of the membrane, showing as unperturbed and pitted areas of the membrane, respectively. **a** × 40 000; **b** × 50 000

exposure in label-fracture preparations, it is clear that the aggregates of gold label occur both in indented, clathrin-coated domains and in flat, coated and non-coated domains of the plasma membrane, and tend to be more closely packed in the former than in the latter. Figure 7a illustrates these typical patterns of LDL receptor distribution as seen in the label-fracture preparations. The purpose of using the sterol-binding agent filipin in these experiments was not to attempt detection of cholesterol (SEVERS and ROBENEK 1983), but to distinguish between clathrin-coated and non-coated regions of the membrane. As with other protein-rich membrane domains, clathrin-coated areas are not perturbed by filipin, irrespective of sterol content (SEVERS and ROBENEK 1983), thus allowing their presence beneath the membrane to be detected as domains free of filipin-induced pits in the en face replica views of the membrane.

These results, and those obtained on fibroblasts manipulated experimentally to remove pre-existing receptors and stimulate insertion of recycled or new receptors (ROBENEK 1989b), suggest that LDL receptors are inserted and displayed in clusters, at least under the experimental conditions we have investigated. This interpretation has, however, been disputed (WOFSY et al. 1985; SANAN et al. 1987, 1989). We therefore designed further experiments to discriminate between the competing views (ROBENEK et al. 1991). To avoid using LDL–gold complexes, which were suggested as a possible cause of artefactual clustering, we used alternative detection systems. These included labelling via anti-apo B-100 antibodies, labelling via anti-LDL receptor antibodies, and direct visualisation of native (unlabelled) LDL molecules bound to the cell surface. The results from all these procedures all reinforce our original conclusion—that LDL receptors are indeed normally displayed in loose aggregates, and not in individually dispersed form (ROBENEK et al. 1991). A recent study, in which LDL receptor distribution and clathrin lattices were simultaneously visualised on membranes torn from the upper surface of cultured cells, reveals the label predominantly in aggregates, though in these experiments the aggregates appear specifically associated with clathrin lattices (SANAN and ANDERSON 1991).

The surface distributions of LDL–gold complexes observed in cultured fibroblasts, smooth muscle cells and hepatocytes are identical, indicating that the cluster display pattern is a characteristic feature of the LDL receptor across cell types.

Experiments comparing the binding patterns of β-VLDL–gold complexes on the fibroblast and hepatocyte plasma membranes further bear out this conclusion, and point to the existence of a cytochemically identifiable receptor for apo E in liver cells. The β-VLDL used in these experiments was obtained from the serum of cholesterol-fed rabbits. When fibroblasts were incubated with β-VLDL–gold complexes for 1 h at 4°C, aggregates of gold label, identical to those observed in the standard LDL–gold experiments, were consistently observed, reflecting binding of β-VLDL, via its apo B and E moieties, to the LDL (apo B/E) receptor. However, when hepatocytes were treated with β-VLDL–gold, again under the same conditions, a different labelling pattern was seen. Aggregates of gold particles were as abundant as in the hepatocyte/LDL–gold experiments, but in addition, a large number of widely dispersed individual gold particles was present. These results are consistent with the idea that the clusters represent the LDL receptor, and that the additional dispersed label represents the apo E receptor, LRP (HERZ et al. 1988, 1990), which is expressed in the hepatocyte but not in the fibroblast (ROBENEK et al. 1991). If this interpretation is correct, then it would seem that LRP, in contrast to the LDL receptor, has a widely dispersed distribution in the plasma membrane.

Using the cytotochemical techniques outlined in Sect. 4, it has been possible to visualise directly the sequences of internalisation and track the subsequent pathways of macromolecules through cellular compartments. Cells internalise diverse receptor–ligand complexes in similar fashion despite difference in initial receptor display patterns and differences in ultimate intracellular fates of ligand and receptor (for review see GOLDSTEIN et al. 1985). The hallmarks of LDL receptor-mediated endocytosis are recycling of internalised receptors and catabolism of LDL in lysosomes.

The events of receptor-mediated endocytosis, extensively characterised over the years (for reviews see MAHLEY and INNERARITY 1983; GOLDSTEIN

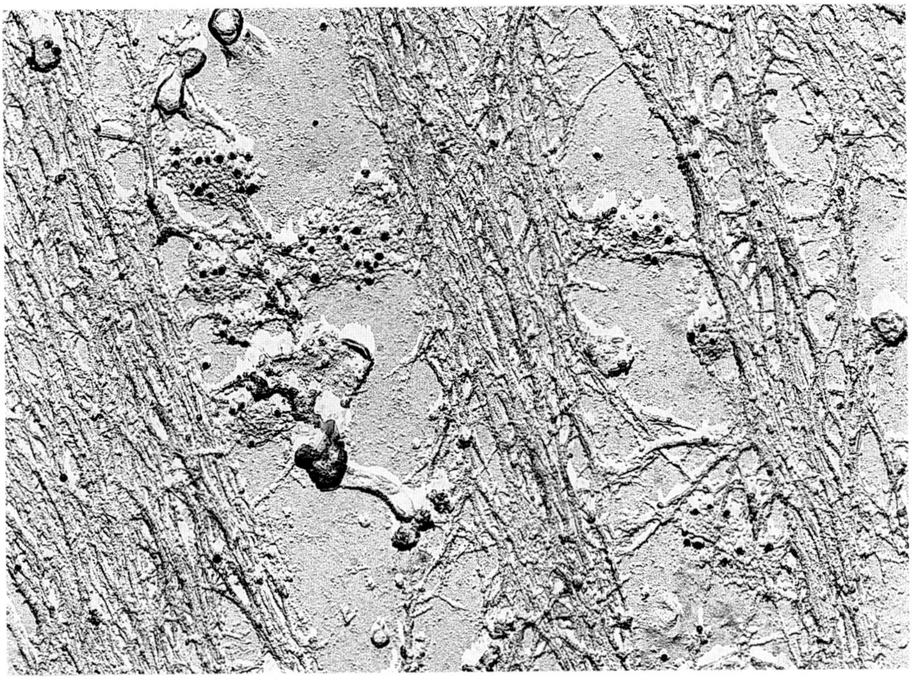

Fig. 8. Immunocytochemical localisation of clathrin on the protoplasmic surface of the fibroblast plasma membrane after lysis squirting. Regions of the "honeycomb" pattern characteristic of clathrin are specifically labelled, using antibodies against clathrin followed by protein A–gold (17 nm). Gold label appears attached to extended, rather flat clathrin sheets found between microfilaments. × 35 000

et al. 1985), are illustrated with dramatic clarity with our labelling techniques (Fig. 5d–f). LDL, via apo B-100, binds to LDL receptors. The receptors operate in concert with a protein, clathrin, that coats the cytoplasmic surface of the receptor-bearing membrane domains. Clathrin is initially organized as flat polygonal lattices beneath the plasma membrane (Fig. 8), interacting with adaptor proteins which in turn interact with the cytoplasmically exposed segments of the receptor molecules. When LDL binds, the clathrin shapes the membrane into a deep invagination and generates forces that pinch it off as a discrete clathrin-coated vesicle (Fig. 5d, e). The adaptor proteins are hypothesised to target the vesicle to the correct destination, which in the case of LDL is the endosomal compartment of the cell. The coat is removed within seconds, allowing the uncoated vesicles to fuse with the endosome. In the low pH environment of the endosome, the LDL and the receptor are uncoupled from one another; the receptor is then recycled back to the cell surface, while the LDL is transported to the lysosomes for degradation (Fig. 5f). This liberates amino acids from apo-B and frees cholesterol from the cholesterol esters present in the lipoprotein. The cholesterol released upon lysosomal hydrolysis of the LDL suppresses both 3-hydroxy-3-methylglutaryl CoA reductase, the rate-limiting step in cholesterol biosynthesis, and synthesis and expression of the receptor. Excess cholesterol not needed for membrane or steroid hormone synthesis is reesterified by acyl CoA: cholesterol acyltransferase (ACAT), which is activated by LDL uptake and stored as cholesteryl oleate in the cytoplasm. It is through these mechanisms that the cells are protected from excessive accumulation of cholesterol or cholesteryl esters, and do not become foam cells (Munro and Cotran 1988; Goldstein and Brown 1979, 1983; Brown and Goldstein 1984).

5.2 Scavenger Receptor and the Macrophage

Macrophages have only limited numbers of LDL receptors of the classical "fibroblast-type," but as outlined in Sects. 2.3 and 2.4, other receptors concerned with lipoprotein uptake are expressed. LDL that has been modified chemically by acetylation (AcLDL) or oxidation (OxLDL) loses the ability to bind to the LDL receptor, but is recognised by a different high-affinity receptor characteristic of the macrophage, the scavenger or AcLDL receptor (Kodama et al. 1990; Rohrer et al. 1990). Localisation of this receptor at the cell surface of a macrophage, as seen by thin-section electron microscopy after exposure of mouse peritoneal cells to AcLDL–gold for 1 h at 4°C, is illustrated in Fig. 9. We have applied labelling techniques to study the surface distribution, dynamics and internalisation of this receptor and its bound ligand. Labelled replicas of cultured mouse peritoneal macrophages exposed to AcLDL–gold complexes for 1 h at 4°C show diffusely distributed gold label, largely confined to a circular band between the central (nuclear) region and the peripheral zone of the plasma

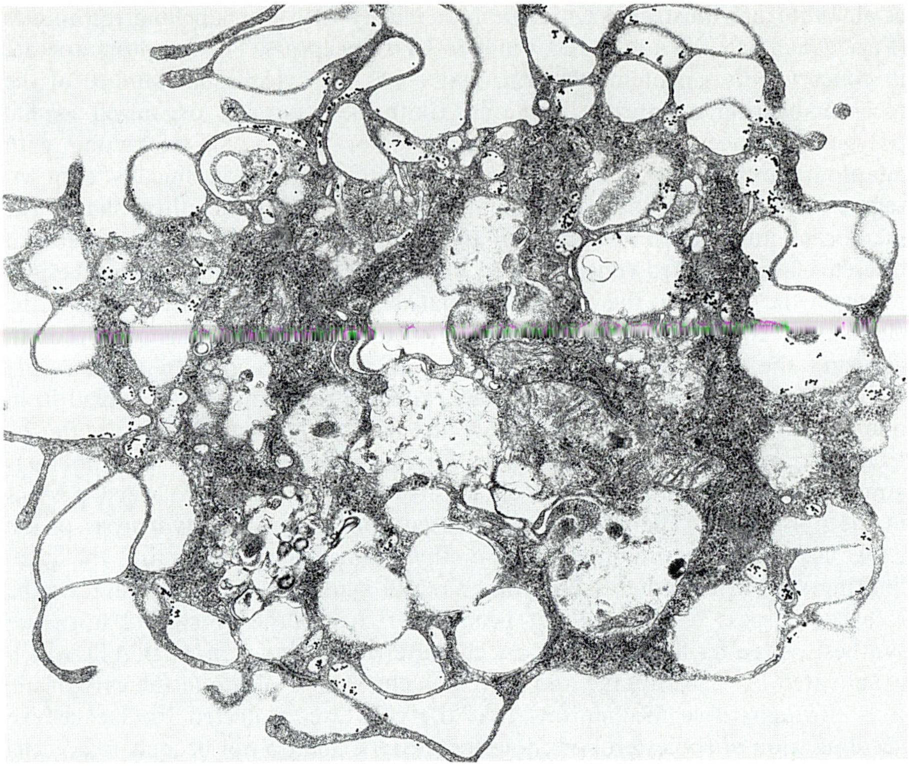

Fig. 9. Thin-section electron micrograph of a cultured mouse peritoneal macrophage treated with AcLDL–gold conjugates for 1 h at 4°C. Gold label is found bound in abundance to the plasma membrane, marking scavenger receptors. × 18 000

membrane. A time-dependent redistribution of receptors occurs on warming the cells to 37°C; by 4 min, most of the gold particles have become aggregated, by 8 min compact clustering in coated pits is observed, and by 15 min virtually all the label has disappeared from the cell surface. Thus, warming leads to progressive coalescence and ultimate endocytosis of the initially diffusely distributed AcLDL–receptor complexes. The distribution and dynamics of AcLDL receptors thus differ markedly from those of LDL receptors. LDL receptors, in contrast to AcLDL receptors, are always confined to presumptive coated pit regions even prior to ligand binding, and do not migrate appreciably in the plane of the membrane.

Receptor-mediated endocytosis of β-VLDL, AcLDL and OxLDL (PATAKI et al. 1992) operate via clathrin-coated pits and vesicles, as with classical LDL receptor-mediated endocytosis. By extending the periods of exposure of cultured macrophages to these labelled lipoproteins, it is possible to follow the process of foam cell formation in vitro. Cultured mouse peritoneal macrophages exposed to AcLdL, OxLDL or β-VLDL for 12–24 h at 37°C develop large multivesicular organelles, 0.5–1.5 μm in diameter. These "foamy organelles" are abundant (4–12 typically being observed per sectional view of cell), and represent a lysosomal compartment of the cell (Fig. 10).

When the macrophages are incubated for a further 6–12 h at 37°C in a lipoprotein-free culture medium, numerous lipid droplets, 0.3–1.5 μm in diameter, appear (typically, 6–15 of these lipid droplets are seen per sectioned cell) (Fig. 11). What happens at the biochemical level is that cholesterol ester from the internalised lipoproteins is hydrolysed in the lysosomes. Cholesterol is then released into the cytoplasm, and re-esterified to form cholesteryl ester lipid droplets. A continuous cycle of re-hydrolysis and esterification then ensues.

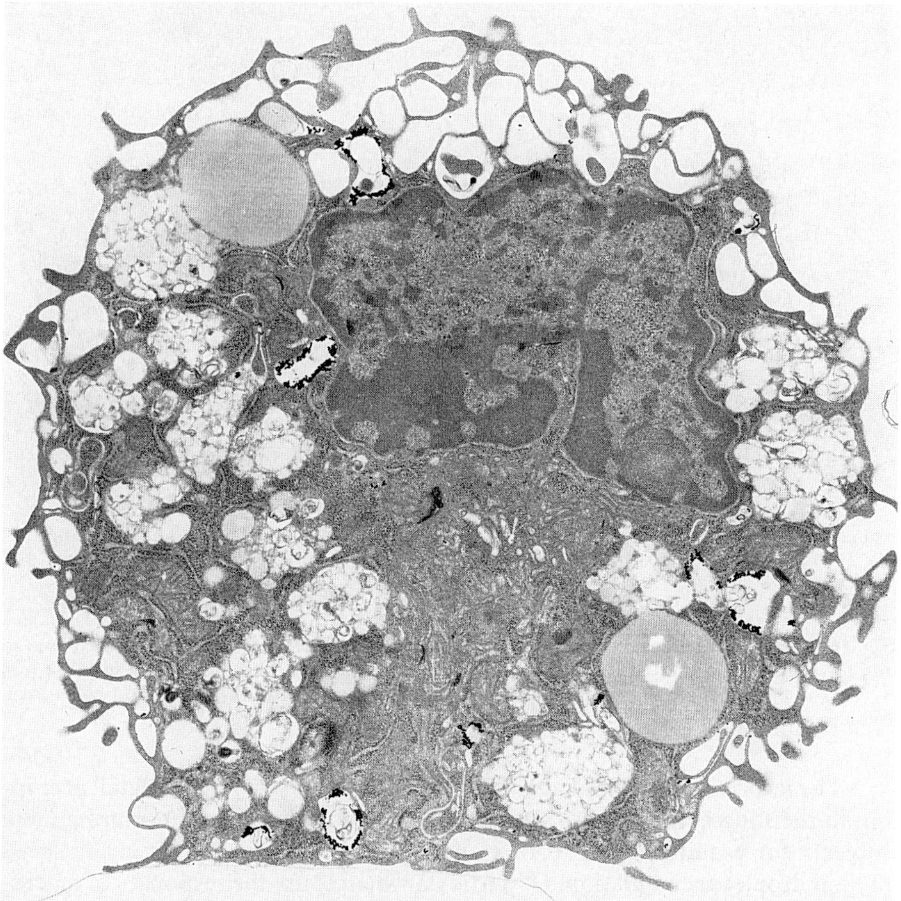

Fig. 10. Thin-section electron micrograph of a cultured mouse peritoneal macrophage cultivated under normal culture conditions for 24 h at 37°C, and then in the presence of 70 μg/ml AcLDL for 12 h at 37°C followed by AcLDL–gold for 15 min. The cytoplasm of the macrophage is filled with numerous large multivesicular organelles the so-called foamy organelles. Gold label has accumulated in some of these foamy organelles, indicating transport of AcLDL–gold to them. × 8500

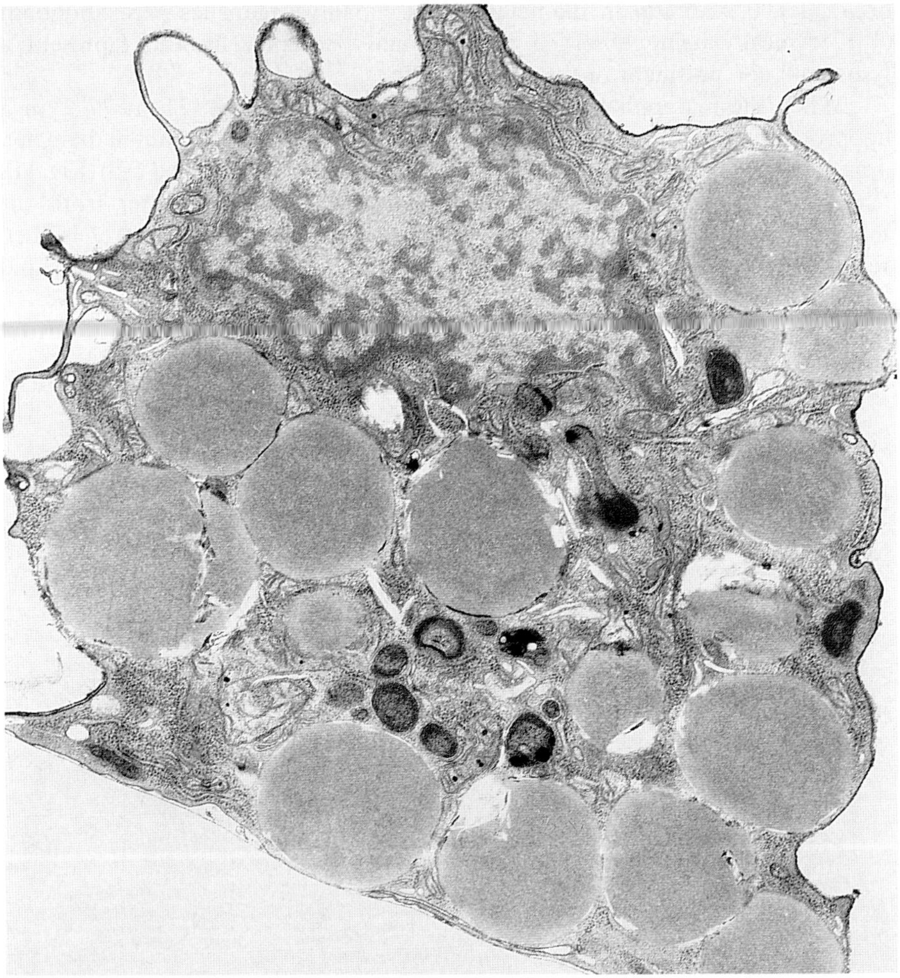

Fig. 11. Thin-section electron micrograph of a cultured mouse peritoneal macrophage exposed to AcLDL (70 μg/ml) for 12 h at 37°C before incubation in the absence of AcLDL for a further 6 h at 37°C. The cytoplasm of the cell is filled with numerous lipid droplets, giving the typical foam cell-like morphology. × 8500

The response of macrophages to feeding with AcLDL differ in detail according to the source of the cells. Macrophages from the plasma of normal human subjects, for example, differ from mouse peritoneal macrophages in the speed of lipid droplet accumulation. Of particular interest are the responses of macrophages from patients with Tangier disease, a rare autosomal recessive disorder characterised by deficiency of HDL and deposition of cholesteryl esters in various organs and tissues.

Under standard culture conditions, the ultrastructure of human control and Tangier macrophages appears broadly similar. The cells contain numerous mitochondria and cisternae of rough endoplasmic reticulum, abundant ribosomes and several vacuoles of variable size. Only occasional single multivesicular bodies, lysosomes and lipid droplets are observed. The Golgi apparatus is well developed, appearing more extensive in the Tangier macrophage than in the control cells. Exposure of cells from both sources to AcLDL for 24 h at 37°C reveals spectacular ultrastructural changes (ROBENEK and SCHMITZ 1991). Control macrophages accumulate abundant small membrane-free lipid droplets, which fill much of the cytoplasm. In Tangier macrophages, fewer cytoplasmic lipid droplets appear, but instead, the cytoplasm becomes packed with distinctive vacuoles not observed in control macrophages. Two types of vacuole, referred to as type I and type II vacuoles, are observed. Type I vacuoles are irregular spheroid or ovoid electron-lucent structures, filled with fine flocculent or fibrillar material, distributed as aggregates in the cell. Type II vacuoles are larger, contain scrolls and lamellae of variable electron opacity, and are filled with more electron-dense material. To determine whether the two vacuole types in Tangier macrophages are forms of lysosome, immunogold cytochemistry was carried out to localise the lysosomal marker enzyme cathepsin D. This was done by post-embedding immunoelectron microscopy using an affinity-purified polyclonal rabbit anti-human cathepsin D antibody. Both type I and type II vacuoles were intensely and specifically labelled, indicating a lysosomal identity for both forms of vacuoles (Fig. 12a). In control macrophages, the size of the lysosomal compartment was much smaller than that of Tangier macrophages, and the individual lysosomes were less intensely stained with the cathepsin D antibody (Fig. 12b).

Whether the two distinct morphological forms of vacuole reflect different stages in maturation of a single type of lysosome or are seperate types of lysosome engaged in different degradative activities is uncertain. Earlier observations suggested that Tangier macrophages are characterised by an abnormal cellular processing of HDL procursors, resulting in their diversion to lysosomes for degradation instead of resecretion, coupled with a dysregulation of cellular lipid metabolism (SCHMITZ et al. 1985a). The presence of a marked accumulation of lysosomes in Tangier macrophages is consistent with a block in the normal mechanism of cholesterol transfer from the lysosomal compartment to storage as lipid droplets. Accompanying this lysosome accumulation, there is a marked hyperplasia of the Golgi apparatus in Tangier macrophages. The Golgi apparatus becomes widely distributed throughout the cell, and develops markedly dilated transcisternae. These changes, not present in control human macrophages exposed to AcLDL, may arise from extra demand for lysosomal enzyme production by the Golgi apparatus under the conditions of blocked cholesterol transfer, or they may reflect overproduction of sphingomyelin and phospholipids (SCHMITZ et al. 1990c).

Tangier disease is thus associated with abnormalities of macrophage intracellular organelles and cellular lipid metabolism which suggest a translocation disorder affecting lysosomal processing and the Golgi apparatus. Interestingly, fibroblasts from Tangier patients exposed to AcLDL show similar changes in

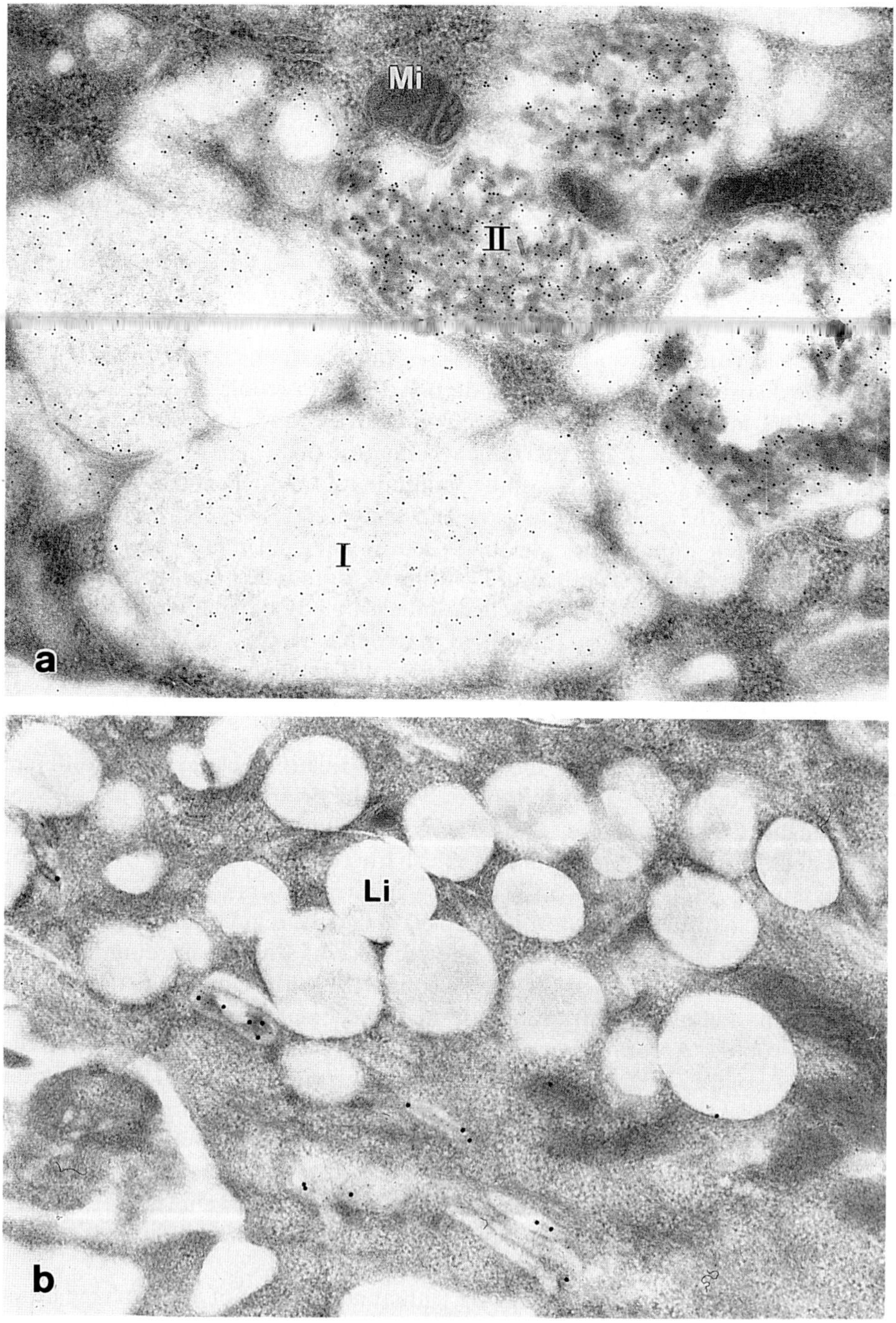
Mi
II
I
a
Li
b

the Golgi apparatus, but not in the lysosomal compartment. This situation may stem from the fundamental difference in the way the two cell types metabolism cholesterol. That a parallel alteration in the Golgi apparatus does occur in the two cell types reinforces the view that this is a fundamental abnormal feature of the disease, and opens the possibility of using fibroblast cell cultures as a model system for investigating the cellular basis of Tangier disease. The advantage of such a system would be the ease of continuous cultivation and the standardisation of experimental conditions on a single, defined cell line.

5.3 Transformation of Smooth Muscle Cells to Scavenger Cells

The micrographs in Figs. 2 and 4 illustrate that in vivo, smooth muscle cells may also become foam cells, even though feeding smooth muscle cells in vitro with chemically modified LDL fails to mimic this process (HOFF et al. 1991). How this transformation process occurs in vivo is poorly understood. One possibility is that altered smooth muscle cells within the plaque start to express scavenger-type receptors. Another possibility is that smooth muscle cells directly acquire scavenger receptors from macrophages. This could occur via intimate associations between macrophages and smooth muscle cells, possibly involving portions of disintegrated macrophage adsorbed onto the plasma membrane of the smooth muscle cell. Evidence that macrophage components can, when brought into close contact with smooth muscle cells in vitro, cause the smooth muscle cells to become foam cell-like in appearance, has come from studies using macrophage-derived cholesteryl ester-rich lipid droplets (WOLFBAUER et al. 1986; MINOR et al. 1986).

In these studies, initial experiments in which medium containing the lipid droplets was added to smooth muscle cell cultures did not result in conversion to foam cells (WOLFBAUER et al. 1986; MINOR et al. 1986). However, when smooth muscle cells grown on coverslips were inverted over the same medium, marked intracellular accumulation of cholesteryl ester occurred. These differences appear to relate to the proximity of the droplets and the cells. Under the standard

◄

Fig. 12a, b. Thin-section electron micrographs showing localisation of cathepsin D in Tangier (**a**) and control macrophages (**b**) cultivated in the presence of 70 μg/ml acetylated LDL for 24 h at 37°C. Cathepsin D was revealed by post-embedding immunoelectron microscopy of Lowicryl sections with monospecific antibodies to cathepsin D plus the protein A–gold technique. **a** In Tangier macrophages both type I (*I*) and type II (*II*) vacuoles are found to be intensely and specifically labelled. Although gold particles (8 nm) are abundant over both types of vacuoles, they appear to be most concentrated over the more electron-dense regions of type II vacuoles. Gold particles are rarely seen over the other organelles such as the nuclei, mitochondria (*Mi*), cisternae of the endoplasmic reticulum, Golgi apparatus, or the cytoplasm. **b** In control macrophages, small pale lysosomes are distributed among the abundant lipid droplets (*Li*). Gold label (12 nm) within these lysosomes is mainly confined to electron-dense fibrillar material within their interiors. The lipid droplets are completely free of label, as are other organelles and the cytoplasm. **a, b** × 43 000

culture conditions, the buoyant lipid droplets float to the surface, and so do not come into direct contact with the cells. When cells are inverted over the droplets, however, close contact is ensured, and this may mimic the in vivo situation. In vivo, lipid droplets released from dying macrophage/foam cells would remain trapped in the arterial wall and become bound to extracellular matrix components, and this might facilitate close contact with the smooth muscle cells.

To explore the effects of macrophage–smooth muscle cell interactions in more detail, we have recently started work on fusing macrophages and their components with smooth muscle cells using polyethylene glycol. The idea behind these experiments is to establish in vitro model systems which permit examination of possible mechanisms by which macrophage scavenger receptors might be acquired by smooth muscle cells, and to investigate how the intrinsic properties of the smooth muscle cell might influence the functional activities of such acquired receptors.

Establishment of a hybrid cell system opens up possibilities for investigating, with the aid of ultrastructural labelling techniques, how the presence of smooth muscle cell nucleus and cytoplasm influences the expression of scavenger receptor properties. Much work needs to be done to develop this model. For example, the fate of the macrophage plasma membrane following its incorporation into the smooth muscle cell will have to be established in detail. Among the many other questions to be addressed are the following. How long does the macrophage plasma membrane remain a distinct entity, and how rapidly do its components intermix with those of the smooth muscle cell plasma membrane? How does the presence of the two nuclei and two cytoplasms originating from different cell types influence the properties of the scavenger receptor? Do hybrids have the ability to transform into foam cells upon exposure to AcLDL, or does the presence of smooth muscle cell-derived components suppress this process? If foam cell formation does occur, do the organelles of the macrophage or those of the smooth muscle cell process internalised AcLDL? And will foam cell formation also occur if macrophage plasma membrane fragments are fused onto smooth muscle cells instead of whole macrophages? All these questions can theoretically be addressed by experimental manipulation of cultured cells combined with ultrastructural labelling by the methods detailed in Sect. 4.

6 Localisation of Apolipoproteins and Lipoproteins in Whole Tissue

In contrast to the cultured cell systems, few cytochemical studies have previously been done on the localisation of lipoproteins in tissue. We report here two investigations in which this has been achieved, namely the localisation of apo A-I in human liver and of various lipoproteins and apolipoproteins in the human atherosclerotic plaque.

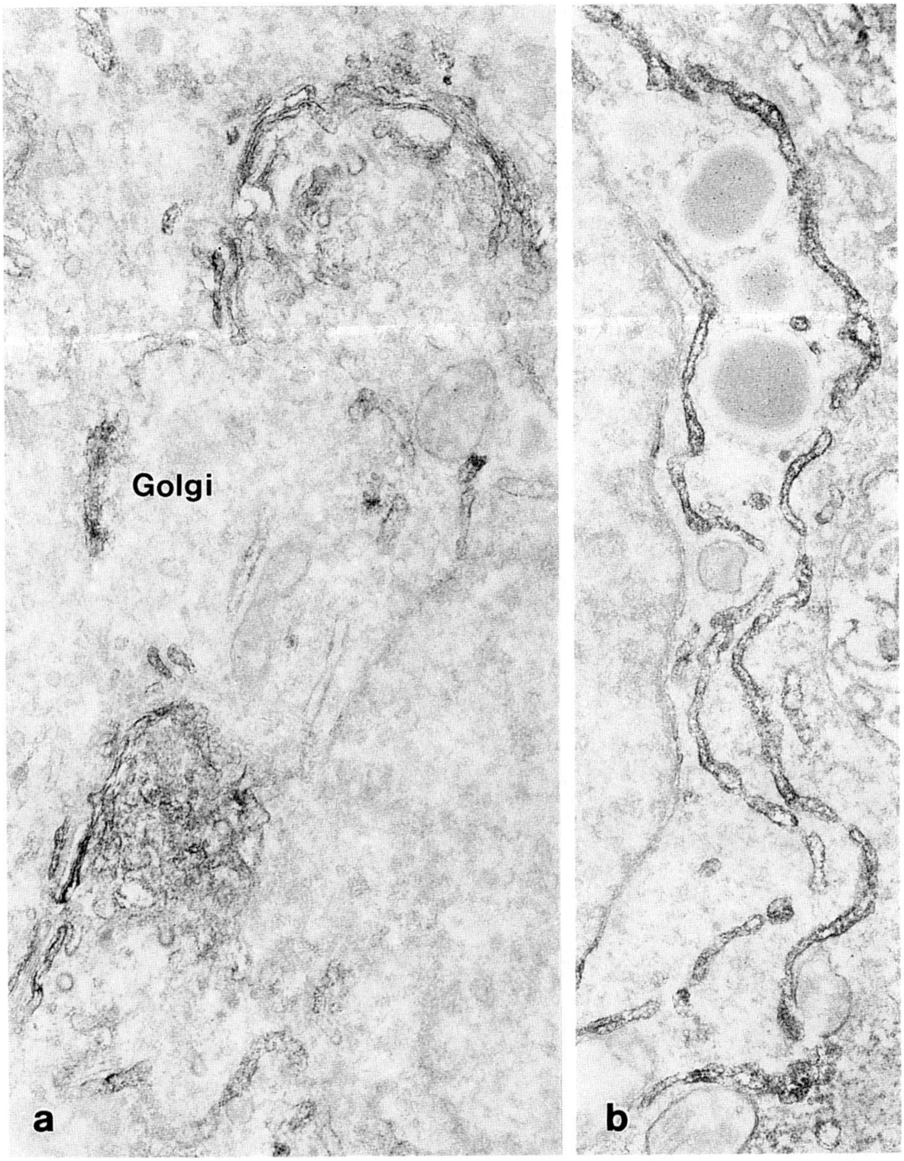

Fig. 13a, b. Transmission electron micrographs of HepG2 cells stained by the indirect pre-embedding immunoperoxidase method for apo A-I. Electron-dense immunoperoxidase reaction products that indicate the antigenic sites for apo A-I are present in **a** the Golgi complex (*Golgi*), **b** cisternae of the rough endoplasmic reticulum and secretion granules. **a** × 11 500; **b** × 17 000

6.1 Localisation of Apolipoprotein A-I in Human Liver

Apo A-I is the major protein constituent of plasma HDL, representing about 60% of its protein mass. In humans, apo A-I is synthesised by intestinal and liver cells, and is secreted as a basic precursor protein which is subsequently processed to more acidic isoproteins found in plasma HDL (ZANNIS et al. 1982). Apo A-I is thought to function as the ligand for the binding of HDL to the HDL receptor (SCHMITZ et al. 1985b, c, 1990b; RIFICI and EDER 1984; FIDGE and NESTEL 1985).

Before conducting experiments on liver tissue, we tested the efficacy of the antibodies for immunocytochemical labelling using HepG2 cells. Standard light microscope immunofluorescence techniques revealed distinct patches of intracellular staining. By applying the pre-embedding immunoperoxidase technique,

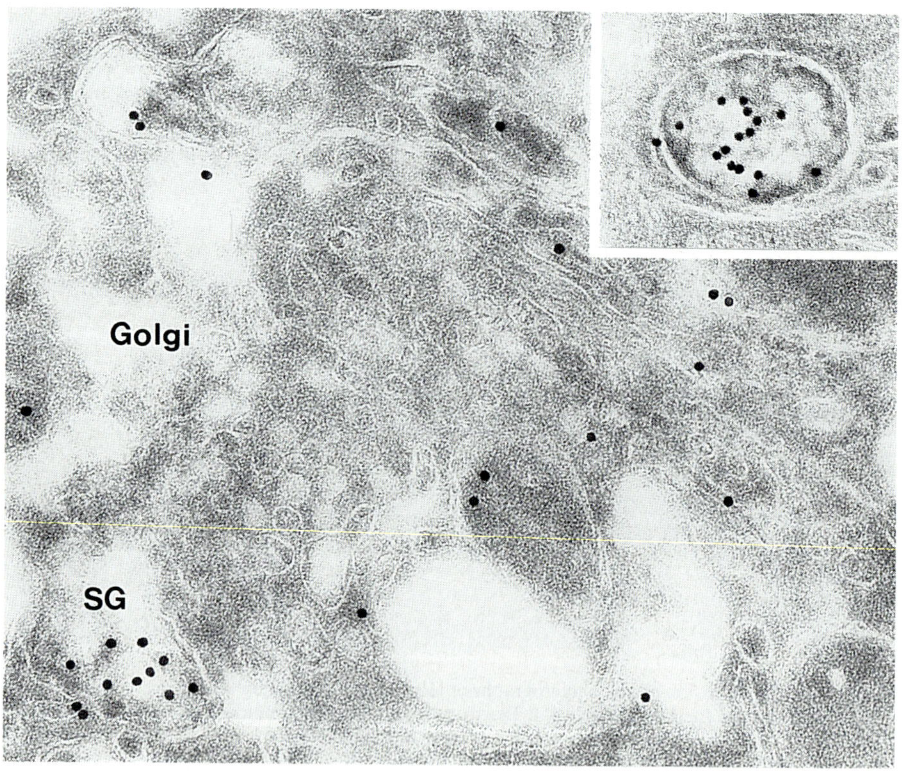

Fig. 14. Transmission electron micrograph of a hepatocyte from human liver stained for apo A-I by post-embedding immunocytochemistry on ultrathin cryosections, using the protein A–gold method. The cisternae of the Golgi complex (*Golgi*) and the secretion granules (*SG*, *inset*) at the trans side of the Golgi complex are strongly labelled, indicating the sites of apo A-I. × 68 000; *inset*: × 61 000

the feasibility of immunolocalising synthesised apo A-I within cells was demonstrated at the ultrastructural level (Fig. 13). Apo A-I was localised in various cellular compartments, especially the Golgi complexes (Fig. 13a), Golgi-associated vesicles and the cisternae of the rough endoplasmic reticulum (Fig. 13b). No positive staining occurred in these organelles in control sections. Other subcellular compartments such as nuclei, mitochondria and lysosomes were consistently negative.

To localise apo A-I in human liver tissue, we used formaldehyde-fixed apo A-I (anti-fix. apo A-I) primary antibodies and protein A–gold on ultrathin cryosections (Fig. 14). Immunolabelling of the Golgi area was marked, and labelling of secretion granules and vacuoles in the trans Golgi network and pericanalicular region was also apparent. Positive labelling was consistently found in the space of Disse. These findings indicate that the synthetic and secretory pathway of apo A-I follows the classical endoplasmic reticulum–Golgi apparatus–secretory granule route, release presumably being mediated by exocytosis of secretory granules.

6.2 Localisation of Lipoproteins in Human Atherosclerotic Plaque

Data on the in situ distribution of lipoproteins within the atherosclerotic plaque have until recently remained retricted to histochemical studies carried out at the light microscopic level (NIENDORF et al. 1990; ROSENFELD et al. 1990; VOLLMER et al. 1991; HABERLAND et al. 1988). Thus little information is available on how different lipoproteins are distributed in the various cellular compartments of the plaque. More precise localisation of these molecules within the lesion would further our knowledge of the composition of the plaque and the role of lipoproteins in progression and regression.

The investigation was carried out on atherosclerotic plaques obtained from human femoral artery. The plaques, characterised as advanced lesions by light microscopy, contained abundant foam cells of macrophage and smooth muscle cell origin embedded in extensive extracellular matrix which contained deposits of crystalline cholesterol. Antibodies against the following were used: LDL, apo B-100, HDL, formaldehyde-modified apo A-I and formaldehyde-modified LDL (two different antibodies). For simultaneous characterisation of the cellular and subcellular constituents of lesions, we used a polyclonal antibody against α-actin to identify smooth muscle cells, and an affinity-purified polyclonal rabbit anti-human cathepsin D antibody to identify lysosomes. In single labelling experiments to detect lipoproteins we used the protein A–gold technique, and in double-labelling experiments for simultaneous identification of other cellular constituents we used protein A–gold followed by protein G–gold (BENDAYAN 1989).

Success was obtained in localising LDL and HDL in the various cellular and extracellular compartments of plaques. Though there were some differences

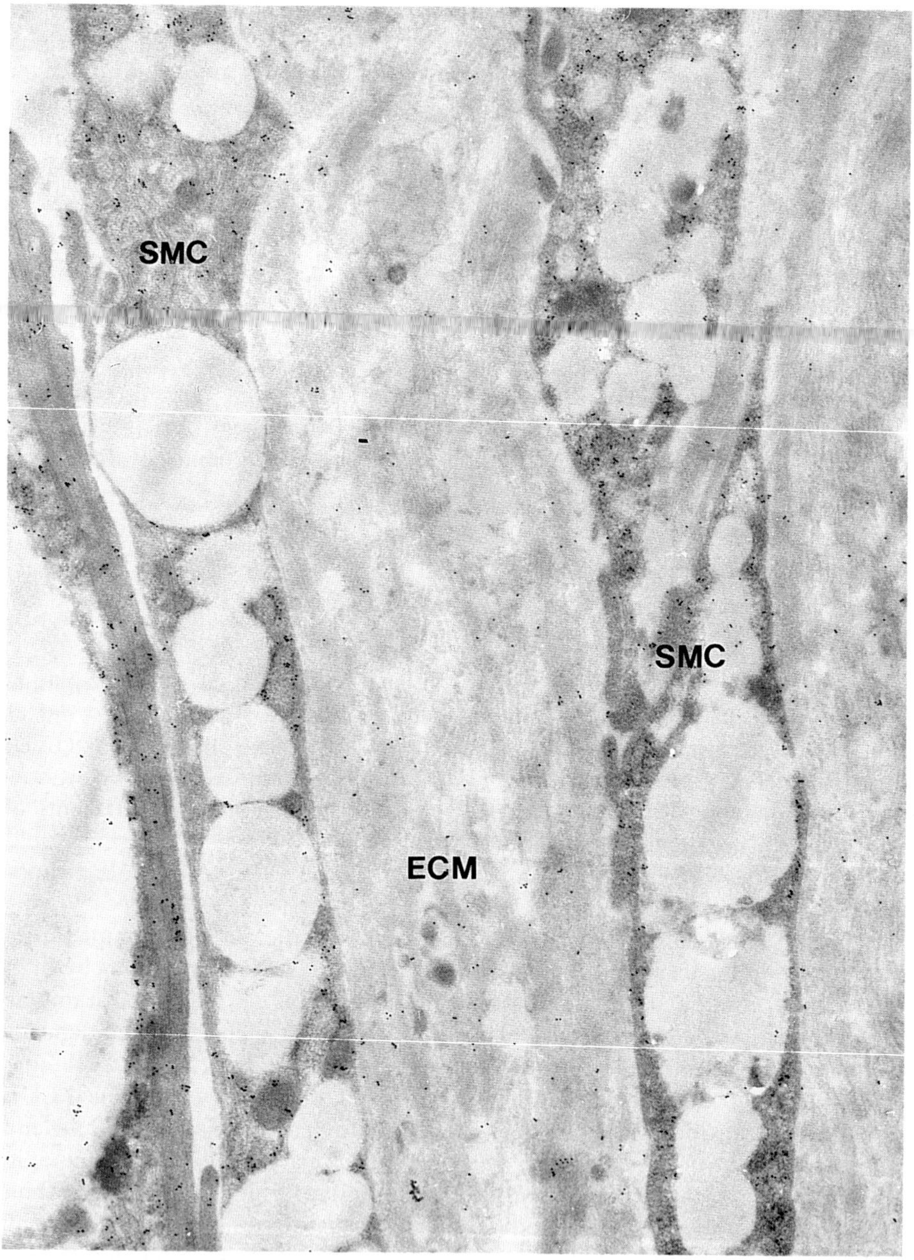

Fig. 15. Transmission electron micrograph of a Lowicryl K4M-embedded atherosclerotic plaque from a human femoral artery stained for LDL by post-embedding immunocytochemistry with anti-fix. LDL antibodies followed by protein A–gold. Gold particles are abundant over the cytoplasm of foam cells derived from smooth muscle cells (*SMC*) as well as in the surrounding extracellular matrix (*ECM*). The lipid droplets and the other organelles are poorly labelled. × 20 000

in labelling efficiency between the different antibodies, consistent results were obtained between antibodies directed against the same lipoprotein. LDL labelling was widely distributed over cells and extracellular matrix; the example in Fig. 15 illustrates portions of smooth muscle cell-derived foam cells in which the cytoplasmic matrix, but not the lipid droplets, is labelled. Although, as shown in Fig. 15, LDL labelling occurs throughout the extracellular matrix, HDL labelling was found predominantly over cellular compartments. Both lipoproteins were abundant in the cytoplasm of macrophages, particularly in electron-dense lamellar organelles identified as lysosomes by cathepsin D antibodies.

Bearing in mind the involvement of lysosomes in the endocytotic pathway, we interpret the intense labelling of LDL and HDL in these organelles as a reflection of active lipoprotein internalisation from the extracellular matrix. Both macrophages and smooth muscle cells within the plaque appear to take up LDL and HDL, and direct them to a lysosomal compartment rich in cathepsin D for hydrolysis. The localisation of LDL and HDL in the same subcellular compartment suggests a common fate for both types of lipoprotein. This conclusion accords with the in vitro biochemical studies of VAN LENTEN and FOGELMAN (1990) and VAN DER WESTHUYZEN et al. (1980), who found that the intralysosomal degradation of lipoproteins, especially apo B, involves an initial limited endoproteolytic attack by cathepsin D.

7 Removal of Cholesterol from Cells and Tissue

Transport of cholesterol is not solely a one-way process leading to deposition within tissues such as the arterial wall; cholesterol may also be transported from peripheral tissues to the liver, a process referred to as "reverse cholesterol transport" (GLOMSET 1968; BADIMORE et al. 1989; HO et al. 1980; SCHMITZ et al. 1990b). From the liver, cholesterol can be eliminated in the bile, via either synthesis of bile acids of secretion of free cholesterol (ZANNIS et al. 1982; RIFICI and EDER 1984).

It is thought that HDL play a central role in reverse cholesterol transport (BIESBROCK et al. 1983; EISENBERG 1984; SCHMITZ et al. 1989; SCHMITZ and ROBENEK 1989), acting as the vehicles for uptake of cholesterol from the tissue and its subsequent transport in the plasma. Cholesterol-enriched HDL may themselves be taken up by receptor-mediated uptake in the liver (NAKAI et al. 1976; SOLTYS et al. 1982; BACHORIK et al. 1982; HOEG et al. 1985; BERNARD et al. 1990; DELAMATRE et al. 1991). Alternatively, the cholesterol picked up by HDL may be transferred via physicochemical exchange mechanisms to other lipoproteins such as VLDL. The VLDL are converted to VLDL remnants and LDL by the action of endothelial lipoprotein lipase, and these lipoproteins can then be cleared by the liver via the LDL receptor.

Further mechanisms, independent of HDL, may also contribute to reverse cholesterol transport. For example, evidence from our experiments suggests that macrophages can release excess cholesterol by direct secretion of lysosome-derived cholesterol and phospholipid-containing "lamellar bodies". We have also found that lipid-laden macrophages can, with appropriate stimulation, be induced to migrate. Foam cells may not, therefore, be inevitably destined to perish in the plaque, but may participate in cholesterol efflux to a variable degree that is determined by external factors.

7.1 Role of the HDL Receptor

High-density lipoprotein is one of the most effective cholesterol accepters known. Like LDL, HDL may undergo oxidative modification, and this abolishes the property of HDL to stimulate efflux of cholesterol (NAGANO et al. 1991). There are still many questions concerning how HDL and its subclasses interact with macrophages and how cholesterol is removed from cells (SCHMITZ et al. 1985b, 1989; FIDGE and NESTEL 1985; SCHMITZ and ROBENEK 1989). It has been hypothesised that the HDL subclass without apo E (low cholesterol content) may absorb unesterified cholesterol by direct interaction with the plasma membrane. The physicochemical mechanisms of cholesterol transfer would be facilitated by a low cholesterol to phosphatidylcholine ratio in the outer surface of the HDL particle compared with that of the plasma membrane. This would lead to an imbalance between cytoplasmic cholesterol and the cholesterol content of the plasma membrane; with re-equilibration, cholesterol from the cytoplasmic pool may replace that lost from the plasma membrane.

Cholesterol accumulation in macrophages stimulates synthesis of large amounts of apo E and secretion of apo E/phospholipid discs, a process independent of HDL (BASU et al. 1981). The current concept of reverse cholesterol transport encompasses the possibility that HDL, during the cytoplasmic cholesterol esterification process mediated by the enzyme lecithin:cholesterol acyltransferase (LCAT), not only absorb unesterified cholesterol from the cell surfaces but also incorporate apo E from extracellular apo E/phospholipid discs. Cholesteryl esters and apo A-I could also be transferred from HDL onto the apo E/phospholipid discs. The net result would be formation of cholesteryl ester-rich and apo E-rich HDL1 (or HDLc) which, upon reaching the liver, would be recognised and internalised via the hepatic apo E receptor (LRP).

We have examined in detail the cellular interaction of HDL and HDL subclasses with cultured mouse peritoneal macrophages (Figs. 16, 17). That HDL receptors are expressed by macrophages and other cells has been demonstrated in a number of studies (SCHMITZ et al. 1987; MURAKAMI et al. 1987; ASSMANN and FUNKE 1990), and using biochemical and morphological methods we have also confirmed that apo A-I-containing apo E-free HDL_3 bind to specific macrophage surface receptors. These HDL receptors can be visualised electron microscopically on the cell surface using gold-labelled HDL and surface replicas (Fig. 6a). When the experiments are carried out at 4°C, the gold-labelled HDL

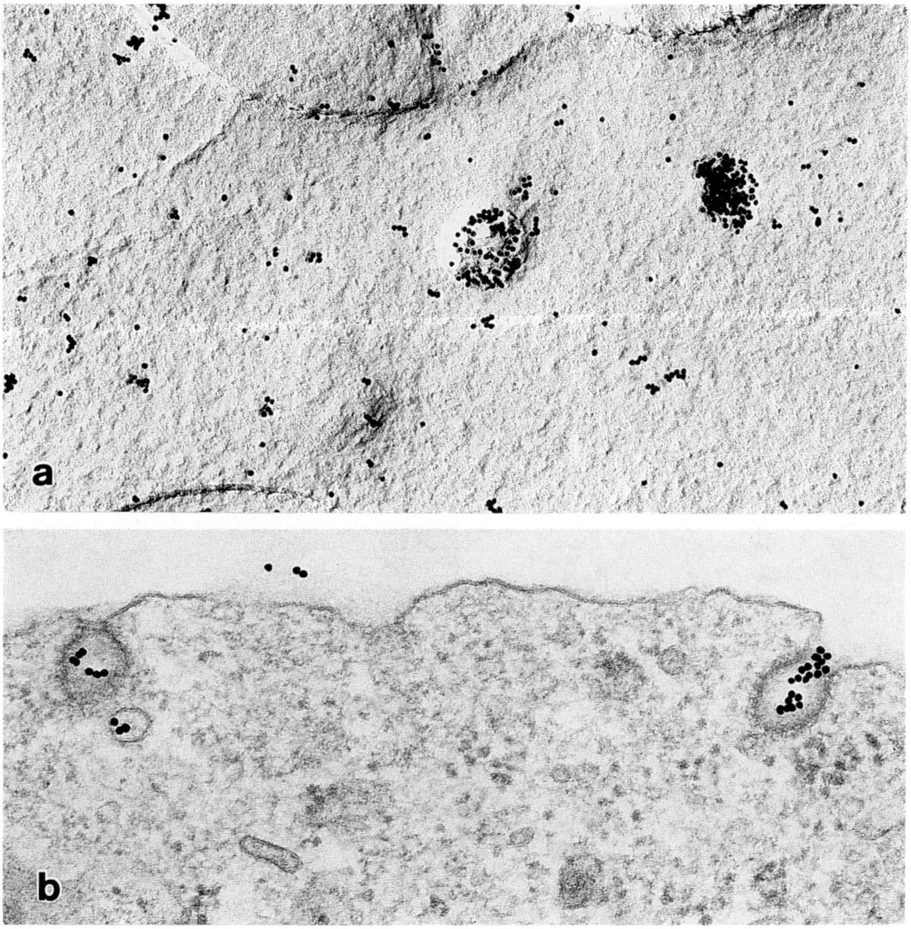

Fig. 16. a Surface replica and **b** thin-section electron micrograph of cultured mouse peritoneal macrophages after exposure to HDL_3–gold conjugates for 1 h at 4°C (**a**) and 5 min at 37°C (**b**). The gold particles, marking positions of HDL_3 receptors, occur in clusters (**a**) and over coated areas (**b**) of the plasma membrane. Between the clusters, individual randomly distributed HDL_3–gold conjugates are observed. **a** × 60 000; **b** × 42 000

particles bind in a combined preclustered and diffusely distributed display pattern. Raising the incubation temperature to 37°C results in rapid concentration of the gold label into aggregates, followed by uptake via coated pits and coated vesicles (Fig. 16b). The internalisation process has been further documented by anti-apo A-I immunoperoxidase staining of thin sections of macrophages prefed native HDL (Fig. 17), and by following the fate of fluorescence-labelled HDL by light microscopy and quantitative flow cytometry. After internalisation, the HDL particles are transported to endosomes, but in contrast to LDL or AcLDL, they are not significantly degraded in lysosomes. On their transcellular

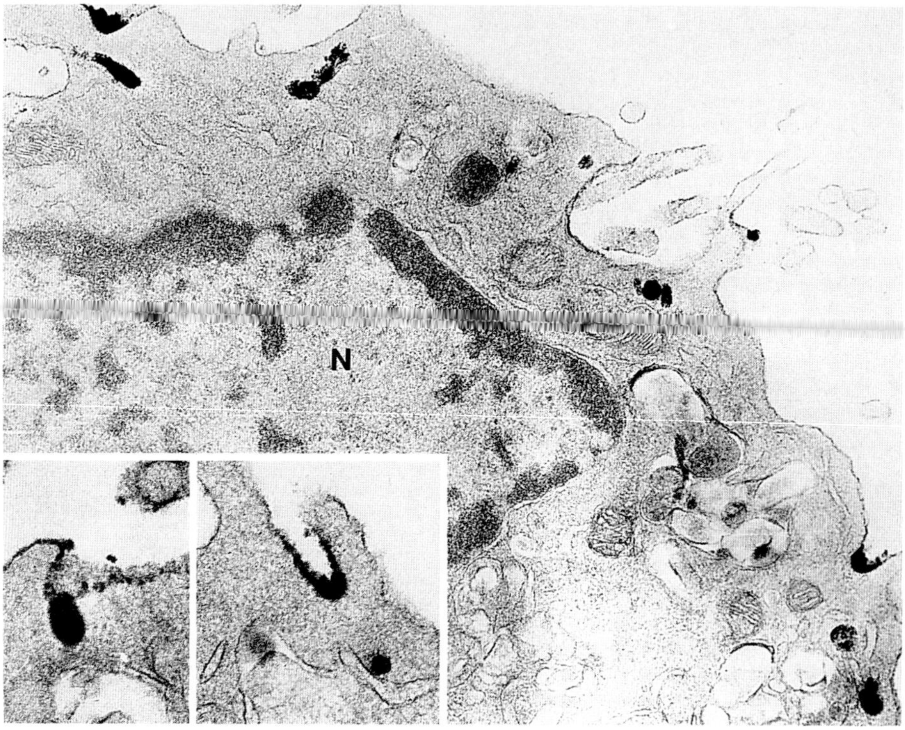

Fig. 17. Cholesterol-loaded macrophage incubated with unlabelled HDL_3 for 1 h at 4°C. The bound HDL_3 molecules were visualised with rabbit-anti apo A-I followed by peroxidase-conjugated goat-anti rabbit IgG F (ab')2. The *insets* show coated pits with peroxidase reaction products. *N*, nucleus. × 27 000; *insets*: × 38 000

route, HDL come into contact with cytoplasmic lipid droplets where they take up cholesterol and apo E. They are then resecreted as intact cholesterol and apo E-rich HDL particles (Schmitz et al. 1987).

The co-ordinate action of lipid-modifying enzymes and physicochemical exchange events results in a series of HDL subclasses differing in density, particle size, charge and protein/lipid composition. Three subpopulations of HDL, with fast, intermediate and slow electrophoretic mobilities, have been identified by preparative free flow isotachophoresis (Schmitz et al. 1990b; Nowicka et al. 1990). The fast migrating HDL particles are rich in apo A-I and phosphatidylcholine. The subpopulation with intermediate mobility is rich in apo A-II, apo E, apo C, cholesteryl esters and sphingomyelin. The slow migrating HDL subpopulation consists of particles rich in apo A-I and apo A-IV, and is associated with high LCAT activity.

The fast migrating HDL particles bind with high affinity to HDL receptors on macrophages, whereas slow migrating HDL particles exhibit high non-specific binding with only a small amount of specific interaction (Schmitz et al. 1990b).

Using the gold-label surface replication technique, we compared the labelling patterns of HDL_3 and fast and slow migrating HDL particles on the surface of macrophages. Gold-labelled HDL_3 and fast migrating HDL particles both showed a pre-clustered distribution with dispersed label in the intervening areas, as described above. The labelling intensity with fast migrating HDL particles was lower than that with HDL_3. The slow migrating HDL particles showed lower binding still and were randomly distributed. These labelling data accord with the binding characteristics determined by biochemical methods. Since both fast and slow migrating HDL subpopulations are good promoters of cholesterol efflux, it may be that the HDL subpopulations rich in apo A-I promote cholesterol efflux via specific interaction with HDL receptors, whereas apo A-VI rich HDL extract cholesterol from the plasma membrane via the action of LCAT during a predominantly non-specific interaction with the cell surface.

7.2 HDL Receptor-Independent Mechanisms

In addition to the above HDL receptor-dependent mechanisms, cholesterol efflux from macrophages may also be facilitated by an HDL receptor-independent secretion of lamellar bodies (Fig. 18). When mouse peritoneal macrophages are cholesterol-loaded, treatment with the Ca^{2+}-antagonist nifedipine inhibits formation of lipid droplets, resulting instead in the production of lamellar bodies within multivesicular foamy organelles of lysosomal origin (Fig. 18a). Prolonged incubation leads to the detachment of membrane-surrounded lamellar bodies from the lysosomes, their movement to the cell periphery and secretion into the surrounding medium (Fig. 18b). This process can occur in the absence of HDL. The lamellar bodies measure 100–300 nm in diameter, and are rich in unesterified cholesterol (68%) and phospholipids (21%), phosphatidylcholine accounting for 70%–80% of the phospholipid. Precisely how the lamellar bodies are released into the extracellular environment is not yet understood. Evidence from intracellular and extracellular lipid analyses and our morphological studies on control and experimentally treated cultures suggests that secretion of the cholesterol-containing lamellar bodies is a naturally occurring process in the macrophage that is enhanced by nifedipine.

A different type of lamellar body, originating from lipid droplets rather than lysosomes, is induced by treatment of macrophages with the ACAT inhibitor octimibate. These lamellar bodies are also bounded by membranes, newly synthesised at the margins of the lipid droplets by elements of the endoplasmic reticulum with which they interact. In contrast to the lamellar bodies induced by Ca^{2+}-antagonist treatment, those originating from lipid droplets after ACAT inhibitor treatment are not secreted. In the absence of HDL, they accumulate in the cytoplasm, but when HDL are added to the medium, these lamellar bodies interact with endosomes containing internalised HDL particles and rapidly decrease in number in parallel with HDL-mediated cholesterol efflux.

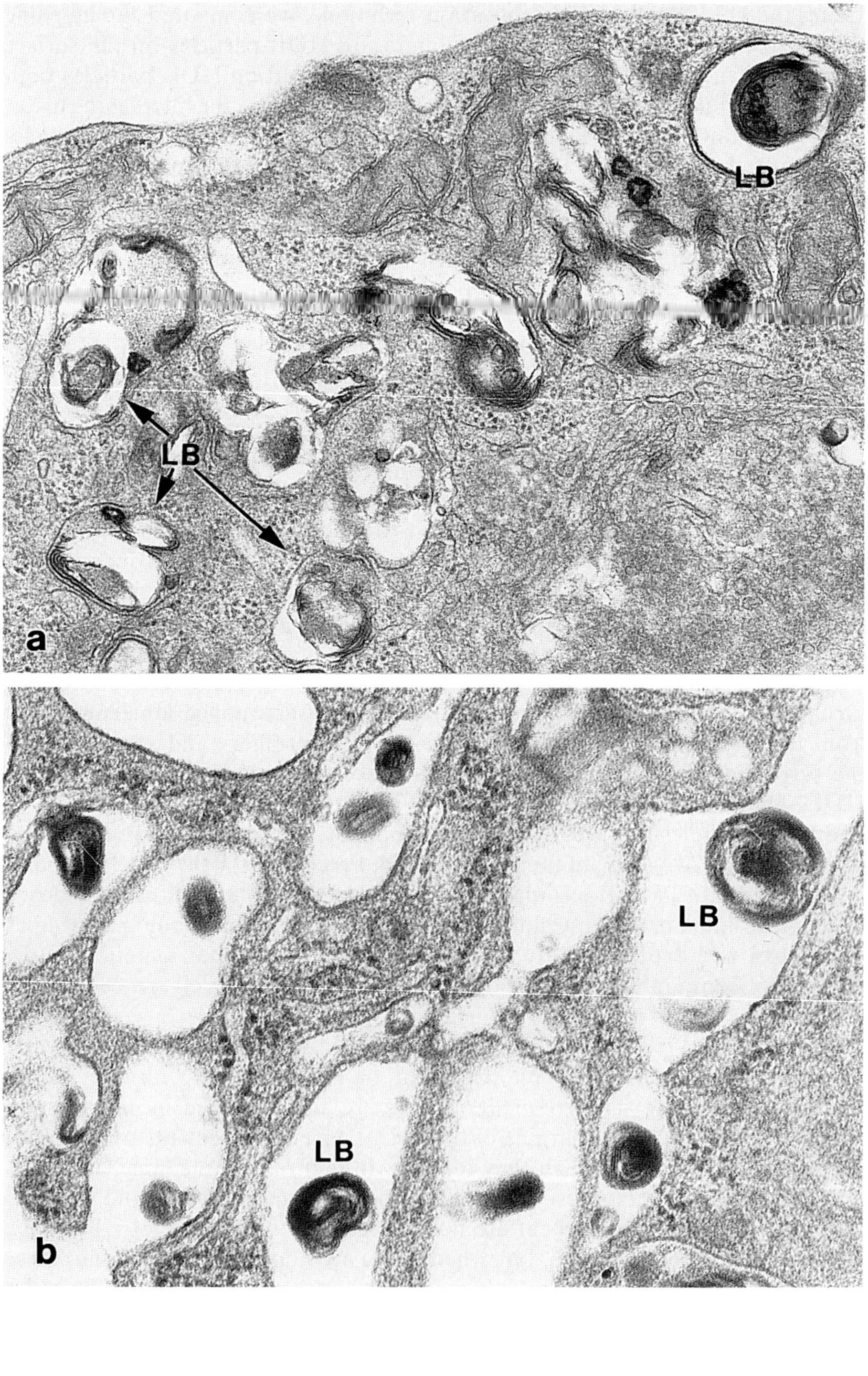
LB
LB
a
LB
LB
b

From biochemical data on cellular cholesterol metabolism, characterisation of the secreted lamellar bodies and other morphological data, we conclude that macrophages release cholesterol by two major pathways; (a) an HDL receptor-mediated release of unesterified cholesterol that is enhanced with ACAT inhibition, and (b) an HDL receptor-independent secretion of cholesterol which can be amplified by Ca^{2+}-antagonists. Both the HDL receptor-dependent and the HDL receptor-independent pathways appear to protect macrophages and possibly other cholesterol-loaded cells from overaccumulation of cholesterol and hence foam cell transformation.

7.3 Macrophage/Foam Cell Mobilisation

Microscopy of fatty streaks and atherosclerotic lesions indicates that foam cells accumulate in the intima, presumably because of cessation of migratory activity. There is, however, experimental evidence that fatty streaks and more advanced lipid-rich lesions may undergo regression, and that foam cell mobilisation is involved in this process (Tucker et al. 1971; Stary et al. 1980; Fritz et al. 1981; Daoud et al. 1981; Small 1988; Dudrick 1987; Wissler and Vesselinovitch 1990). In animal models involving lipid feeding, several authors have reported that a significant decrease in the number of lipid-laden macrophages in intimal lesions occurs after a couple of months' regression died (Daoud et al. 1985; Gerrity 1981b; Gerrity and Naito 1980). Moreover, micrographs suggesting the departure of foam cells from lesions have been presented (Gerrity 1981b; Gerrity and Naito 1980). A monocyte-macrophage lipid clearance mechanism, in which the numbers of macrophage/foam cells in a lesion are determined by the balance between monocyte entry into the arterial wall and departure of foam cells from it, may therefore exist in vivo. However, whether immobile foam cells of established human atherosclerotic plaques retain a latent capacity to migrate is not known.

We have investigated the capacity of foam cells to undergo migration, and examined how lipid uptake and cholesterol accumulation affect this process (Pataki et al. 1992). The system we used involved lipid-loading mouse peritoneal macrophages with AcLDL, and then measuring their motility in an in vitro

Fig. 18a, b. Thin-section electron micrographs of peritoneal mouse macrophages cultured in the presence of 70 μg/ml acetylated LDL for 12 h at 37°C and sequentially in the presence of 70 μg/ml acetylated LDL and 2 μmol/l nifedipine for 8 h at 37°C (**a, b**). Under these conditions, the macrophages develop foamy organelles containing a large number of membrane-bound vacuoles, which exhibit multiple layers of membrane arranged in concentric whorls. With longer exposure time these lamellar bodies (*LB*) become increasingly condensed. The foamy organelles exhibit a progressive fragmentation into single lamellar bodies that move towards the cell periphery. **b** The lamellar bodies (*LB*) are released by the cells into the extracellular space and either remain in intimate contact with the cell membrane or lie free in the extracellular environment. The lamellar bodies released by the cells have a diameter of about 100–300 nm. **a** × 69 000; **b** × 72 000

migration assay in the presence or absence of the chemotactic agent, zymosan-activated mouse serum (ZAMS).

The migration assay was carried out in Petri dishes containing agar medium. Seven small holes were made in each agar plate, and 10^5 macrophages transferred to each hole. The cells were maintained under standard conditions, and after attachment, an aliquot of medium with 10% fetal calf serum was added to one plate as a control, and similar aliquots of medium supplemented with 50 μg/ml oxidised LDL were poured onto the remaining plates. After 24 hours' incubation with oxidised LDL, a 10 × dilution of ZAMS or mouse serum was added to the oxidised LDL containing medium, and the cells were incubated for a further 24 h. The agar plates were then fixed with glutaraldehyde, and the cells adherent to the plastic dish stained with Wright's Giemsa solution for 60 min. The individual areas of migration were magnified through a photomagnifier and measured.

Using this system, we confirmed that foam cells produced by incubating macrophages with oxidised LDL are significantly less mobile than control macrophages. However, the presence of ZAMS caused a significant enhancement of mobility in lipid-laden macrophages to levels matching those of controls. Immunofluorescence microscopy using antibodies against actin revealed that ZAMS-activated resumption of motility is associated with reorganisation of the cytoskeleton. The identities of the active factors, and whether they originate from ZAMS itself or are produced by the macrophages in response to treatment, remain to be determined. Nevertheless, the results show that the immobilisation of foam cells associated with accumulation of oxidised LDL can be reversed. If foam cells in lesions in vivo can similarly be stimulated to migrate, then approaches to lesion regression based on this strategy may ultimately become possible.

8 Concluding Remarks

Modern ultrastructural cytochemical techniques have opened up a new era in the study of the mechanisms underlying the diverse interactions of lipoproteins with cells. One of the major contributions of these techniques is the way they allow the direct testing of hypotheses derived from other experimental approaches. To the pathologist, the opportunity to visualise directly how different cultured cell types detect and respond to lipoproteins, and to be able to track them to their intracellular destinations and follow their fates, provides lessons that are directly applicable to the understanding of pathogenetic mechanisms in vivo.

Acknowledgements. We thank our colleagues, Drs. A. Hesz, G. Schmitz, and H. Dieplinger, for their numerous contributions. The experimental results from our laboratories include those from work carried our by members of our teams, in particular Drs. B. Harrach, R. Semich, M. Pataki, F. Robenek, and N.S. Peters, Dipl.-Biol. B. Kaesberg, and S. Rothery and J. Reckless. For excellent technical assistance we thank S. Otter, K. Schlattmann, and M. Opalka. We thank M. Rohe for outstanding secretarial support.

Studies were carried out with the aid of grants from the Deutsche Forschungsgemeinschaft (SFB 223, SFB 310, H. Robenek), and British Heart Foundation (N.J. Severs). Both authors are supported by a NATO Collaborative Research Grant (CRG. 910122).

References

Anderson RGW, Brown MS, Goldstein JL (1977) Role of coated endocytic vesicle in the uptake of receptor-bound low density lipoprotein in human fibroblasts. Cell 10:351–364

Anderson RGW, Brown MS, Beisiegel U, Goldstein JL (1982) Surface distribution and recycling of the low density lipoprotein receptor as visualized with antireceptor antibodies. J Cell Physiol 93:523–531

Aquel NM, Bell RY, Walmann H, Mitchinson MJ (1985) Identification of macrophages and smooth muscle cells in human atherosclerosis using monoclonal antibodies. J Pathol 146:197–204

Assmann G (1982) Lipid metabolism and atherosclerosis. Schattauer, Stuttgart, p 1

Assmann G, Funke H (1990) HDL metabolism and atherosclerosis. J Cardiovasc Pharmacol 16:15–20

Bachorik PS, Franklin FA, Virgil DG, Kwiterovich PO (1982) High-affinity uptake and degradation of apolipoprotein E free high-density lipoprotein and low-density lipoprotein in cultured porcine hepatocytes. Biochemistry 21:5675–5684

Badimore JJ, Badimore L, Galvez A, Dische R, Fuster V (1989) High density lipoprotein plasma fractions inhibit aortic fatty streaks in cholesterol-fed rabbits. Lab Invest 60:455–461

Basu SK, Brown MS, Ho YK, Havel JR, Goldstein JL (1981) Mouse macrophages synthesize and secrete a protein resembling apo E. Proc Natl Acad Sci USA 78:7545–7549

Bendayan M (1984) Protein A-gold electron microscopic immunocytochemistry: methods, applications and limitations. J Electron Microsc Tech 1:243–270

Bendayan M (1989) Protein A-gold and protein G-gold post-embedding immunoelectron microscopy. In: Hayat MA (ed) Colloidal gold: principles, methods and applications, vol 1. Academic, New York, pp 33–94

Bernard DW, Rodriguez A, Rothblat GH, Glick JM (1990) Influence of high density lipoprotein on esterified cholesterol stores in macrophages and hepatoma cells. Arteriosclerosis 10:135–144

Biesbrock R, Oram JF, Albers JJ, Biermann EL (1983) Specific high-affinity binding of high density lipoproteins to cultured human skin fibroblasts and arterial smooth muscle cells. J Clin Invest 71:525–539

Bradley WA, Gianturco SH (1988) Lipoprotein receptors in cholesterol metabolism. In: Yeagle PL (ed) Biology of cholesterol. CRC, Boca Raton, pp 95–120

Brown D (1981) Polyvinyl coating—an improvement of the freeze-fracture technique. J Microsc 121:283–287

Brown D (1989) Low-temperature embedding and cryosectioning in the immunocytochemical study of membrane recycling. In: Plattner H (ed) Electron microscopy of subcellular dynamics. CRC, Boca Raton, pp 179–197

Brown MS, Goldstein JL (1983) Lipoprotein metabolism in the macrophage: implications for cholesterol deposition in atherosclerosis. Ann Rev Biochem 52:223–261

Brown MS, Goldstein JL (1984) How LDL receptors influence cholesterol and atherosclerosis. Sci Am 251:58–66

Brown MS, Goldstein JL, Krieger M, Ho YK, Anderson RGW (1979) Reversible accumulation of cholesteryl esters in macrophages incubated with acetylated lipoproteins. J Cell Physiol 82:597–613

Campbell GR, Campbell JH (1990) The phenotypes of smooth muscle expressed in human atheroma. Ann NY Acad Sci 598:143–158

Campbell JH, Black MJ, Campbell GR (1989) Replication of smooth muscle cells in atherosclerosis and hypertension. In: Meyer P, Marche P (eds) Blood cells and arteries in hypertension and atherosclerosis. Raven, New York, pp 15–33

Daoud AS, Jarmolych J, Augustyn JM, Fritz KE (1981) Sequential morphologic studies of regression of advanced atherosclerosis. Arch Pathol Lab Med 105:233–239

Daoud AS, Fritz KE, Jarmolych J, Frank AS (1985) Role of macrophages in regression of atherosclerosis. 454:101–114

DeLamatre JG, Carter RM, Hornick CA (1991) Evidence for extralysosomal hydrolysis of high density lipoprotein cholesteryl esters in rat hepatoma cells (Fu 5AH): a model for delivery of high density lipoprotein cholesterol. J Cell Physiol 146:18–24

Doerr-Schott J (1989) Colloidal gold for multiple staining. In: Hayat MA (ed) Colloidal gold: principles, methods and applications, vol 1. Academic, New York, pp 145–190

Draeger A, Amos WB, Ikebe M, Small JV (1990) The cytoskeletal and contractile apparatus of smooth muscle: contraction bands and segmentation of the contractile elements. J Cell Physiol 111:2463–2473

Dudrick SJ (1987) Regression of atherosclerosis by the intravenous infusion of specific biochemical nutrient substrates in animals and humans. Ann Surg 206:296–315

Eisenberg S (1984) High density lipoprotein metabolism. J Lipid Res 25:1017–1058

Ellsworth JL, Fong LG, Kraemer FB, Cooper AD (1990) Differences in the processing of chylomicron remnants and β-VLDL by macrophages. J Lipid Res 31:1399–1411

Fan J, Yamada T, Tokunaga O, Watanabe T (1991) Alterations in the functional characteristics of macrophages induced by hypercholesterolemia. Virchows Arch [B] 61:19–27

Fidge NH, Nestel PJ (1985) Identification of apolipoproteins involved in the interaction of human high density lipoprotein$_3$ with receptors on cultured cells. J Biol Chem 260:3570–3575

Fogelman AM, Shechter I, Seager J, Hokom M, Child JS, Edwards PA (1980) Malondialdehyde alteration of low density lipoproteins leads to cholesteryl ester accumulation in human monocyte-macrophages. Proc Natl Acad Sci USA 77:2214–2218

Fogelman AM, Van Lenten BJ, Warden C, Haberland ME, Edwards PA (1988) Macrophage lipoprotein receptors. J Cell Sci Suppl 9:135–149

Frens G (1973) Controlled nucleation for the regulation of particle size in mono-dispersed gold solutions. Nature 241:20–22

Fritz KE, Augustyn JM, Jarmolych J, Daoud AS (1981) Sequential study of biochemical changes during regression of swine aortic atherosclerotic lesions. Arch Pathol Lab Med 105:240–246

Gerrity RG (1981a) The role of the monocyte in atherogenesis. I. Transition of blood-borne monocytes into foam cells in fatty lesions. Am J Pathol 103:181–190

Gerrity RG (1981b) The role of the monocyte in atherogenesis. II. Migration of foam cells from atherosclerotic lesions. Am J Pathol 103:191–200

Gerrity RG, Naito HK (1980) Lipid clearance from fatty streak lesions by foam cell migration. Artery 8:215–219

Glomset JA (1968) The plasma lecithin: cholesterol acyltransferase reaction. J Lipid Res 9:155–167

Goldstein JL, Brown MS (1974) Binding and degradation of low density lipoproteins by cultured human fibroblasts. Comparison of cells from a normal subject and from a patient with homozygous familial hypercholesterolemia. J Biol Chem 249:5153–5162

Gooldstein JL, Brown MS (1977a) Atherosclerosis: the low-density lipoprotein receptor hypothesis. Metabolism 26:1257–1265

Goldstein JL, Brown MS (1977b) The low-density lipoprotein pathway and its relation to atherosclerosis. Ann Rev Biochem 46:897–930

Goldstein JL, Brown MS (1979) The LDL receptor locus and the genetics of familial hypercholesterolemia. Ann Rev Genet 13:259–289

Goldstein JL, Brown MS (1983) Familial hypercholesterolemia. In: Stanbury JB, Wyngarden JB, Fredrickson DS (eds) The metabolic basis of inherited disease, McGraw-Hill, New York, pp 672–712

Goldstein JL, Anderson RGW, Brown MS (1979a) Coated pits, coated vesicles and receptor-mediated endocytosis. Nature 279:679–685

Goldstein JL, Ho YK, Basu SK, Brown MS (1979b) Binding site on macrophages that mediates uptake and degradation of acetylated low density lipoprotein, producing massive cholesterol deposition. Proc Natl Acad Sci USA 76:333–337

Goldstein JL, Ho YK, Brown MS, Innerarity TL, Mahley RW (1980) Cholesteryl-ester accumulation in macrophages resulting from receptor-mediated uptake and degradation of hypercholesterolemic canine β-very low density lipoprotein. J Biol Chem 258:1839–1848

Goldstein JL, Brown MS, Anderson RGW, Russel DW, Schneider WJ (1985) Receptor-mediated endocytosis: concepts merging from the LDL receptor system. Ann Rev Cell Biol 1:1–39

Gordon S (1988) Macrophage plasma membrane receptors: structure and function, J. Cell Sci Suppl 9:1–211 The Company of Biologists Ltd., Cambridge

Gordon S, Perry VH, Rabinowitz S, Chung L-P, Rosen H (1988) Plasma membrane receptors of the mononuclear phagocyte system. J Cell Sci Suppl 9:1–26

Haberland ME, Fong D, Cheng L (1988) Malondialdehyde-altered protein occurs in atheroma of Watanabe heritable hyperlipidemic rabbits. Science 241:215–218

Hajjar DP (1991) Viral pathogenesis of atherosclerosis: impact of molecular mimicry and viral genes. Am J Pathol 139:1195–1211

Handley DA (1989a) Methods for synthesis of colloidal gold. In: Hayat MA (ed) Colloidal gold: principles, methods and applications, vol 1. Academic, New York, pp 13–32

Handley DA (1989b) The development and application of colloidal gold as a microscopic probe. In: Hayat MA (ed) Colloidal gold: principles, methods and applications, vol 1. Academic, New York, pp 1–12

Harrach B, Robenek H (1990) Polyclonal antibodies against formaldehyde-modified apoliproprotein A-I. An approach to circumventing fixation-induced loss of antigenicity in immunocytochemistry. Arteriosclerosis 10:564–576

Heinecke JW, Snits AG, Aviram M, Chait A (1991) Phagocytosis of lipase-aggregate low density lipoprotein promotes macrophage foam cell formation: sequential morphological and biochemical events. Arteriosclerosis Thromb 11:1643–1651

Henson DA, St. Clair RW, Lewis JC (1989) β-VLDL and acetylated-LDL binding to pigeon monocyte macrophages. Atherosclerosis 78:47–60

Herz J, Hamann U, Rogne S, Myklebost O, Gausepohl H, Stanley KK (1988) Surface location and high affinity for calcium of a 500 kD liver membrane protein closely related to the LDL-receptor suggest a physiological role as lipoprotein receptor. EMBO J 7:4119–4127

Herz J, Kowal RC, Goldstein JL, Brown MS (1990) Proteolytic processing of the 600 kd low density lipoprotein receptor-related protein (LRP) occurs in a trans-Golgi compartment. EMBO J 9:1769–1776

Ho YK, Brown MS, Goldstein JL (1980) Hydrolysis and excretion of cytoplasmic cholesteryl esters by macrophages: stimulation by high density lipoproteins and other agents. J Lipid Res 21:391–398

Hobbs HH, Russel DW, Brown MS, Goldstein JL (1990) The LDL receptor locus in familial hypercholesterolemia: mutational analysis of a membrane protein. Ann Rev Genet 24:133–170

Hobot JA (1989) Lowicryls and low temperature embedding for coloidal gold methods. In: Hayat MA (ed) Colloidal gold: principles methods and applications, vol 2. Academic, New York, pp 75–115

Hoeg JM, Demosky SJ Jr, Edge SB, Gregg RE, Osborne JC JR, Brewer HB JR (1985) Characterization of a human hepatic receptor for high density lipoproteins. Arteriosclerosis 5:228–237

Hoff HF, Pepin JM, Morton RE (1991) Modified low density lipoprotein isolated from atherosclerotic lesions does not cause lipid accumulation in aortic smooth muscle cells. J Lipid Res 32:115–124

Holund B, Clausen PP, Clemmensen I (1981) The influence of fixation and tissue preparation on the immunohistochemical demonstration of fibronectin in human tissues. Histochemistry 72:291–299

Huff MW, Evans AJ, Sawyez CG, Wolfe BM, Nestel PJ (1991) Cholesterol accumulation in J774 macrophages induced by triglyceride-rich lipoproteins. Comparison of very low density lipoprotein in subjects with type II, IV and V hyperlipoproteinemias. Arteriosclerosis Thromb 11:221–233

Hurt E, Camejo G (1987) Effect of arterial proteoglycans on the interaction of LDL with human monocyte-derived macrophages. Atherosclerosis 67:115–126

Innerarity TL, Arnold KS, Weisgraber KH, Mahley RW (1986) Apolipoprotein E is the determinant that mediates the receptor uptake of beta-very low density lopoproteins by mouse macrophages. Arteriosclerosis 6:114–122

Jaakkola O, Ylä-Herttuala S, Särkioja T, Nikkari T (1989) Macrophage foam cells from human aortic fatty streaks take up β-VLDL and acetylated LDL in primary culture. Atherosclerosis 79:173–182

Jones EY, Stuart DI (1990) The structure of tumour necrosis factor—implications for biological function. J Cell Sci Suppl 13:11–18

Joris I, Zand T, Nunnari JJ, Krolikowski FJ, Majno G (1983) Studies on the pathogenesis of atherosclerosis. I. Adhesion and emigration of mononuclear cells in the aorta of hypercholesterolemic rats. Am J Pathol 113:341–358

Kargacin GJ, Cooke PH, Abramson SB, Fay FS (1989) Periodic organization of the contractile apparatus in smooth muscle revealed by the motion of dense bodies in single cells. J Cell Physiol 108:1465–1475

Klurfeld DM (1985) Identification of foam cells in human atherosclerotic lesions as macrophages using monoclonal antibodies. Arch Pathol Lab Med 109:445–449

Kodama T, Freeman M, Rohrer L, Zabrecky J, Matsudaira P, Krieger M (1990) Type I macrophage scavenger receptor contains α-helical and collagen-like coiled coils. Nature 343:531–535

Law SKA (1988) C3 receptors on macrophages. J Cell Sci Suppl 9:67–97

Libby P, Hansson GK (1991) Involvement of the immune system in human atherogenesis: current knowledge and unanswered questions. Lab Invest 64:5–15

Luc G, Fruchart J-G (1991) Oxidation of lipoproteins and atherosclerosis. Am Clin Nutr 53:206–209

Mahley RW, Innerarity TL (1983) Lipoprotein receptors and cholesterol homeostasis. Biochim Biophys Acta 737:197–222

Massagué J (1990) The transforming growth factor family. An Rev Cell Biol 6: 597–641

Massmann J (1979) Mononuclear cell infiltration of the aortic intima in domestic swine. Exp Pathol 17:110–112

McLean IW, Nakane PK (1974) Periodate lysine paraformaldehyde fixative. A new fixative for immunoelectron microscopy. J Histochem Cytochem 22:1077–1083

Mellman I, Koch T, Healey G, et al. (1988) Structure and function of Fc receptors on macrophages and lymphocytes. J Cell Sci Suppl 9:45–65

Meloan SN, Barton BP, Puchtler H, Waldrop ES, Hobbs JL (1984) Effects of formaldehyde and methacarn fixation on prekeratin. Georgia J Sci 42:31

Minor LK, Glick JM, Rothblat GH (1986) Smooth muscle cells in culture: uptake of artificial lipid inclusions. Arteriosclerosis 6:523a

Moore LK, Beyer EC, Burt JM (1991) Characterization of gap junction channels in A7r5 vascular smooth muscle cells. Am J Physiol Cell Physiol 260:C975–C981

Mühlpfordt H (1982) Preparation of colloidal gold particles using tannic acid as an additional reducing agent. Experientia 38:1127–1128

Munro JM, Cotran RW (1988) Biology of disease. The pathogenesis of atherosclerosis: atherogenesis and inflammation. Lab Invest 58:249–261

Murakami M, Horiuchi S, Takata K, Morino Y (1987) Distinction in the mode of receptor-mediated endocytosis between high density lipoprotein and acetylated high density lipoprotein: evidence for high density lipoprotein receptor-mediated cholesterol transfer. J Biochem 101:729–749

Nagano Y, Arai H, Kita T (1991) High density lipoprotein loses its effect to stimulate efflux of cholesterol from foam cells after oxidative modification. Proc Natl Acad Sci USA 88:6457–6461

Nakai T, Otto PS, Kennedy DL, Whayne FF Jr (1976) Rat high density lipoprotein HDL_3 uptake and catabolism by isolated rat liver parenchymal cells. J Biol Chem 251:4914

Nermut MV (1989) Strategy and tactics in electron microscopy of cell surfaces. Electron Microsc Rev 2:171–196

Newman GR, Hobot JA (1989) Role of tissue processing in colloidal gold methods. In: Hayat MA (ed) Colloidal gold: principles, methods and applications, vol 2. Academic, New York, pp 33–73

Nicol A, Nermut MV, Doeinck A, Robenek H, Wiegand C, Jockusch BM (1987) Visualization of cytoskeletal elements at the ventral plasma membrane of fibroblasts by gold immunolabeling. J Histochem Cytochem 35:499–506

Niendorf A, Rath M, Wolf K, Peters H, Arps U, Beisiegel U, Dietel M (1990) Morphological detection and quantification of lipoprotein (a) deposition in atheromatous lesions of human aorta and coronary arteries. Virch Arch [A] 417:105–111

Nowicka G, Brüning T, Böttcher A, Kahl G, Schmitz G (1990) The macrophage interaction of HDL subclasses separated by free flow isotachophoresis. J Lipid Res 31:1947–1963

Palinski W, Rosenfeld ME, Ylä-Herttuala S, Gurtner GC, Socher SS, Butler SW, Parthasarathy S, Carew TE, Steinberg D, Witztum JL (1989) Low density lipoprotein undergoes oxidative modification in vivo. Proc Natl Acad Sci USA 86:1372–1376

Parthasarathy S (1987) Oxidation of low-density lipoprotein by thiol compounds leads to its recognition by the acityl LDL receptor. Biochim Biophys Acta 917:337–340

Parthasarathy S, Printz DJ, Boyd D, Joy L, Steinberg D (1986) Macrophage oxidation of low density lipoprotein generates a modified form recognized by the scavenger receptor. Arteriosclerosis 6:505–510

Pataki M, Lusztig G, Robenek H (1992) Reversibility of oxidized LDL-induced migration inhibition in macrophage-derived foam cells in vitro. A mechanism for the regression of atherosclerosis? Arteriosclerosis Thromb 12:936–944

Pathak RK, Merkle RK, Cummings RD, Goldstein JL, Brown MS, Anderson RGW (1988) Immunocytochemical localization of mutant low density lipoprotein receptors that fail to reach the Golgi complex. J Cell Physiol 106:1831–1841

Pathak RK, Yokode M, Hammer RE, Hofmann SL, Brown MS, Goldstein JL, Anderson RGW (1990) Tissue-specific sorting of the human LDL receptor in polarized epithelia of transgenic mice. J Cell Physiol 111:347–359

Penn A, Garte SJ, WArren L, Nesta D, Mindich B (1986) Transforming gene in human atherosclerotic plaque DNA. Proc Natl Acad Sci USA 83:7951–7955

Pinto da Silva P, Kan FWK (1984) Label-fracture: a method for high resolution labeling of cell surfaces. J Cell Physiol 99:1156–1161

Polacek D, Byrne RE, Scanu AM (1989) Modification of low density lipoproteins by polymorphonuclear cell elastase leads to enhanced uptake by human monocyte-derived macrophages via the low density lipoprotein receptor pathway. J Lipid Res 29:797–808

Ravetch JV, Kinet J-P (1991) Fc receptors. Annu Rev Immunol 9:457–492

Rifici VA, Eder HA (1984) A hepatocyte receptor for high-density lipoproteins specific for apolipoprotein A-I. J Biol Chem 259:13814–13818

Robenek H (1989a) Topography and internalization of cell surface receptors as analyzed by affinity- and immunolabeling combined with surface replication and ultrathin sectioning techniques. In: Plattner H (ed) Electron microscopy of subcellular dynamics. CRC, Boca Raton, pp 141–163

Robenek H (1989b) Distribution and mobility of receptors in the plasma membrane. In: Hui SW (ed) Freeze-fracture studies of membranes. CRC, Boca Raton, pp 61–86

Robenek H, Schmitz G (1985) Receptor domains in the plasma membrane of cultured mouse peritoneal macrophages. Eur J Cell Biol 39:77–85

Robenek H, Schmitz G (1988) Ca^{++} antagonists and ACAT inhibitors promote cholesterol efflux from macrophages by different mechanisms. II. Characterization of intracellular morphological changes. Arteriosclerosis 8:57–67

Robenek H, Schmitz G (1991) Abnormal processing of Golgi elements and lysosomes in Tangier disease. Arteriosclerosis Thromb 11:1007–1020

Robenek H, Rassat J, Hesz A, Grünwald J (1982) A correlative study on the topographical distribution of the receptors for low density lipoprotein (LDL) conjugated to colloidal gold in cultured human skin fibroblasts employing thin section, freeze-fracture, deep-etching, and surface replication techniques. Eur J Cell Biol 27:242–250

Robenek H, Schmitz G, Assmann G (1984) Topography and dynamics of receptors for acetylated and malondialdehyde-modified low-density lipoprotein in the plasma membrane of mouse peritoneal macrophages as visualized by colloidal gold in conjunction with surface replicas. J Histochem Cytochem 32:1017–1027

Robenek H, Schmitz G, Greven H (1987) Cell surface distribution and intracellular fate of human β-very low density lipoprotein in cultured peritoneal mouse macrophages: cytochemical and immunocytochemical study. Eur J Cell Biol 43:110–120

Robenek H, Harrach B, Severs NJ (1991) Display of low density lipoprotein receptors is clustered, not dispersed, in fibroblast and hepatocyte plasma membranes. Arteriosclerosis Thromb 11:261–271

Rohrer L, Freeman M, Kodama T, Penman M, Krieger M (1990) Coiled-coil fibrous domains mediate ligand binding by macrophage scavenger receptor type II. Nature 343:570–572

Rosenfeld ME, Palinski W, Ylä-Herttuala S, Butler S, Witztum JL (1990) Distribution of oxidation specific lipid-protein adducts and apolipoprotein B in atherosclerotic lesions of varying severity from WHHL rabbits. Arteriosclerosis 10:336

Ross R (1986) The pathogenesis of atherosclerosis—an update. N Engl J Med 314:488–500

Ross R, Masuda J, Raines EW, et al. (1990) Localization of PDGF-β protein in macrophages in all phases of atherogenesis. Science 248:1009–1012

Roth J (1982) The protein A-gold (pAg) technique—a qualitative and quantitative approach for antigen localization on thin sections. In: Bullock GP, Petrusz P (eds) Techniques in immunocytochemistry, vol 1. Academic, London, pp 107–133

Sanan DA, Anderson RGW (1991) Simultaneous visualization of LDL receptor distribution and clathrin lattices on membranes torn from the upper surface of cultured cells. J Histochem Cytochem 39:1017

Sanan DA, Van der Westhuyzen DR, Gevers W, Coetzee GA (1987) The surface distribution of low density lipoprotein receptors on cultured fibroblasts and endothelial cells. Histochemistry 86:517–523

Sanan DA, Van der Westhuyzen DR, Gevers W, Coetzee GA (1989) Early appearance of dispersed low density lipoprotein receptors on the fibroblast surface during recycling. Eur J Cell Biol 48:327–336

Schmitz G, Robenek H (1989) Significance of the interaction between lipoprotein subfractions and macrophages for reverse cholesterol transport. In: Klör HU (ed) Recent developments in lipid and lipoprotein research. Lipoprotein subfractions omega-3 fatty acids. Springer, Berlin Heidelberg New York, pp 82–87

Schmitz G, Assmann G, Robenek H, Brennhausen B (1985a) Tangier disease: a disorder of intracellular membrane traffic. Proc Natl Acad Sci USA 82:6305–6309

Schmitz G, Niemann R, Brennhausen B, Krause R, Assmann G (1985b) Regulation of high density lipoprotein receptors in cultured macrophages: role of acyl CoA: cholesterol acyltransferase. EMBO J 4:2773–2779

Schmitz G, Robenek H, Lohmann U, Assmann G (1985c) Interaction of high density lipoproteins with cholesteryl ester-laden macrophages: biochemical and morphological characterization of cell surface receptor binding, endocytosis and resecretion of high density lipoproteins by macrophages. EMBO J 4:613–622

Schmitz G, Robenek H, Assmann G (1987) Role of the high density lipoprotein receptor cycle in macrophage-cholesterol metabolism. In: Gotto A (ed) Atherosclerosis reviews. Raven, New York, pp 95–107

Schmitz G, Robenek H, Beuck M, Krause R, Schurek A, Niemann R (1988) Ca^{++} antagonists and ACAT inhibitors promote cholesterol efflux from macrophages by different mechanisms. I Characterization of intracellular lipid metabolism. Arteriosclerosis 8:46–56

Schmitz G, Brennhausen B, Robenek H (1989) Regulation of macrophage cholesterol homeostasis. In: Steinmetz A, Kaffarnik H, Schneider J (eds) Recent developments in lipid and lipoprotein research. Cholesterol transport systems and their relation to atherosclerosis. Springer, Berlin Heidelberg New York, pp 22–31

Schmitz G, Beuck M, Fischer H, Robenek H (1990a) Regulation of phospholipid biosynthesis during cholesterol influx and high density lipoprotein-mediated cholesterol efflux in macrophages. J Lipid Res 31:1741–1752

Schmitz G, Brüning E, Williamson E, Nowicka G (1990b) The role of HDL in reverse cholesterol transport and its disturbances in Tangier disease and HDL deficiency with xanthomas. Eur Heart J 11 [Suppl E]:197–211

Schmitz G, Fisher H, Beuck M, Hoecker K-P, Robenek H (1990c) Dysregulation of phospholipid synthesis in Tangier monocyte-derived macrophages. Arteriosclerosis 10:1010–1019

Schneider WJ, Beisiegel U, Goldstein JL, Brown MS (1982) Purification of the low density lipoprotein receptor, an acidic glycoprotein of 164,000 molecular weight. J Biol Chem 257:2664–2673

Scott J (1989) Thrombogenesis linked to atherogenesis at last? Nature 341:22–23

Semich R, Robenek H (1990) Organization of the cytoskeleton and the focal contacts of bovine aortic endothelial cells cultured on type I and III collagen. J Histochem Cytochem 38:59–67

Semich R, Gerke V, Robenek H, Weber K (1989) The p36 substrate of pp60 src kinase is located at the cytoplasmic surface of the plasma membrane of fibroblasts; an immunoelectron microscopic analysis. Eur J Cell Biol 50:313–323

Severs NJ (1989) Freeze-fracture cytochemistry: review of methods. J Electron Microsc Tech 13:175–203

Severs NJ, Robenek H (1983) Detection of microdomains in biomembranes: an appraisal of recent developments in freeze-fracture cytochemistry. Biochim Biophys Acta 737:373–408

Small DM (1988) Progression and regression of atherosclerotic lesions. Insights from lipid physical biochemistry. Arteriosclerosis 8:103–129

Soltys PA, Portman OW, O'Malley JP (1982) Binding properties of high density lipoprotein subfractions and low-density lipoproteins to rabbit hepatocytes. Biochim Biophys Acta 713:300

Sparrow CP, Parthasarathy S, Steinberg D (1989) A macrophage receptor that recognizes oxidized low density lipoprotein but not acetylated low density lipoprotein. J Biol Chem 264: 2599–2604

Stary HC (1987) Macrophages, macrophage foam cells, and accentric intimal thickening in the coronary arteries of young children. Atherosclerosis 64:91–108

Stary H (1989) Evolutional progression of atherosclerotic lesions in coronary arteries of children and young adults. Arteriosclerosis 9 [Suppl 1]:19–32

Stary HC, Strong JP, Eggen DA (1980) Differences in the degradation rate of intracellular lipid droplets in the intimal smooth muscle cells and macrophages of regressing atherosclerotic lesions of primates. In: Gotto AM, Smith LC, Allen B (eds) Atherosclerosis V. Springer, Berlin Heidelberg New York, pp 753–756

Steinberg D, Parthasarathy S, Carew TE, Khoo JC, Witztum JC (1989) Beyond cholesterol: modifications of low-density lipoprotein that increase its atherogenicity. N Engl J Med 320:915–924

Tokuyasu KT (1980) Immunocytochemistry on ultrathin frozen sections. Histochem J 12:381–403

Travo P, Weber K, Osborn M (1982) co-existence of vimentin and desmin type intermediate filaments in a subpopulation of adult rat vascular smooth muscle cells growing in primary culture. Exp Cell Res 139:87–94

Tucker CF, Catsulis C, Strong JP, Eggen DA (1971) Regression of early cholesterol-induced aortic lesions in rhesus monkeys. Am J Pathol 65:493–502

Van Bergen en Honegouwen PMP (1989) Immunogold labelling of ultrathin crysections. In: Hayat MA (ed) Colloidal gold: principles, methods and applications, vol 1. Academic, New York, pp 191–216

Van der Westhuyzen DR, Gevers W, Coetzee GA (1980) Cathepsin-D-dependent initiation of the hydrolysis by lysosomal enzymes of apoprotein B from low-density lipoproteins. Eur J Biochem 112:153–160

Van Lenten BJ, Fogelman AM (1990) Processing of lipoproteins in human monocyte-macrophages. J Lipid Res 31:1455–1466

Vijayagopal P, Srinivasan SR, Jones KM, Radhakrishnamurthy B, Berenson GS (1985) Complexes of low-density lipoproteins and arterial proteoglycan aggregates promote cholesteryl ester accumulation in mouse macrophages. Biochim Biophys Acta 837:257–267

Vollmer E, Roessner A, Bosse A, et al. (1991) Immunohistochemical double labeling of macrophages, smooth muscle cells and apolipoprotein E in the atherosclerotic plaque. Pathol Res Pract 187:184

Völker W, Frick B, Robenek H (1985) A simple device for low temperature polymerization of Lowicryl K4M resin. J Microsc 138:91–93

Watanabe T, Hirata M, Yoshikawa, Nagafuchi Y, Toyoshima H (1985) Role of macrophages in atherosclerosis. Lab Invest 53:80–90

Watanabe T, Tokunaga O, Fan J, Shimokama T (1989) Atherosclerosis and macrophages. Acta Pathol Jpn 39:473–486

Wissler RW, Vesselinovitch D (1990) Can atherosclerotic plaques regress? Anatomic and biochemical evidence from nonhuman animal models. Am J Cardiol 65:33–40

Wofsy C, Echavarria-Heras H, Goldstein B (1985) Effect of preferential insertion of LDL receptors near coated pits. Cell Biophys 7:197–204

Wolfbauer G, Glick JM, Minor LK, Rothblat GH (1986) Development of the smooth muscle foam cell: uptake of macrophage lipid inclusions. Proc Natl Acad Sci USA 83:7760–7764

Wolpe SD, Cerami A (1989) Macrophage inflammatory proteins 1 and 2: members of a novel superfamily of cytokines. FASEB J 3:2565

Yin HL, Hartwig JH (1988) The structure of the macrophage actin skeleton. J Cell Sci Suppl 9:169–184

Zannis VJ, Kurnit DM, Breslow JL (1982) Hepatic apo-A-I and intestinal apo-A-I are synthesized in precursor isoprotein forms by organ cultures of human fetal tissues. J Biol Chem 257:536–544

In Situ Localization and Distribution Pattern of Apolipoproteins in Arterial Walls: A Comparative Study in Atherosclerosis and Renal Transplant Arteriopathy*

E. VOLLMER and A. ROESSNER

1 Introduction

Disorders of lipid metabolism are among the main risk factors for atherosclerosis, others being cigarette smoking, hypertension, diabetes mellitus, and age. In recent years, the impact of lipid metabolic disorders on the development of arteriosclerotic disease has been defined in greater detail by biochemical, genetic, clinical, and epidemiologic studies on the physiology and pathophysiology of lipid metabolism in general, and on the particular role of lipids and lipoproteins in atherogenesis. According to epidemiologic results, cholesterol plays a major part in this context: experimental studies of animals and clinical observations in humans have confirmed that the mere increase in cholesterol levels in the blood, i.e., without concurrent risk factors, is liable to provoke atherosclerotic changes.

Today, the responsible atherogenic lipoprotein fractions have been identified as "low-density lipoproteins" (LDL), which transport most of the cholesterol, and also "very low-density lipoproteins" (VLDL), consisting predominantly of triglycerides and carrying only a minor amount of the cholesterol. It is also known that "high-density lipoproteins" (HDL) are negatively correlated with coronary heart disease.

The physiology of lipid metabolism is governed by surface receptors on cells of the liver and peripheral organs. Besides their lipid fractions, plasma

*This chapter is dedicated to Prof. Dr. K. M. MÜLLER, Bochum

Current Topics in Pathology
Volume 87, Vollmer/Roessner (Eds.)

lipoproteins contain certain proteins that act as specific binding proteins for such receptors, whereby the lipoproteins are directed toward definite targets. Cell surface receptors and their (plasma) apolipoproteins play a decisive role in the homeostasis of lipid metabolism. Cholesterol uptake is triggered by binding of LDL to specific receptors of the cell surface (GOLDSTEIN and BROWN 1977). The receptor recognizes LDL by its main structural component, apolipoprotein B (apo B).

Like the main structural components of HDL (apo A-I and A-II), apo B is synthesized in the bowel and liver. To date, two subtypes of apo B have been distinguished: apo B-100 (MW 549000) and apo B-48 (MW 265000), the latter being identified as a structural protein of chylomicrons. Apo B-100 is the structural protein not only of LDL but also of VLDL and intermediate-density lipoprotein (IDL); it is known to interact with so-called apo B/E receptors of peripheral cells and the corresponding receptors of hepatocytes, effecting uptake and catabolization of LDL in the cells. In this connection, apo E is seen as a key protein for modulating the metabolism of highly atherogenic, apo B-loaded lipoproteins (GETZ et al. 1988).

High-density lipoprotein-binding cholesterol contains the highest amount of all lipoproteins and consists of two main fractions, HDL_2 and HDL_3, the latter bearing the strongest negative association with atherosclerosis. Another fraction, HDL_1 (HDLc), contains apo E as its dominant protein component and is actually induced by cholesterol. HDL is supposed to act as an effective acceptor of cholesterol which is able to carry excess cholesterol back from the periphery into the liver by way of reverse cholesterol transport (BROWN and GOLDSTEIN 1985); in the liver, it is eventually excreted as bile acids.

According to the latest lipid theory, the genesis and progression of atherosclerotic change are influenced not only by the absolute quantity of cholesterol-bearing lipoproteins circulating in the plasma, but also by their respective proportions: apo A-bearing HDL has a protective effect against atherosclerosis, apo B-bearing LDL a promoting effect. Recently, increased attention has been given to another factor, lipoprotein (a), which, although known since about 1963, has only recently been identified as an antigenic plasma variant of LDL carrying a high risk of atherosclerosis (HEGELE 1989).

We learn from many publications that renal transplantation is frequently impaired by subsequent iatrogenic disorders of the lipid metabolism (KOBAYASHI et al. 1983; HARRIS et al. 1986; KASISKE and UMEN 1987; LOWRY et al. 1987; VATHSALA et al. 1989). These are a major risk factor for transplant patients with regard to the ensuing obliterative vascular changes and concomitant cardiovascular complications. In transplantation-related disease, too, the risk factors of "conventional" atherosclerosis (CAS) are of additional and decisive importance (KASISKE 1988).

However, most of the aforementioned studies concern only the plasma levels of LDL and HDL; very few investigations have dealt with their actual distribution within the tissue of atherosclerotic lesions or of renal transplant arteriopathy (RTA), which share many morphogenetic similarities. We therefore attempted to define the extent to which this distribution is reflected in the vascular lesion proper. The demonstration of lipoproteins in the vascular wall was achieved by identifying their respective typical structural components—apo B as well as apo A-I and A-II. We also wanted to identify the cells involved in that process and possibly in secretion of apo E. Both investigations were performed in CAS and in chronic rejection of renal transplants in order to demonstrate the potential parallelism between the two diseases with regard to the role of lipoproteins, and thereby to elucidate arteriosclerotic alterations in general.

2 Materials and Methods

The study covered 32 aortas (elastic-type vessels) and 23 coronary arteries (muscular type), and also large and medium-sized arteries from 22 transplanted kidneys in chronic rejection. One part of the examination comprised a qualitative and descriptive analysis of apolipoprotein distribution with special regard to subendothelial foam cells and advanced intimal fibrosis. The other part consisted in semiquantitative vessel analysis to define the distribution and composition of the main structural proteins of LDL and HDL in both CAS and RTA. The criteria for semiquantitative classification of apolipoprotein contents in vascular walls and for staging CAS (using roman numerals) have been detailed in a previous paper (VOLLMER et al. 1991c). For RTA, staging (using arabic numerals) was adapted to the degree of luminal obliteration in medium-sized arteries of renal parenchyma (Aa. interlobulares et arcuatae), which is crucial for the loss of renal function (SALINAS-MADRIGAL et al. 1988). RTA has a decisive effect on the sufficiency of renal circulation wherever the lumen is reduced to less than 17.5% of the vascular surface (ALEXANDER 1984). If the proportion of the lumen exceeds this limit, functional criteria assume stage 1 of RTA. Lumen percentages between 4% and 17% are subsumed under stage 2 (transplant arteriopathy of medium severity), while stage 3 describes the final stage of complete or nearly complete luminal obliteration with a remaining lumen proportion of 4% to 0%.

Immunocytochemical and histologic workup was performed on formol-fixed, paraffin-embedded material; ultrastructural studies were carried out on tissues subjected to either chemical fixation or cryofixation. In the latter case, optimal cryopreparation of samples was ensured by subsequent cryosubstitution (HUMBEL and SCHWARZ 1989; SJÖSTRAND 1990). The material was embedded in apolar, hydrophilic synthetic media (Lowicryl resins) at temperatures between − 50° and − 35°C. We also applied a modified ultracryosection technique according to TOKUYASU (1984), using 2.3 *M* sucrose as cryoprotectant. Immunolabeling in light microscopy was performed using alkaline phosphatase and peroxidase methods (VOLLMER et al. 1991a–c). At the ultrastructural level, secondary gold-coupled antibodies or a protein A–gold technique was used. The primary antibodies applied in this study have been characterized in detail in previous publications (VOLLMER et al. 1991a–c).

3 Results

3.1 Atherosclerosis

In contrast to the normal pattern of unaltered vascular segments (Fig. 1a), microscopic evidence of apolipoprotein antigens is already found in the early stage of atherosclerosis, manifested in scanty granular deposits in the extracellular matrix of intimal areas near the lumen (Fig. 1b). Hardly any apo lipoprotein deposits are found in this early stage, either in subendothelial foam cells or other locally stable cells. With increasing intimal thickening and swelling of the intimal matrix, apolipoprotein deposits are found in deeper layers of the intima (Fig. 1c), and with advancing atherosclerosis, further layers of the whole wall are affected (Fig. 1d, e). The distribution pattern of apolipoproteins (A-I, A-II, and B) is distinctly altered at such advanced stages.

Apolipoprotein deposits are not evenly distributed over all the strata of the vascular wall; rather they appear in varying densities in the intimal, medial, and adventitial layers (Table 1). The number and amount of apolipoprotein deposits in these layers increase with the progressive development of the atherosclerotic lesion: the amount of apolipoprotein deposits is generally lowered from intima to media, apo A-I being the dominant type. Within the media, there is hardly any evidence of apo B, while the adventitia holds less apo B than A. In this layer, too, apolipoprotein deposits fail to show any correlation with the stage of atherosclerosis, owing to certain peculiarities of tissue preparation. It

Table 1. Semiquantitative distribution of apolipoproteins in the progressing stages of atherosclerosis

	Stage I			Stage II			Stage III		
	A–I	A–II	B	A–I	A–II	B	A–I	A–II	B
Intima	+	+	+	+ + +	+ +	+ +	+ + + +	+ + +	+ + +
Media	–	–	–	+ +	+	–	+ + +	+ +	+
Adventitita	+ +	+	+	+ + +	+ +	+	+ + +	+ + +	+ +

Number of apolipoprotein deposits: – none; + few; + + moderate number; + + + many; + + + + abundant (For reasons of clarity the minor differences between the distributions of apo A–I and A–II mentioned in the text with regard to elastic and muscular types of arteries have not been considered in this table; cf. text and VOLLMER et al. 1991c).

Fig. 1a–e. Aorta in progressive stages of CAS. **a** Unchanged segment of a vessel without apolipoprotein deposits. × 100. **b** Early stage of atherosclerosis with a few granular deposits of apo A-I in the intima, adjacent to the lumen. × 100. **c** Increasing intimal thickening and apo A-I deposits in deeper layers of the intima × 100. **d** Advanced atherosclerosis, stage of complicated lesion with calcification and wall splicing (*right*) and advanced deposition of apo A-II in the vascular wall. × 60. **e** Advanced atherosclerosis with apo B deposits and formation of needle-like negative patterns of cholesterol crystals (*center*). × 80

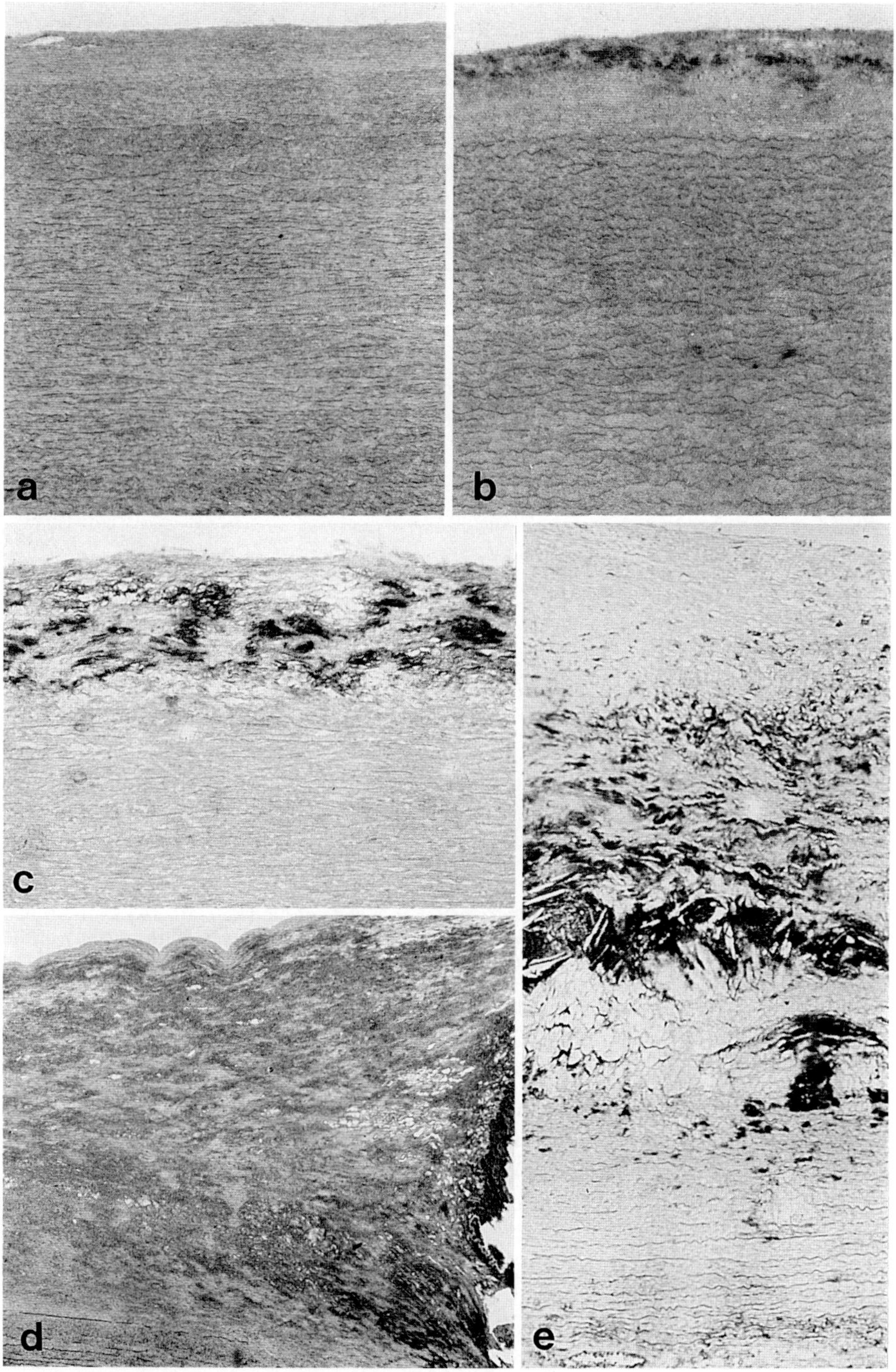
a
b
c
d
e

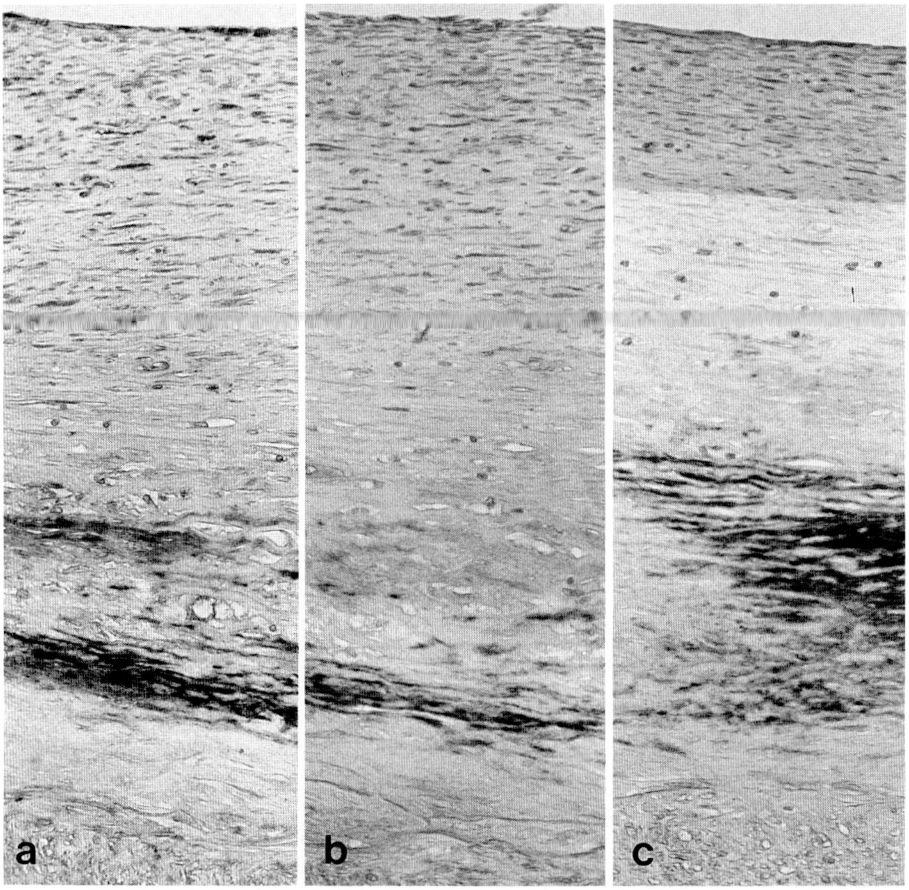

Fig. 2a–c. Consecutive sections of a coronary artery in a state of moderate atherosclerotic transformation with distinct apolipoprotein accumulation in deeper intimal layers in the vicinity of the lamina elastica interna (*lower margin*) and manifestation of foam cells. **a** Extra- and intracellular deposits of apo A-I in spindle as well as foam cell elements. **b** Apo A-II deposits of a similar pattern, but lower intensity. **c** Exclusively extracellular manifestation of apo B. **a–c**, × 300

is interesting to note that coronary arteries (muscular type) reveal deposits of apo A-I and A-II at an earlier stage, or distinctly more of them at the same stage, than do aortas (elastic type). This remarkable difference is not found with regard to apo B; it is not represented in Table 1 for reasons of clarity (cf. VOLLMER et al. 1991c).

In the fibrous intimal thickening of stage II, accumulations of apo A-I, A-II, and B appear mainly in the basal parts of the lesions near the lamina elastica interna (Fig. 2a–c). Besides extracellular accumulations, intracellular deposits of apo A are present in spindle and foam cell elements of the fibrous cap (Figs. 2a, b, 3a). Occasionally, such apolipoprotein deposits are also found in smooth muscle

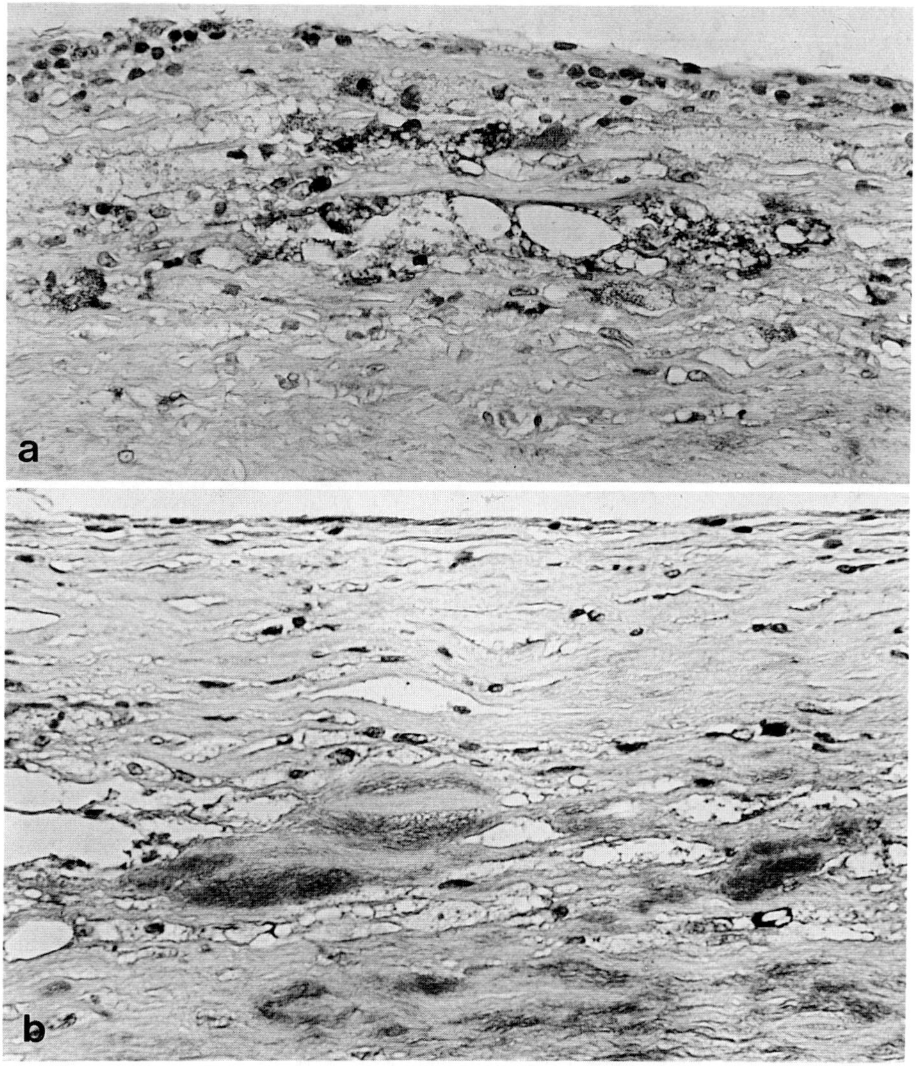

Fig. 3a, b. Progressing atherosclerotic changes of the wall **a** Numerous intracellular apo A-I deposits in foam cells (mainly in the *center*) and some isolated extracellular deposits (*lower right margin*). × 400. **b** Exclusively extracellular apo B deposits (*lower third*); no immunohistochemical staining of foam cells, in contrast to **a**. × 400

cells of the media (Fig. 5). In contrast, deposits of apo B are almost exclusively extracellular at this stage (Fig. 3b).

On the basis of histogenetic criteria, the so-called foam cells are subdivided into a myogenic (Fig. 4a) and a histiocytic type (Fig. 4b, c). The latter predominates in the early stages of atherosclerosis, whereas myocytes in foamy transformation are mostly found in advanced atherosclerotic lesions. That the majority of apolipoprotein-bearing foam cells are indeed of histiocytic origin, at least during the early and middle states, can be verified by immunohistochemical double-labeling against both exclusively histiocytic cell elements and apolipoproteins (Fig. 5). When this technique is applied, foam cells reveal an intense mixed coloring, especially in the part of the fibrous cap adjacent to the lumen; in

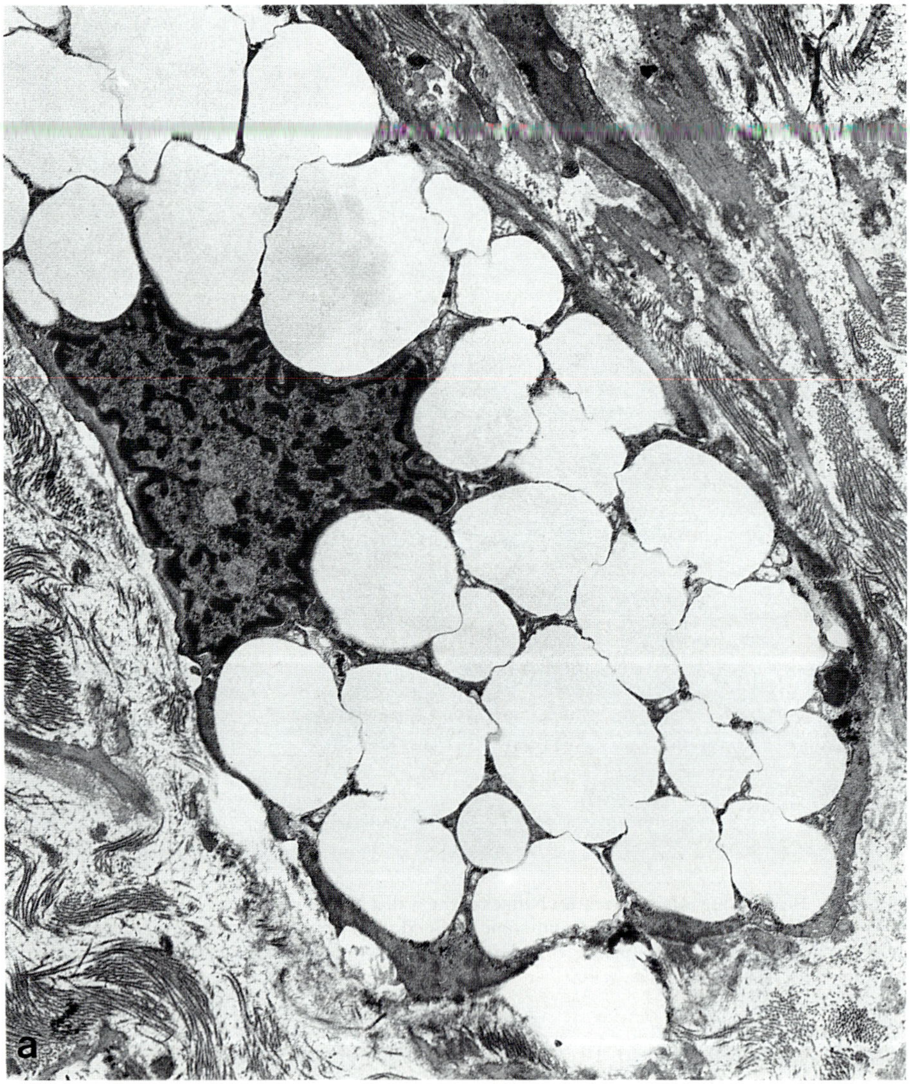

Fig. 4a–c. Ultrastructural representation of various foam cell subtypes with numerous lipid vesicles. **a** Foam cell of myogenic type. × 8000. **b** Incipient foamy transformation of a macrophage with numerous intracytoplasmic vesicles with lipid minidroplets. × 14 000. **c** Foam cell of histiocytic type with many confluent intracytoplasmic vacuoles containing coarse lipid droplets, but still intact cytoplasmic membrane. × 17 000

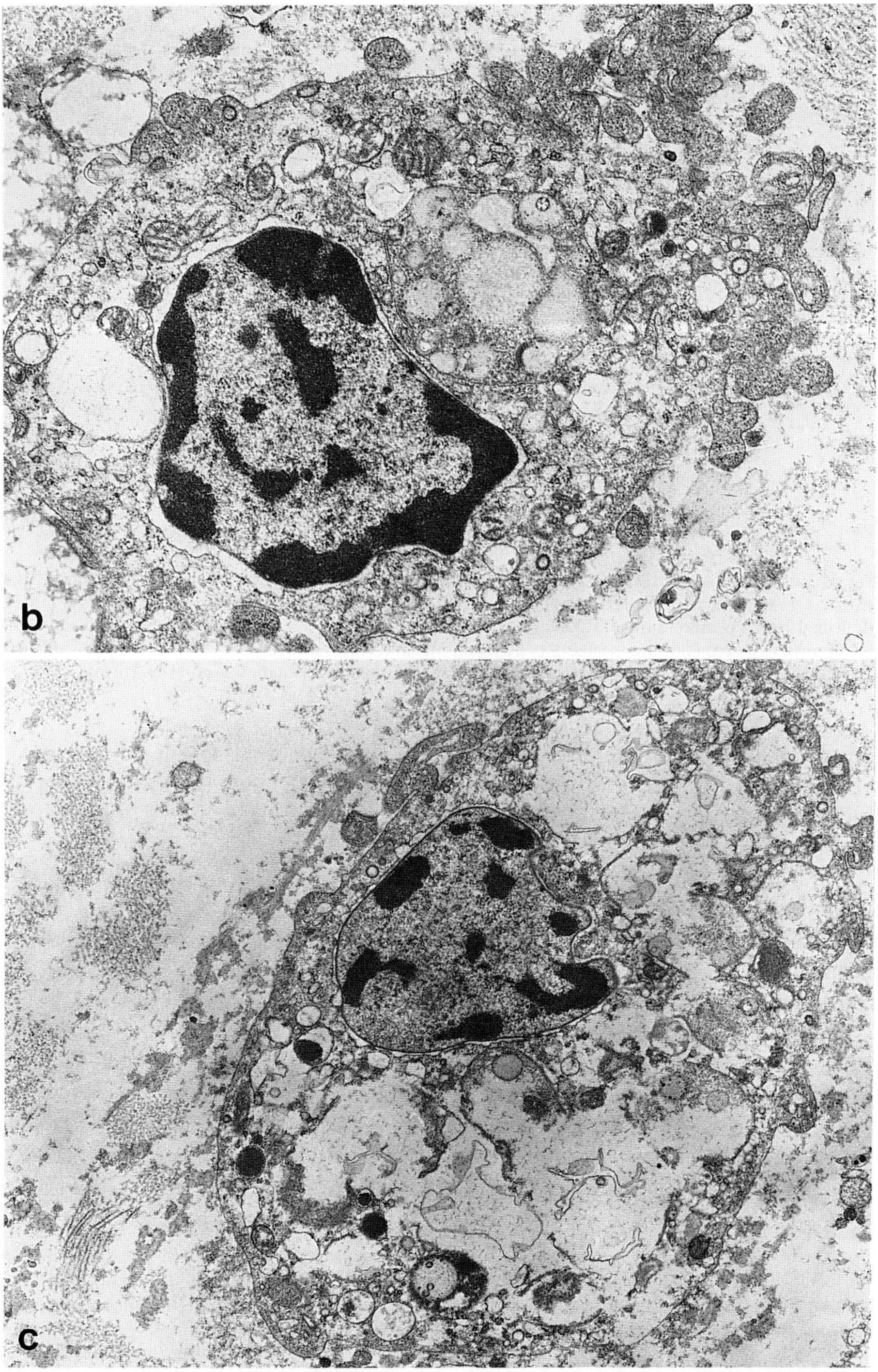
b
c

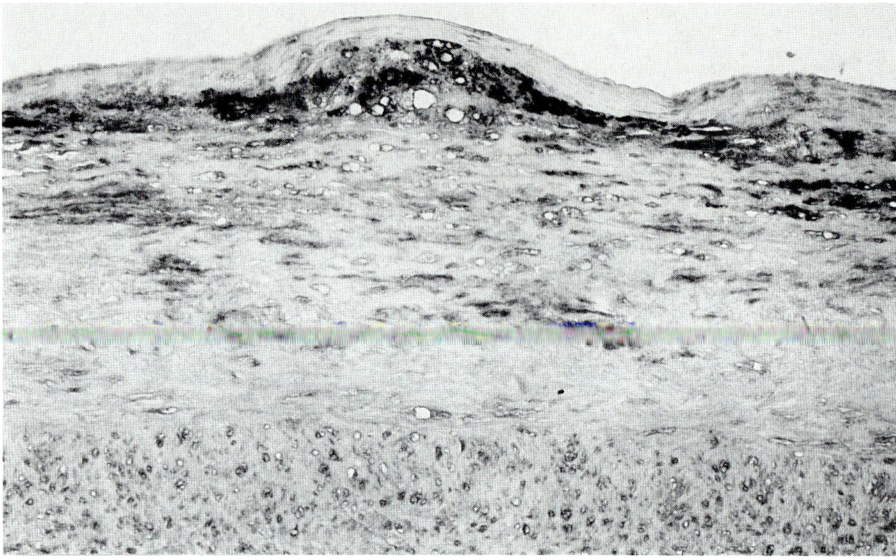

Fig. 5. Immunohistochemical double labeling indicating the histiocytic origin of foam cells and the intra- and extracellular deposits of apo A-I. Note the well-stained intimal foam cells near the lumen identified by a specific marker against mature tissue macrophages, and containing additional apo A-I deposits. Minor staining intensity is observed in non-macrophage-associated deposits in intimal spindle-shaped mycocytes as well as in extracellular and also in medial (*lower part*) locations. × 300

contrast, sheer deposits of apo A-I in deeper layers of the wall will show a much weaker coloring. These are found in the intimal layer, in extracellular spaces, and in spindly myocytes; in the media, numerous myocytes will also carry this apolipoprotein.

During the progression of atherosclerosis, basal apolipoprotein deposition is further extended (Fig. 1d, e); sometimes a necrotic zone will be formed in the depth of the plaque, with sedimentation of cholesterol crystals, and actual calcification is frequently observed. These phenomena involve apo A-I, A-II, and B. However, while apo A-I and A-II occur in both intra- and extracellular locations, apo B is seen but very rarely in an intracellular location, and then only in some foam cells of advanced lesions. The occasional presence of apolipoproteins in the adventitia must be interpreted as the result of torn vasa vasorum during preparation, that is, of apolipoprotein diffusion from these disrupted vessels. It occurs independently of, and thus cannot be correlated with, the stage of atherosclerosis (cf. VOLLMER et al. 1991c). As adventitial tissue

Fig. 6a–c. Ultrastructural presentation of apo A-I. **a** Intracellular apolipoprotein depositis, predominantly in the electron-dense organelles of a macrophage, and some extracellular deposits (*below*). Lipid droplets (*arrows*) remain largely unlabeled. × 45000. **b** Apo A-I in extracellular matrix. × 65000. **c** Intracellular evidence of apo A-I in a myocyte of synthesizing type with an immunohistochemically negative lipid vacuole (*arrow*). × 45000

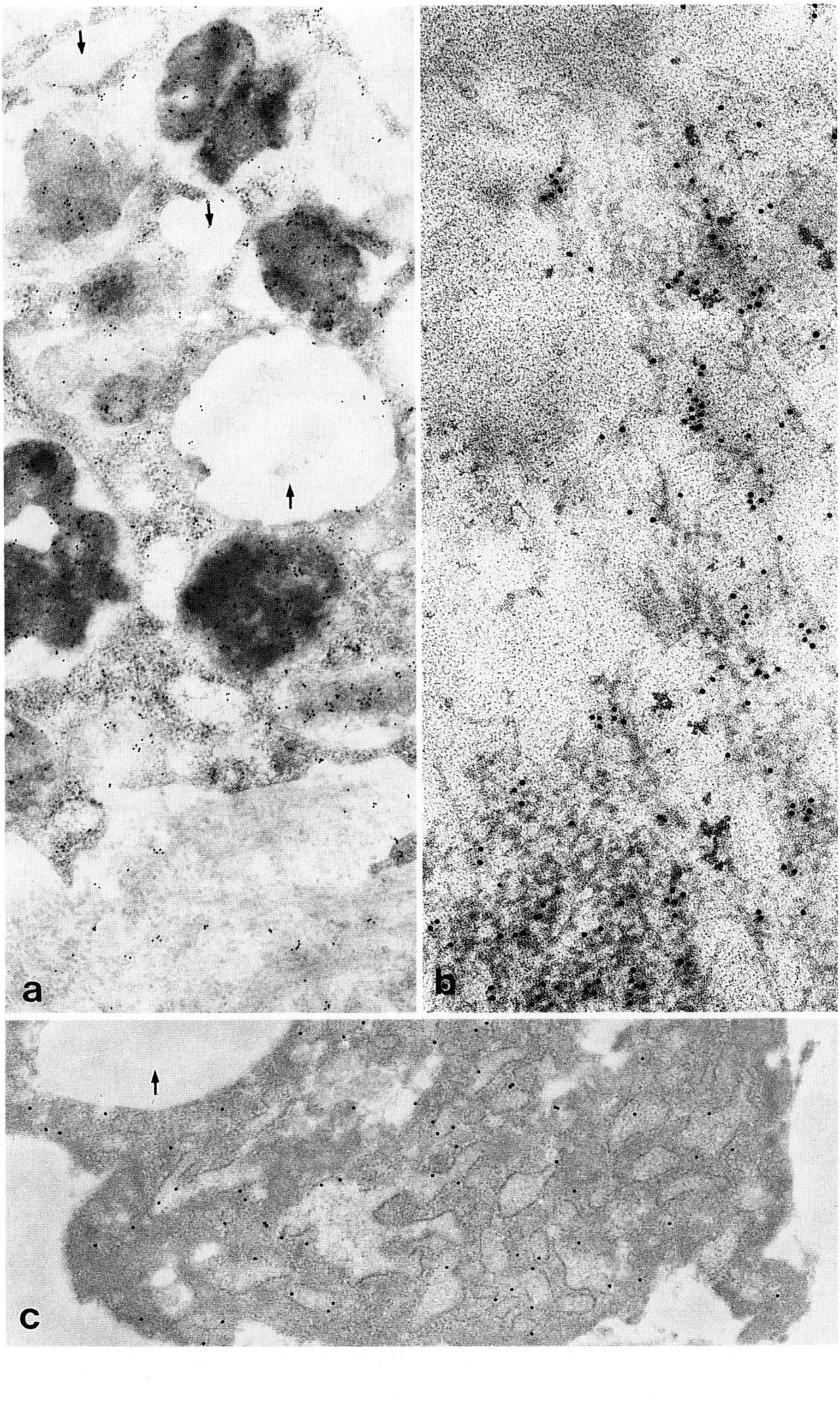
a
b
c

is much less tightly coherent than the media, apolipoproteins from the serum spread much more readily in that layer.

Immunoelectron microscopic investigations facilitated the clear ultrastructural classification and localization of apo types and confirmed previous light microscopic findings. Apo A was found in both extra- and intracellular locations in macrophages and smooth muscle cells (Fig. 6a–c). Areas with a rather low intracytoplasmic labeling for apo A-I are identified predominantly in the zone surrounding the synthetic apparatus; areas with strong cytoplasmic apo A-I labeling are found in electron-dense, partly lamellar cell organelles. Lipid droplets are often unlabeled or show comparatively less labeling. Extracellular apo A-I is situated between components of the extracellular matrix, the amount rising in parallel with advancing atherosclerosis. The pattern of apo A-II is similar.

On the ultrastructural level, extracellular demonstration of apo B (like that of apo A) is possible between components of the extracellular matrix and in parallel with the advancing stages of atherosclerosis (Fig. 7b). Intracellular evidence is found only in the more advanced stages, where foam cell macrophages show distinct apo B accumulation especially in electron-dense, partly lamellar cell organelles (Fig. 7a), with mostly unlabeled lipid droplets. These electron-dense organelles are mainly of lysosomal origin, as confirmed by cytochemical studies with cathepsin D, a lysosomal marker (Fig. 7c). No apo B, however, could be found in smooth muscle cells that were morphologically intact (Fig. 7d). Only in myocytes with high-grade regressive changes in a very advanced stage of atherosclerosis was there some ultrastructural evidence of diffuse but sparse apo B labeling, which, however, could not be attributed to definite cell structures and depended on the grade of regresion (Fig. 8a–d). Distinctly altered areas will show a stronger, although equally diffuse labeling than areas with lesser changes. The membrane surface of such regressively altered myocytes may comprise certain defects that may be interpreted as openings where apo B may diffuse from the extracellular spaces into the cells.

From these results we may deduce the very important role of foam cells in the local lipid metabolism. In vitro studies confirmed that under an overload of cholesterol, macrophages and other cells (e.g., hepatocytes) will increase their production of apo E. The actual rate of synthesis seems to depend on the amount of free cholesterol within the cell, and is responsible for modulating the metabolism of highly atherogenic apo B. Subsequent investigations were intended to determine whether such in vitro findings might be transferred to the vascular wall in atherosclerosis. Strong positive reactions with antibodies against apo E were observed predominantly in foam cells of the so-called fatty streaks, but in complicated lesions as well (Fig. 9a).

To determine the origin of such foam cells, we performed histologic double labelings with monoclonal antibodies against macrophages and myocytes and against apo E. The majority of the foam cells revealed intense mixed coloring when the markers for histiocytes and apo E were applied (Fig. 9b). In contrast, there were but a few spindle cell elements of myogenic origin, some of which

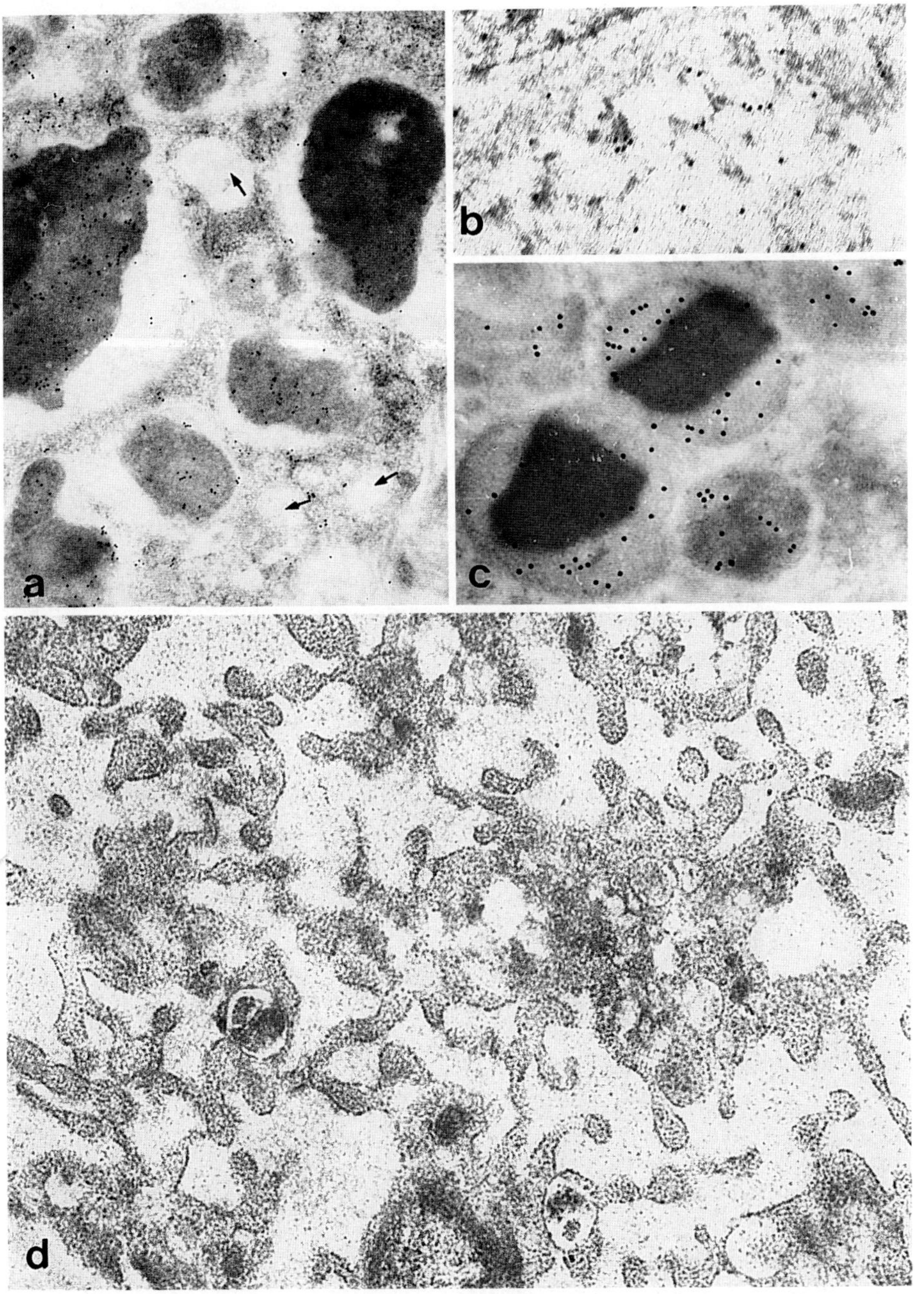

Fig. 7a–d. Ultrastructural presentation of apo B. **a** Macrophage labeled for apo B predominantly in electron-dense organelles; lipid droplets (*arrows*) are mostly unlabeled. × 40 000. **b** Apo B deposits in the extracellular matrix. × 50 000. **c** Cathepsin D, a lysosomal marker, is found in partly electron-dense intracytoplasmic organelles. × 45 000. **d** Granular endoplasmic reticulum in a morphologically intact myocyte without any immunocytochemical evidence of apo B. × 50 000

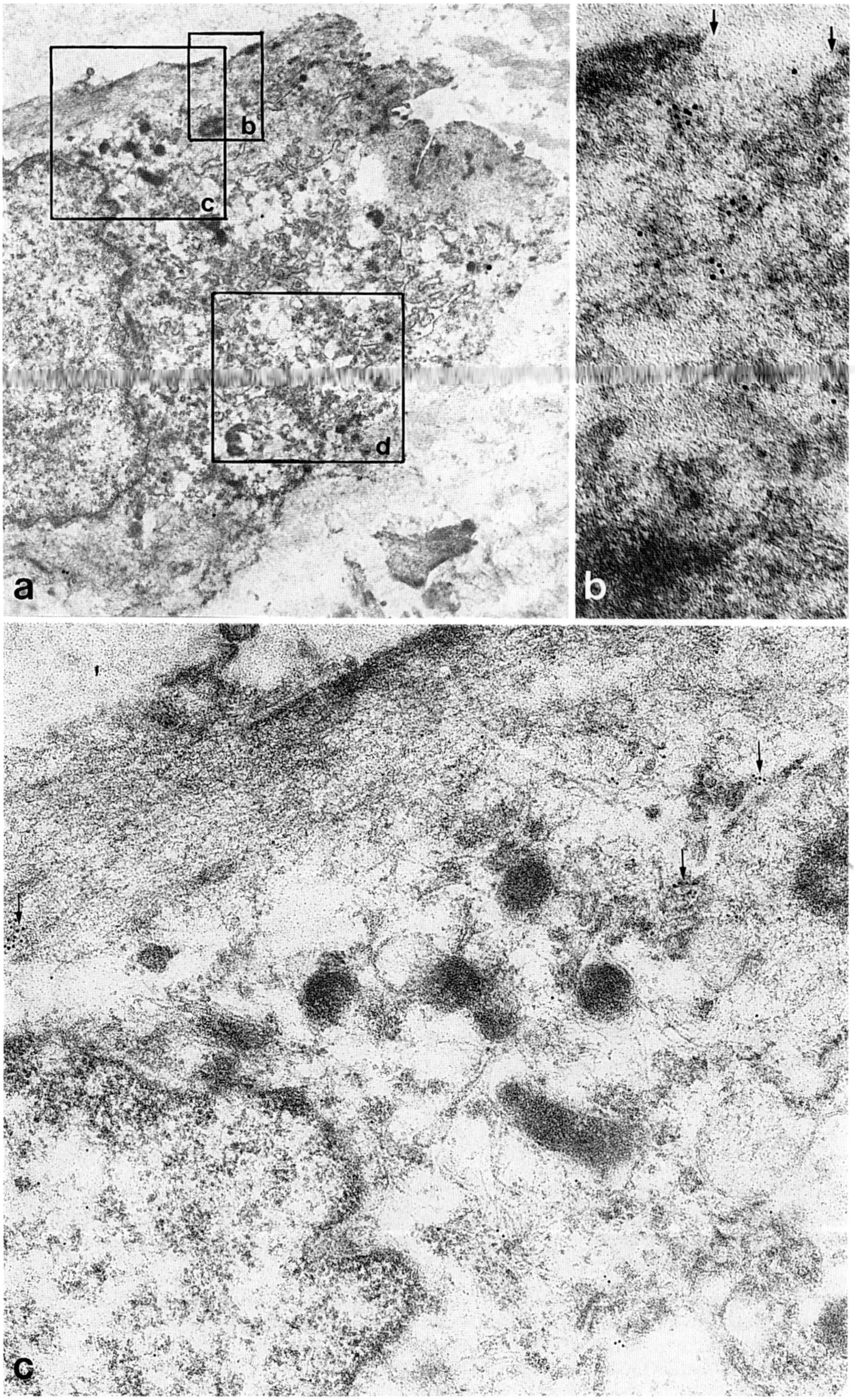
b
c
d
a
b
c

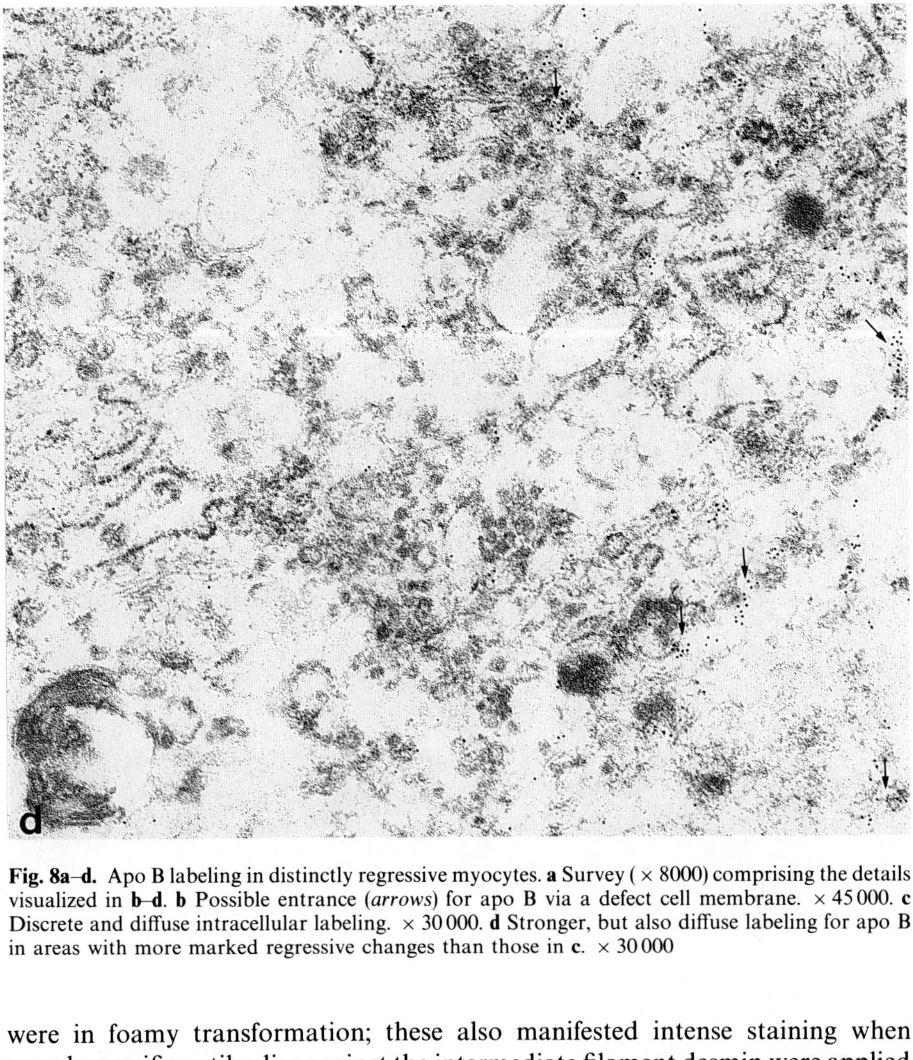

Fig. 8a–d. Apo B labeling in distinctly regressive myocytes. **a** Survey (× 8000) comprising the details visualized in **b–d**. **b** Possible entrance (*arrows*) for apo B via a defect cell membrane. × 45 000. **c** Discrete and diffuse intracellular labeling. × 30 000. **d** Stronger, but also diffuse labeling for apo B in areas with more marked regressive changes than those in **c**. × 30 000

were in foamy transformation; these also manifested intense staining when muscle-specific antibodies against the intermediate filament desmin were applied simultaneously with antibodies against apo E (Fig. 9c). Obviously, the majority of apo E-bearing foam cells in such lesions can be traced back to macrophages and do not originate from smooth muscle cells.

3.2 Renal Transplant Arteriopathy

In transplanted kidneys, a similar correlation was observed between the severity of the lesion and the extent of HDL- or LDL-associated apolipoprotein accumulation in the vascular walls involved. Apolipoprotein deposits are found in

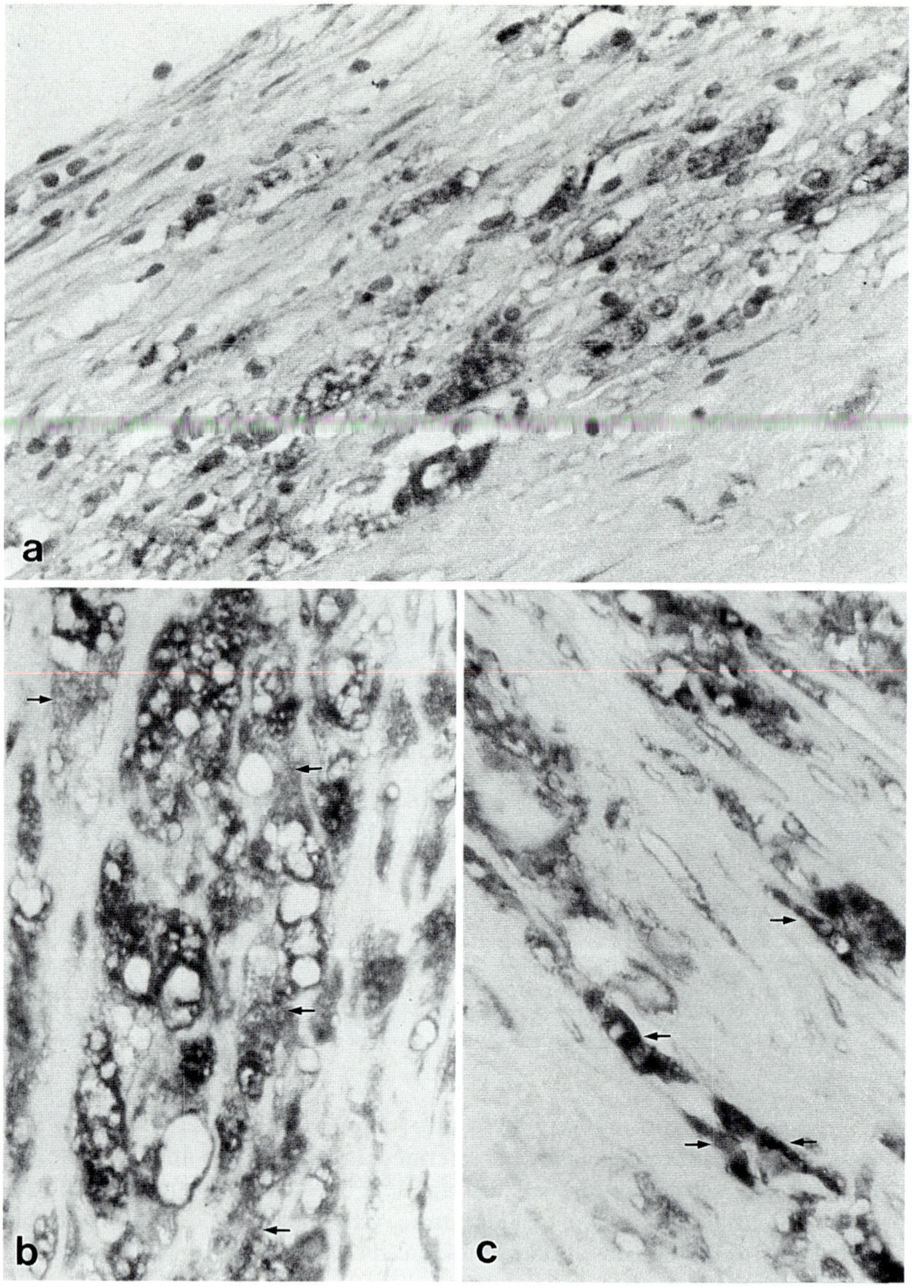

Fig. 9a–c. Immunohistochemical presentation of apo E. **a** Foam cells in the atherosclerotic plaque of an aorta containing apo E. × 550. **b** In Immunohistochemical double labeling with an antibody against so-called mature tissue macrophages and another antibody against apo E, the majority of foam cells show intense staining. Only a few foam cells (*arrows*) containing no apo E are labeled with the macrophage marker alone. × 550. **c** Immunohistochemical double labeling with antibodies against desmin and against apo E reveals evidence of the latter only in a few spindle cells staining intensely (*arrows*), which are thereby identifiable as smooth muscle cells. The remaining spindle-shaped cells, comparatively less well labeled, are only desmin positive and so classified as smooth muscle cells devoid of apo E. × 550

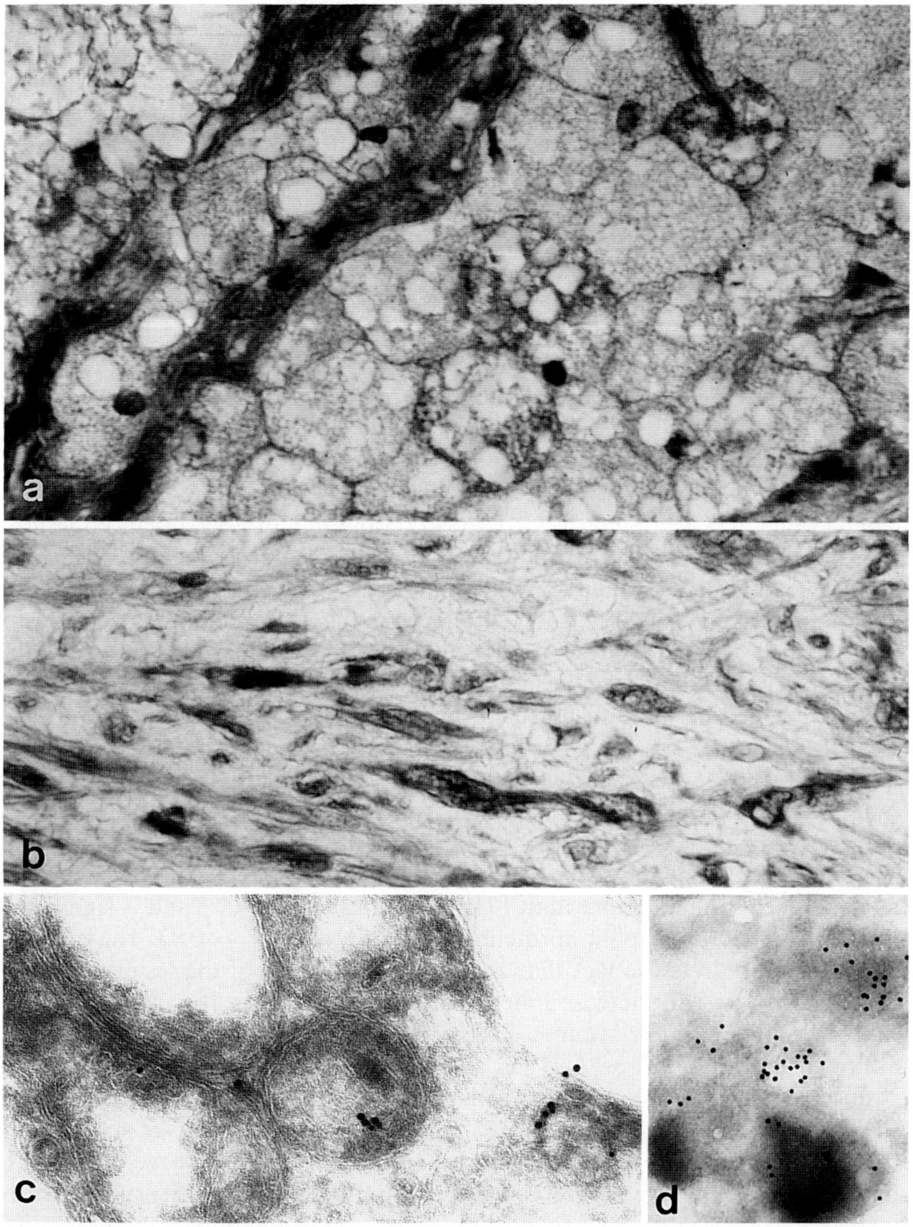

Fig. 10a–d. Representation of apo A in RTA. **a** Apo A-I in an extracellular location as well as in foam cells. × 450. **b** Manifestation of apo A-II in advanced RTA, observed in spindle-shaped cells of the media. × 550. **c, d** Ultrastructural evidence of apo A-I in mainly electron-dense cell organelles. **c** × 45 000; **d** × 35 000

intra- and extracellular locations, predominantly in the intima; the media holds much smaller deposits, mainly in very advanced lesions. Subsequent to initially extracellular accumulation, apo A-I and A-II occur with increasing frequency within cells (mostly foam cells; Fig. 10a) as lumen obliteration progresses. However, their extracellular accumulation will also increase with progression of RTA, especially in cell-depleted necrotic zones. As in CAS, we were able to demonstrate by immunohistochemical double labeling that the majority of apolipoprotein-bearing foam cells are of histiocytic rather than myogenic origin. With the progress of RTA, apo A deposits will spread to the media, where they are also evident in spindle-shaped myocytes (Fig. 10b). The accumulation pattern of apo A-II corresponds largely to that of Apo A-I, though the latter is always present in greater quantities. As in CAS, on the ultrastructural level apo A is found in electron-dense cell organelles, while lipid droplets remain mostly unlabeled (Fig. 10c, d).

The accumulation of apo B is predominantly extracellular in all grades of obliteration, especially in cell-depleted necroses, where the internal elastic lamina often acts as a kind of barrier (Fig. 11a). Only in very advanced lesions does the honeycomb-like cytoplasm of some histiocytic foam cells also hold apo B; such cells are often found in the vicinity of numerous extracellular apolipoprotein deposits (Fig. 11b). Ultrastructurally, extracellular apo B deposits appear closely interwoven with the elements of extracellular matrix (Fig. 11c). In contrast the myocytes, even in foamy transformation, hardly ever show apo B, as confirmed by immuno-histochemical double labeling.

On the whole, extra- and intracellular apolipoprotein deposits are much more distinct in the vascular walls of medium-sized renal parenchymal arteries (Aa. arcuatae and interlobulares) than in those of preceding or subsequent arteries. With increasing luminal obliteration the number of intimal apolipoprotein deposits increases correspondingly (Fig. 12). This increasing concentration affects stages 1 (lumen more than 17%) and 3 (lumen 4%–0%) and is significant in respect of all three apolipoprotein types at a level of $P = 0.02$. The mode of presentation reflects the fact that at an advanced stage of the lesion, apolipoprotein deposits will increase much more rapidly than in the initial phase of development. The shape of curves is generally similar in all apolipoprotein types, although the curve of apo A-II lies somewhat closer to the abscissa than that of apo A-I. Both these apolipoproteins seem to have a similar mode of entering the intima, but the amount of apo A-I gaining access to that layer is obviously higher than that of apo A-II. Compared to the A types, the curve of apo B is flatter in the early stage of RTA, but the amount of apo B deposits subsequently increases so markedly as to equal that of apo A-I in the final stage of luminal obliteration, or even to surpass it to a minor extent. This trend is reflected in Fig. 13, demonstrating the quantity of apolipoprotein deposits per field of vision in the different stages of RTA. In stage 1, when 20% of vessels already bear strong deposits of apo A-I, no vessel shows apo B deposits of similar number. In contrast, in stage 3 abundant apo B deposits are present in 60% of the vessels,

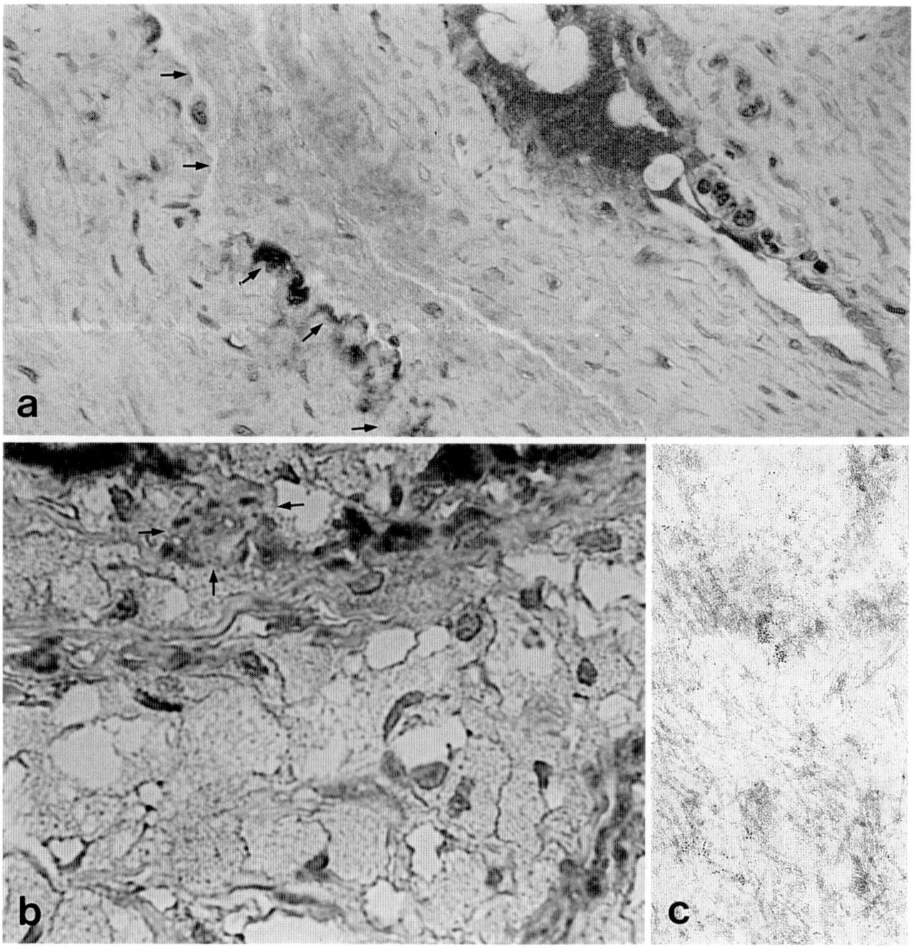

Fig. 11a–c. Representation of apo B in RTA. **a** Predominantly extracellular apo B deposits, especially in cell-depleted areas of necrosis; the lamina elastica interna (*arrows*) is often acting as a kind of barrier. × 50. **b** A very few foam cells (*arrows*) near massive extracellular deposits of apo B manifest that same apo B in their cytoplasm; the majority of the foam cells (*lower part*) show no evidence of apo B. × 450. **c** Ultrastructural evidence of apo B interwoven with elements of the extracellular matrix. × 12000

this figure actually exceeding that for apo A-I (58%), as well as the much lower figure for apo A-II (33.3%).

To recapitulate: apo A-I and A-II primarily accumulate in the intima, preferably in an intracellular location (Fig. 14). With regard to apo A-I accumulation in stage 1 of RTA, 89% of involved vessels belong to the group with extracellular deposition of apo A-I. As in the case of CAS, ultrastructural analysis of RTA revealed apo A deposits predominantly within electron-dense organelles

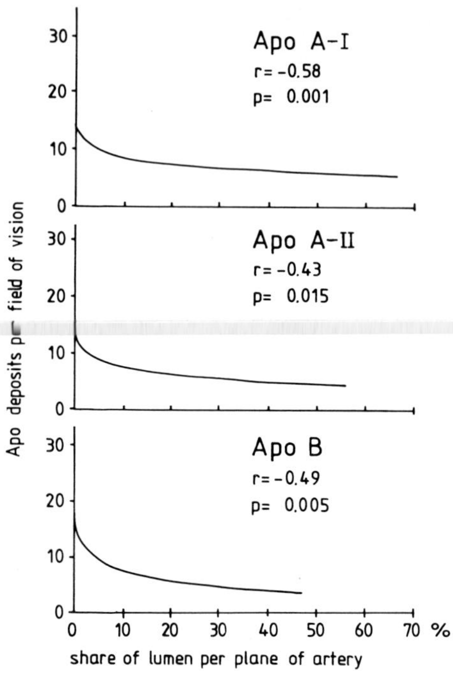

Fig. 12. Regression curves displayed with the distributions of apo A-I, A-II, and B deposits (arithmetic means) in the intima of medium-sized renal arteries during obliterative RTA; note the accelerated increase of deposits in the later stage of the lesion

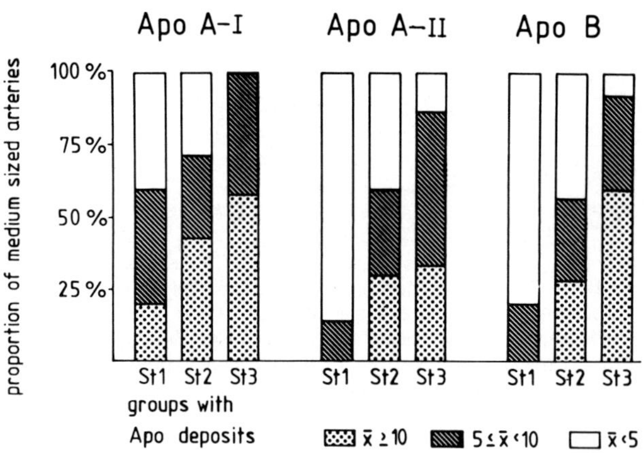

Fig. 13. Comparison of apolipoprotein contents during the consecutive stages (*St*) of obliterative RTA of medium-sized arteries, after statistical evaluation of total intimal deposits of A-I, A-II, and B in intra- *and* extracellular locations

(cf. Figs. 10c,d,6a); in the course of luminal obliteration, extracellular deposits also increase. The affinity of apo A-I for intracellular accumulation surpasses that of apo A-II (cf. Fig. 14). The developmental pattern of apo B is reversed: apo B shows a distinct preference for extracellular accumulation; its entrance into the cytoplasm is exceptional (Fig. 15) and, if it occurs at all, involves the

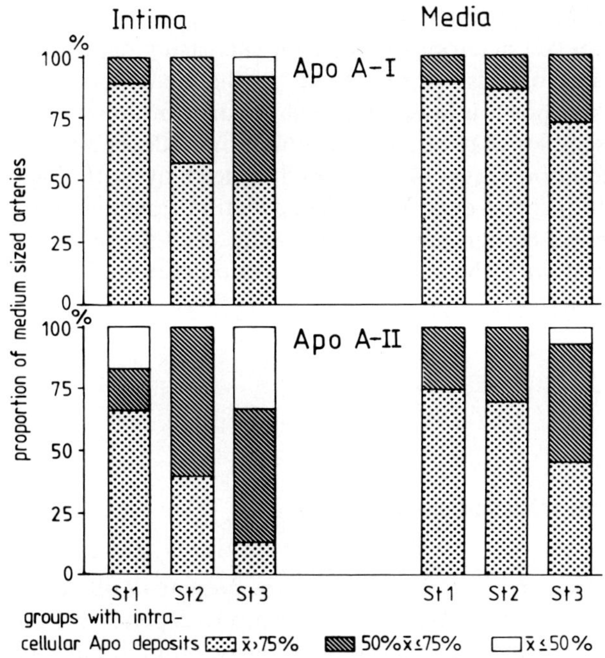

Fig. 14. Proportion of vessels with intracellular deposits of apo A-I and A-II in the intima and media of medium-sized arteries during the stages (*St*) of obliterative RTA

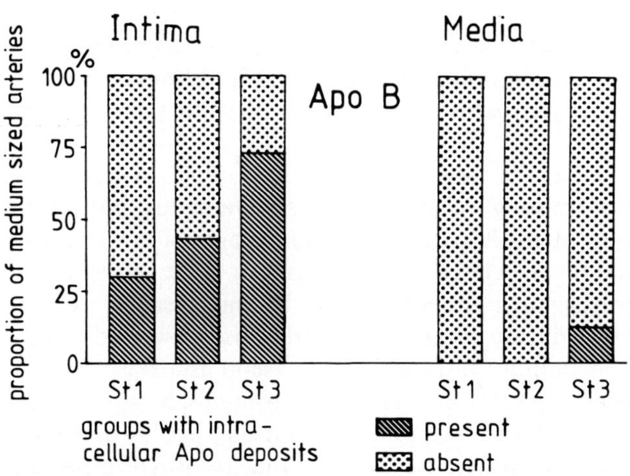

Fig. 15. Proportion of vessels with intracellular deposits of apo B in the intima and media of medium-sized arteries during the stages (*St*) of obliterative RTA.

so-called foam cell macrophages. In general, there is a positive correlation between the presence of foam cell macrophages and the increasing deposits of A-I, A-II, and B in the intima, but also in the media. In the media, however, the number of apolipoprotein deposits is lower, although the distribution pattern of apo A-I, A-II, and B resembles that observed in the intima, depending on the grade of luminal obliteration (Figs. 14,15). Un-influenced by pathologic changes in the vessels, apolipoprotein deposits in the adventitia resemble those seen in CAS and seem to reflect certain preparatory conditions. Obviously, no correlation can be established with the stage of luminal obliteration, i.e., the progress of the vascular lesion.

4 Discussion

4.1 Intramural Apolipoprotein Distribution in Arteries

According to our observations, apo A-I, A-II, and B are present in all stages of the atherosclerotic lesion. The quantity of accumulations depends on the stage of the individual lesion: the more advanced an atherosclerotic lesion, the higher the intramural content of apolipoproteins. This increase in apolipoprotein deposits is most marked in the intima and media, and the morphologic changes of atherosclerosis are most visible in these layers. They are also supplied by diffusion from the lumen, in contrast to the adventitia, which is much less affected by morphologic changes even in the final stage of atherosclerosis. Obviously, the stronger increase in apolipoproteins in the intima and media reflects certain local metabolic alterations. Such changes are also seen in obliterative RTA in medium-sized renal arteries, especially in the intimal layer. The media of these renal arteries is less strongly affected than that of the larger A. renalis and is also less markedly affected than in CAS, although morphological similarities between these diseases are evident (despite their different etiologies).

In view of the different effects of varying plasma levels of apo A-I and A-II (protective) and apo B (promoting sclerosis), the simultaneous intramural increase in all three apolipoproteins in parallel to lesion progression was rather an unexpected finding: If HDL-associated lipoproteins, like those in the serum, exert a protective function against atherosclerosis in the vascular wall, a decrease in apo A-I and A-II during progression of the disease would appear more likely, whereas the concomitant intramural increase in apo B is as would be expected. Our results regarding HDL-associated lipoproteins, however, agree well with those of Carter et al. (1987), who pointed out that apo A-I found in the lesion need not have the same protective effect as that recorded in plasma. Recent studies by Rath et al. (1989) also suggested that no significant correlation could be established between serum levels of apo B and apo(a) and their levels in aortic tissue. These data confirm that apolipoprotein accumulation depends primarily on morphologic changes in the vascular wall with subsequent functional disorders of the altered cells, whereas their role in blood plasma conditions is rather secondary.

The intra- and extracellular co-localization of A-I and A-II could have been anticipated, given that both of these apolipoproteins are structural components of HDL, and such co-localization has been supported by the fluorescence microscopic studies of BEDOSSA et al. (1989). However, even apo B, which is LDL associated, was evident in both intra- and extracellular locations in vascular walls— although the intracellular manifestation of apo B is such lower, and restricted to foam cell macrophages. These findings agree with the immunohistochemical studies of other authors who used the appropriate apolipoprotein components to label HDL and LDL (HOFF et al. 1975a, b; CARTER et al. 1987; MORA et al. 1987; NIENDORF et al. 1990a, b; VOLLMER et al. 1989b, 1991c). The claim by YOMANTAS et al. (1984) that intracellular evidence of apo B exists only in the aorta, and not in coronary arteries, was not confirmed in our studies, but this discrepancy is obviously due to the differing material of his and our studies.

The accumulation of apolipoproteins in the arterial wall can be principally attributed to three possible mechanisms:

1. Insudation and transcytosis of lipoproteins from the plasma into the vascular wall
2. Neosynthesis of lipoproteins or only of apolipoproteins in the wall proper, effected by local cells or others immigrating during the progress of arteriosclerosis
3. Discharge of intracytoplasmic lipoproteins from necrotic cells in the vascular wall

The strongest structural changes, even with respect to lipoprotein distribution, are observed in the intima during the progression of CAS and RTA. In the normal intima of vascular segments adjacent to arteriosclerotic lesions, no morphologic evidence could be found for the presence of both LDL and HDL. This, too, agrees with the results of other immunohistochemical studies (HOFF et al. 1975a, b; YOMANTAS et al. 1984; CARTER et al. 1987) and was confirmed by electron microscopy (HOFF and GAUBATZ 1975, 1977). FELDMAN et al. (1984), however, had recorded intimal evidence of apo B prior to the development of a lesion, but only in areas of thicker or edematous intima—a status that was classified as stage I (=early lesion) of CAS in our study. The fluorescence microscopic demonstration of extracellular apo B reported by SHEKHONIN et al. (1990) in normal intima could not be confirmed by our own observations.

Despite the lack of evidence for the presence of LDL or HDL in normal intima in our own immunohistologic investigations, there must be a certain transfer of cholesterol-bearing lipoproteins in these normal tissues. Minor quantities of lipoproteins and related apolipoproteins have indeed been isolated from extracts of normal intimal tissue (SMITH and STAPLES 1980; NICOLL et al. 1981; LINDEN et al. 1986; YLÄ-HERTTUALA et al. 1987) and interpreted as lipoprotein insudates from the plasma. This potential physiologic exchange, however, escapes any immunohistochemical method of analysis. Obviously, the cholesterol content of normal intima is regulated by a well-adapted influx and efflux mechanism and by the metabolism of lipoproteins, which prevents the accumulation of cholesterol in larger quantities.

The preferential localization of LDL and HDL in the immediate subendothelial intimal layer, as observed in the early stages of CAS in our study, suggests a mechanism of insudation or transcytosis from the lumen into the subendothelium of the vessel. The almost exclusively extracellular location of apolipoproteins in these early stages would in fact permit no other conclusion than that such insudation from the lumen occurs not only in CAS but also in the renal arteries of rejected renal transplants. However, medium-sized renal arteries (Aa. arcuatae and interlobulares) showing much more pronounced luminal obliteration than larger vessels already bear intracellular apolipoprotein deposits, indicating an active metabolic involvement of such cells.

With regard to apo A-I and A-II, the relative percentage of vessels with intracellular deposits in the intima and also the media decreases in favor of those with extracellular deposits in a continuous slope until complete obliteration. The pattern is reversed for apo B, but the total amount of apo A-I, A-II, and B increases concomitantly with the progression of the lesion. Obviously, the lipoproteins in or near the lesion are fixed by elements of ground substance, synthesized in increasing quantity, and are prevented from rediffusion into the vascular lumen (Srinivasan et al. 1986). The same trend is illustrated by our immunoelectron microscopic data and the results reported by More et al. (1989) from a rabbit model.

Among the elements of newly synthesized ground substance, proteoglycans seem to be responsible for the retention of lipoproteins. Sulfated glycosaminoglycans in particular are able to bind LDL, forming regular LDL-glycosaminoglycan complexes extractable from arterial tissues (Mawhinney et al. 1978; Nakashima et al. 1985; Radhakrishnamurthy et al. 1990; Camejo et al. 1990; Bondjers et al. 1990). Immunohistologic demonstration of the co-localization of apo B with sulfated glycosaminoglycans in atherosclerotic lesions was reported by Yutani et al. (1987). These LDL–proteoglycan complexes are known to enhance LDL catabolism in macrophages (Salisbury et al. 1985), whereas HDL is thought not to form such complexes (Vijayagopal et al. 1981). Ylä-Herttuala et al. (1987), however, suppose that HDL is captured in the intima by another mode of retention. According to their studies, the contents not only of apo B but also of apo A-I depend on the amount of sulfated glycosaminoglycans. These authors discuss a kind of molecular sieve as the mechanism responsible for HDL retention, whereby macromolecules would be unable to pass the 5-nm pores of proteoglycans. In addition, the extracellular space, which increases in the course of atherosclerosis (due to continuous introduction of, for example, sulfated glycosaminoglycans into the extracellular matrix), is seen as an additional space offered for the retention of HDL. Our own observations in respect of medium-sized renal parenchymal vessels seem to concur with this concept: in RTA the ratio of intra- to extracellular deposits of apo A-I and A-II decreases as obliteration increases, whereas the reverse trend was evident for apo B.

In the further progress of atherosclerosis, the distribution of lipoproteins over the intima is not even, but rather preferentially localized in the basal parts of the plaque. Even in a condition of increased endothelial permeability that would permit massive invasion into the intima, lipoproteins seem unable to freely join the fluid stream directed from the lumen towards the peripheral or adventitial layer of the vessel wall. Equally unable to pervade the media, they will accumulate especially in the basal strata of the intima. Along with other authors (SMITH and STAPLES 1980; SMITH 1990), we feel entitled to interpret the lamina elastica interna as a barrier against the deeper intrusion of lipoproteins. Our morphometric data gathered especially in RTA offer convincing proof that this barrier is maintained and is often still functional untill complete luminal obliteration. Moreover, the fibrotic zone above basal lipoprotein deposits is rendered thicker and denser by the quantitative increase in smooth muscle cells and their synthesis of extracellular matrix during the development of the atheromatous plaque. This, too, impairs the efflux of lipoproteins towards the lumen simply by lengthening the pathways of diffusion.

Thus, insudated lipoproteins are actually incarcerated in the basal strata of developing atheromas, and accumulated massively, as illustrated by the numerous apolipoprotein deposits in our samples of advanced lesions. The cytotoxicity of high cholesterol levels, together with increasing hypoxia caused by enhanced fibrosis from impaired diffusion pathways, may be the ultimate cause of eventual necrosis in the plaque basis. Many cases of stage III CAS show not only numerous apolipoprotein deposits in these areas, but also calcium salt sedimentation, reflecting the complete failure of metabolic homeostasis in the arterial wall and indicating the metabolism of cholesterol and cholesterol-bearing lipoproteins. While the extracellular accumulation of apo A-I, A-II, and B increases almost evenly in our cases of atherosclerosis, the total amount of apo A-I and A-II deposits is augmented by an intracellular component. Our findings in RTA call for a similar explanation. Corrospondingly, the relative increase in renal vessels with intracellular deposits of apo B would reflect the failure of lipid metabolism during progressing luminal obliteration.

The results described so far permit the following conclusions:

1. The effects of apolipoproteins (known from plasma measurements to be protective in the case of apo A-I and A-II, and sclerosis promoting in the case of apo B), their relative proportions, and their patterns of distribution must be re-evaluated with regard to their presence in the arterial wall.
2. Only with the inception of a vascular lesion will these apolipoproteins enter the lumen-adjacent layers of that wall (intima and media) by means of insudation or transcytosis.
3. In this process, the invading apolipoproteins are fixed by extracellular ground substance while the lamina elastica interna acts as a barrier against diffusion.

4. Some (transitory) active lipid metabolism occurs in situ since an additional intracellular component is obviously developing for apo A-I and A-II; it eventually fails due to the equally increasing presence of intracellular apo B deposits in the progressing lesion.

The potential scope of local lipid metabolism and the kind of cell involved in it are discussed in the following sections.

4.2 HDL Metabolism In Vitro and In Vivo

The accumulation of HDL apolipoproteins within the cells becomes morphologically discernible, unlike its early extracellular manifestation, at a somewhat advanced stage of atherosclerosis. Only near the end of stage I were some single cells bearing apo A-I andA-II seen under light microscopy. They were mostly situated within the areas of extracellular accumulation.

Cells with larger HDL deposits were mainly classified as foam cells with the (immuno) morphologic characteristics of the macrophage. Some minor additional evidence of such apolipoproteins was seen in endothelial and smooth muscle cells. This same pattern is also found in RTA, in which it is even more strongly manifested since the relevant morphologic changes are particularly evident in the walls of medium-sized renal arteries. Here, too the majority of foam cells storing apo A-I and A-II are known to originate from histiocytes. According to current knowledge, the myogenic genesis of foam cells appears less important, especially in the early stage of atherosclerosis (MITCHINSON et al. 1990; VOLLMER et al. 1991c). It should be mentioned, however, that one relatively recent publication (GENDRA and BOUNADER-BECHENNEC 1989) did put forward the opposite interpretation again.

The facts that macrophages contain hardly any HDL apolipoproteins in the initial phase of atherosclerosis and that a discernible amount is seen with advancing lipid accumulation during progressive lesion development suggest a system of counterregulation for an increasing lipid overload, especially of cholesterol. The compensatory mechanism against increasing cholesterol is found in the intramural macrophages, namely the uptake of HDL, a cholesterol acceptor, from the extracellular deposits and the subsequent mobilization and transfer of cholesterol upon this protein. In vitro investigations have shown that lipid or cholesterol overload can be checked by macrophages if HDL is added to the culture medium (HO et al. 1980).

One current model of cholesterol transport from peripheral cells back to the liver proposes that, during intracytoplasmic esterification by lecithin-cholesterol acyltransferase (LCAT), HDL take up apo E from apo E/phospholipid disks or from apo E-rich plasma lipoproteins. An alternative model claims that cholesterol esters and apo A-I are transferred from HDL to apo E/phospholipid disks (for details, see below). This might lead to cholesterol esters and apo E-rich

HDL being able to transport secreted cholesterol towards the liver. In vitro assays with murine peritoneal macrophages and human monocytes/macrophages have shown that HDL without apo E can bind to specific surface receptors on the macrophage (SCHMITZ et al. 1985a, b, 1987). HDL identified by such receptors will be internalized by so-called coated pits and coated vesicles. During intracellular activity, HDL are carried by endosomes through the cell, come into contact with lipid droplets, take up unesterified cholesterol, and finally are secreted from the cell as cholesterol-laden HDL particles. Certain observations suggest that the availability of unesterified cholesterol is an essential prerequisite for receptor-mediated cholesterol reflux. Normally, lysosomal HDL degradation plays only a minor role, but this pattern changes if increased cholesterol uptake provokes an imbalance in the required enzyme activities, such as neutral cholesterol ester hydrolase (NCEH) and cholesterol acyltransferase (ACAT).

Our ultrastructural analyses have shown, especially in CAS, that areas with low intracytoplasmic labeling for apo A-I are often preferentially located near the synthetic apparatus in smooth muscle cells as well as in macrophages. Lipid droplets, if present, mostly remain unlabeled, as also shown by recent studies of HARRACH and ROBENEK (1990). Any stronger cytoplasmic labeling of apo A-I is to be found in electron-dense, partly lamellar organelles which are often of lysosomal origin. Observed in vitro, macrophages reveal two main pathways, in addition to normal physicochemical degradation, for eliminating excess cholesterol: Firstly, formation of cholesterol- or phospholipid-bearing, lamellar corpuscles, derived from lysosomes and moving to the cell periphery, where they bind to the membrane, releasing their lipid particles into the extracellular medium or into the cell membrane proper. This mechanism of intracellular cholesterol release is promoted by HDL particles rich in apo A-I/apo A-IV-LCAT with a preference for unspecific binding to the cell membrane (so-called low-affinity binding).

The second pathway implies a cholesterol reflux mediated by HDL receptors: apo A-I-rich HDL binds specifically to a 110-kDa HDL-binding protein of macrophages. These apo A-I-rich HDL particles are internalized into a nonlysosomal compartment where they can take up cholesterol from lamellar organelles that have been formed by cytoplasmic lipid droplets after adherence to endoplasmic reticulum or released from the trans-Golgi apparatus. The latter mechanism is promoted by ACAT inhibitors provoking an increase in free intracellular cholesterol (SCHMITZ et al. 1990).

Our own apolipoprotein antibodies are obviously unable to identify more than the final step in the intracellular HDL metabolic pathway, since they reflect only an immunocytochemical labeling inside electron-dense organelles that are frequently of lysosomal origin. The technique is still inadequate for defining the previous steps, which means that our in situ data can merely indicate a kind of metabolism of HDL apolipoproteins in the cells of the vascular wall which, so far, has not been characterized by other authors either.

Apo E plays a major role in the maintenance of cellular cholesterol homeostasis. Monocytes/macrophages are active secretory cells able to produce apo

E, as shown in cell culture studies (BASU et al. 1981, 1982); smooth muscle cells are also thought to possess this ability (DRISCOLL and GETZ 1984). Apo E secretion by macrophages may be stimulated by incubation with acetylated LDL and certain other sources of cholesterol. Under a maximum cholesterol overload, synthesized apo E represents more than 10% of the overall protein secretion in these macrophages (BROWN and GOLDSTEIN 1983). The direct, apo E-mediated pathway via the "reverse cholesterol transport" towards the human liver implies about 11% of HDL cholesterol (WEISGRABER and MAHLEY 1980). In addition, apo E plus HDL seem to supply cholesterol to peripheral cells with low cholesterol levels, by way of a reallocation process (SCHMITZ et al. 1990). Our studies of apo E labeling, which were successful in foam cells of histiocytic but also of myocytic origin, indicate that, in analogy to previous in vitro results, these metabolic pathways, and especially the reverse cholesterol transport pathway, also play an important role in vascular tissues undergoing atherosclerotic changes (VOLLMER et al. 1991a).

Apo A-I has been identified as the chief ligand for HDL receptor binding in various cell systems (KASHYAP 1989). Such receptors are expressed on the cell surface in response to cholesterol overload, thereby initiating or mediating cellular cholesterol release from peripheral cells via reverse cholesterol transport. The mechanism itself, however, is still not fully explained (FRANCONE and FIELDING 1990). It even seems to work differently in different cell systems (SLOTTE 1990). In human fibroblasts and in bovine aortic endothelial cells, for instance, HDL seem to be specifically bound to the cell surface, which induces a shift of intracellular cholesterol towards the cell membrane, whence it is eventually taken up by HDL particles (STEINMETZ and KAFFARNIK 1989). Macrophages in vitro undergo an additional cholesterol loading of HDL after it is taken into the cell, with subsequent resecretion (SCHMITZ et al. 1985a, 1987). According to our in situ findings, the same mechanism occurs in macrophages and possibly even in smooth muscle cells of the arterial wall in the presence of atherosclerotic change.

Findings recorded in obliterative RTA point in the same direction. In addition, the possibility of neosynthesis cannot be excluded. The number of HDL-storing cells will continually increase with advancing atherosclerosis. The percentage of arteries bearing intracellular depositis of apo A-I and A-II in the intima and media will decrease somewhat in favor of extracellular accumulation. This does not contradict the findings in CAS, which also indicate an increase in the overall quantity of both apolipoproteins. Thus, the apparent decrease in intracellular apo A-I and A-II is a relative phenomenon due to higher accumulation in extracellular spaces.

The main conclusions to be drawn from these observations are:

1. In the vascular wall, HDL is metabolized by macrophages as well as by smooth muscle cells to an immunocytochemically identifiable degree.
2. In macrophages, this obviously acts as a compensatory mechanism only when a cholesterol overload is present.

3. Although to date only the final step in intracellular metabolic pathway is recognizable in situ, it often suggested a lysosomal type of metabolism.
4. In a vessel undergoing arteriosclerotic change, the so-called reverse cholesterol transport obviously offers another possibility; evidence of apo E is found in histiocytic as well as in myogenic foam cells.

4.3 LDL Metabolism In Vitro and In Vivo

In contrast to HDL-associated apolipoproteins, intracellular deposits of apo B (signaling LDL) were only rarely found in the foam cells of advanced-stage CAS. In obliterative RTA, too, apo B was very seldom found in foam cells; when it was present, it was usually within foam cells of histiocytic origin in advanced lesions.

If apo B was seen in smooth muscle cells at all, it appeared only in strongly regressive cells. According to our immunoelectron microscopic investigations, it was then diffusely present, without any clear association with intracytoplasmic structures. The surface of the cells concerned showed frequent defects, with enhanced intracytoplasmic deposits of apo B in the vicinity. The ultrastructural picture suggests a merely passive diffusion of apo B from extracellular spaces into the cellular interior of dying or dead smooth muscle cells. In morphologically intact myocytes there was never specific intracellular evidence of apo B, in contrast to the picture in macrophages.

In foam cells of histiocytic origin, apo B is accumulated in electron-dense organelles, quite similar to HDL-associated apo A-I. Labelling with antibodies against cathepsin D, a lysosomal marker, enabled us to identify the lysosomal origin of many, though not all, of these organelles. Previous studies by Amanuma et al. (1986) point in a similar direction. The optically void lipid droplets contain hardly any immunocytochemically discernible apo B, and it can be concluded that, in a sclerotic vessel, LDL is taken up from the surrounding tissue for metabolism by macrophages. Since these macrophages appear loaded with fat, the process must be effected either directly by phagocytosis or possibly by an alternative metabolic (receptor) pathway. Our in situ findings and their interpretation are supported by recent in vitro studies by Haberland et al. (1990) that resulted in parallel conclusions. Normal cells, when confronted by high concentrations of LDL, will present specific receptors for counterregulation, thereby avoiding excess fat uptake.

The apparent predisposition of macrophages to take up fat and undergo transformation into foam cells may be explained by certain particularities in their lipid metabolism as reported by Brown and Goldstein (1983). Macrophages possess a specific LDL receptor ("scavenger" or acetyl receptor) which allows for unlimited cholesterol uptake on account of its mode of synthesis: unlike the synthesis of specific LDL receptors in other cell types, it does not undergo automatic counterregulation when the cholesterol level is rising.

According to current knowledge, macrophages are not the only cells to display an alternative LDL metabolism: in fact indirect, cell-mediated LDL modification may take place in endothelial and smooth muscle cells (STEINBERG et al. 1989). The latter process entails the oxidation of multiple unsaturated fatty acids in LDL lipids, whereby the LDL molecule undergoes distinct structural and functional alterations. Such changes include fragmentation of apo B (which, compared to native LDL, contains a reduced set of certain amino acids) and chemotaxis for circulating monocytes, and will ultimately lead to foam cell formation due to increased fat uptake via the scavenger receptor. It might be expected that specific evidence for apo B would also be found in smooth muscle cells, but in fact such evidence exists only in macrophages.

We feel that any ultrastructural apo B labeling, low and diffuse as it is, and occurring only in functionally impaired myocytes, should be interpreted as a mere diffusion phenomenon balancing the disparity between the apo B concentration in the cell interior and its extracellular abundance. It must also be considered whether our antibodies against apo B may fail to recognize altered apo B epitopes in metabolized LDL cholesterol. This tentative idea is supported by light microscopic studies performed by PALINSKI et al. (1989, 1990): In Watanabe heritable hyperlipidemic (WHHL) rabbits, aortic tissue was investigated with specific antibodies against oxidatively modified apo B and native apo B. Both antibodies showed an approximately similar distribution pattern in extracellular spaces. The antibody against oxidatively modified apo B, however, showed distinct intracytoplasmic staining in macrophages, whereas the other antibody evoked hardly any intracellular reaction. Nevertheless, the fact that apo B can be specifically demonstrated in macrophages by our serum militates against this interpretation. Moreover, consideration must also be given to the possibility that foam cell macrophages, unlike smooth muscle cells, might contain sufficient unmodified apo B epitopes in their LDL to enable our marker to remain binding. The results of HASHIMOTO et al. (1988) regarding cholesterol demonstration in smooth muscle cells agree with this interpretation.

Recent studies (HOFF et al. 1990) indicate aggregation of LDL when it is present in the high concentration observed in extracellular locations in cases of advanced atherosclerosis. The aggregation is probably effected by intermolecular linking with aldehydes released during oxidation of LDL particles. In contrast to another group showing only smaller monomeric LDL particles, and which is internalized via scavenger receptors the larger aggregates are swallowed by phagocytosis, a mechanism independent of LDL or the scavenger receptor system. Smooth muscle cells, however, are unable to take up such aggregates. In addition, LDL aggregates may join the larger components of the plaque, or may form insoluble complexes with smaller aggregates that may also be phagocytosed. These results of HOFF et al. (1990) may be readily correlated with our results from specific macrophage staining.

We may thus infer that the morphologic methods presently available can demonstrate only the type of apo B that represents the common terminal step in intracellular metabolism, that is, lysosomal digestion. In all preceeding steps the apo B concentration is obviously too low to permit immunomorphologic assessment. In addition to alterations of the apo B epitope, this may be due either to the rapidity of previous steps of the metabolic pathway and/or to problems in the workup of tissue for morphologic examination. Potential alternatives are sought in the raising of antibodies against modified, e.g., oxidated LDL (STEINBERG et al. 1989) and against prefixed antigens (HARRACH and ROBENEK 1990) for use in ultracryosectioning (HARRACH et al. 1989). Further promising techniques are cryofixation and cryosubstitution, which will not only preserve protein components but also maintain lipids in their original location within the tissue in a way that is not possible with routine methods of preparation (HUMBEL and SCHWARZ 1989). With these pioneer techniqes, our team has obtained some promising initial results in this field (VOLLMER and ROESSNER 1990).

In the course of the development of atherosclerosis, mechanisms of unregulated cholesterol uptake in macrophages finally lead to fat overloading. However, according to the findings of GERRITY (1981a,b) and WATANABE et al. (1985), some of the macrophages are capable of remigrating into the vascular lumen, thereby retransferring the lipids ingested from the lesion into the blood. These experimental findings are said to be applicable to human conditions, too (STARY 1987b). Thus, the role of macrophages in the vascular wall would be that of a lipid clearance system: monocytes/macrophages entering the atherosclerotic lesion from the blood to phagocytize accumulated lipids will eventually return into the lumen from where they are eliminated together with the incorporated lipids. This would explain the protective effect of macrophages—at least in the early stages of lesion development—which seems to delay the progress of atherosclerosis. Similar mechanisms are postulated for RTA.

Foam cells retained within the lesion are ultimately overburdened with intracytoplasmic lipid deposits and will succumb necrosis. According to STARY (1983, 1987a,b, 1990a,b), macrophages will thus make up the majority of the necrotic material found at the base of atherosclerotic plaques. This has been confirmed in recent investigations by ROSENFIELD et al. (1990): using specific antibodies against native and oxidated LDL, they found both LDL components in the extracellular matrix of advanced, relatively macrophage-depleted lesions. If the macrophages are destroyed, the previously ingested cholesterol is released and may, like the simultaneously released lysosomal enzymes, additionally damage the surrounding tissue of the arterial wall. A further mechanism involved in such damage is the secretion of factors promoting the migration of smooth muscle cells from the media into the intima, thereby hastening the development of lesions not only in CAS but also in RTA (ROGERS et al. 1986; ROSS 1986, 1990; GLENN and ROSS 1981; MUNRO and COTRAN 1988.

To recapitulate the main points in this context:

1. In the arterial wall, macrophages obviously ingest increasing amounts of LDL from the surrounding tissue, and proceed to lysosomal metabolism in a demonstrable degree.

2. This unregulated LDL uptake induces fat overloading and is effected in situ by phagocytosis and/or by alternative (receptor-mediated) metabolic pathways.
3. In the early phase of arteriosclerotic changes in the vascular wall, macrophages may thus serve as a transitory lipid clearance system.
4. Along with the progression of the vascular lesion, the protective mechanism against excess cholesterol uptake increasingly fails; macrophages will perish, and atherogenic lipids will be accumulated in the arterial wall in addition to those deposited by insudation and transcytosis.
5. In situ, macrophages play a leading role in local LDL metabolism within the arterial wall.

5 Summary, Conclusions, and Outlook

In CAS, as in RTA, it has been established that lipids and their metabolism by various local or immigrating cells play a decisive role in the very complex interrelations involved in the development of arteriosclerosis. Particular importance is attributed to the application of modern functional morphologic techniques on the light and electron microscopic level which have helped to elucidate in situ the local lipid metabolism of the involved cells in both diseases. This is of particular interest since previous information on cholesterol-bearing lipoproteins had been based mainly on plasma levels and in vitro investigations, whereas their distribution in situ, i.e., in the affected arterial walls, had hardly been ascertained.

Under normal conditions, all pathways of lipoprotein metabolism are closely interrelated, and their fine tuning and interdependence is similarly observed in the vascular walls. A grave change occurs under pathologic conditions (Fig. 16): Hyperlipidemia, due to whichever etiologic factor, may lead to endothelial dysfunction even without the presence of any other risk factor. Atherogenic LDL and the opposing HDL are both capable of increasingly permeating the vascular wall, by both transcytosis and insudation. In this context, apo B represents the main structural component of LDL and is found almost exclusively in extracellular locations in advanced vascular lesions of both CAS and RTA. It is subsequently found in foam cells of mostly histiocytic origin. In contrast, apo A-I and A-II, the main structural components of HDL, are also found intracellularly in smooth muscle cells at a very early stage of the lesion.

Apolipoprotein deposits accumulate in deeper intimal layers of the extracellular matrix where the lamina elastica interna obviously acts—especially in RTA—as a kind of barrier to prevent the intrusion of apolipoprotein deposits into the media, at least for some time. In advanced lesions, the deposits will reach the deeper medial layers, too.

Normally, LDL serve to supply cholesterol to the cells of the arterial wall, and are taken up in well-regulated fashion mainly via LDL receptors. This

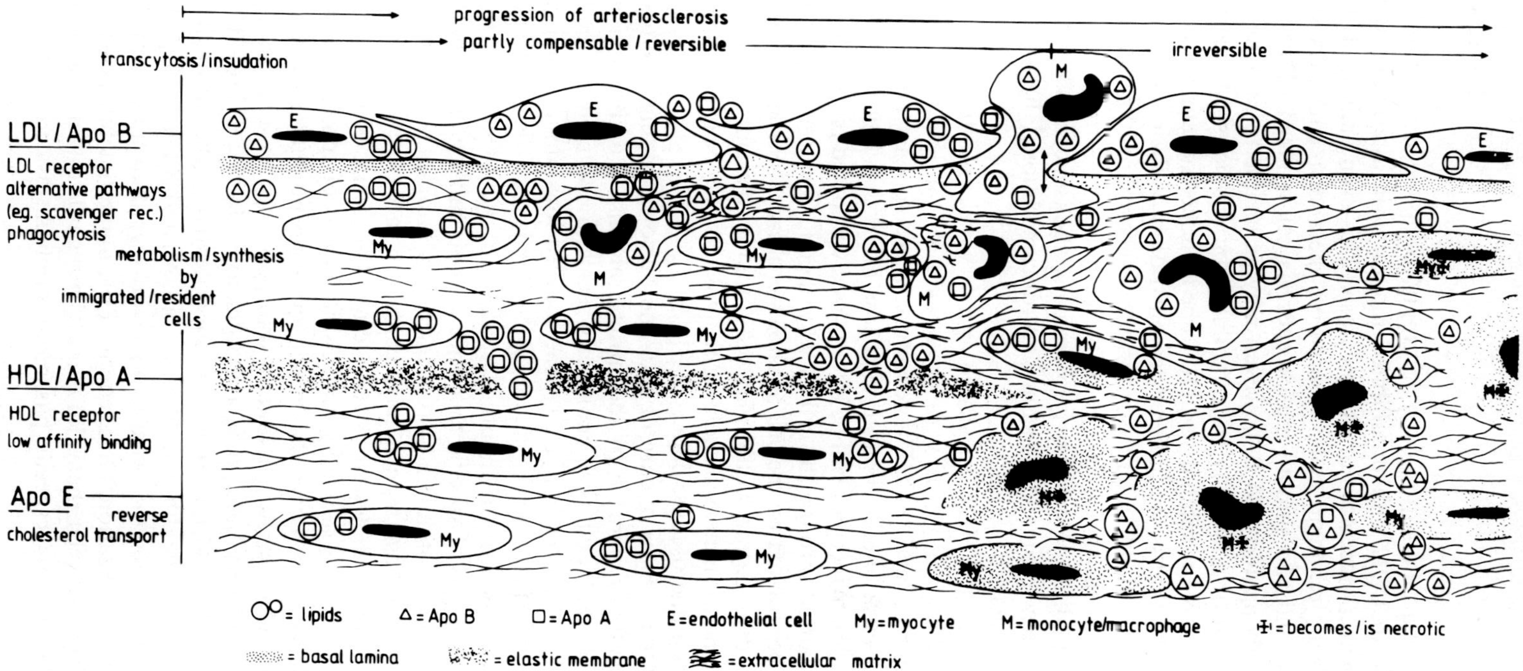

Fig. 16. Lipid metabolism of the vascular wall in CAS and RTA

mode of accumulation does not apply to monocytes/macrophages, which will taken up LDL with uninhibited intensity via alternative pathways such as "scavenger" receptors or phagocytosis. This eventually leads to the formation of histiocytic foam cells. Alternative metabolic pathways of LDL exist in endothelial and smooth muscle cells via cell-induced LDL modification. Our antibody against apo B, however, may be unable to recognize apo B epitopes provoked or altered by LDL modification. Obviously, foam cell macrophages still possess enough native LDL to be identified immunocytochemically by our antibody, that is, by indirect demonstration of their main component, apo B. We feel entitled to infer from our ultrastructural results that monocytes/macrophages are in fact capable of synthesizing apo B in the vascular wall itself. Our in situ findings confirm the lysosomal metabolism of apo B in these cells, because when they ultimately become necrotic, additional lipid deposits appear in extracellular locations.

Currently, HDL-associated apo A, which is initially found extracellularly and subsequently (i.e., with progression of the lesion) also intracellularly, is thought to bind via HDL receptors where apo A-I and A-II serve to release excess intracellular cholesterol. Those HDL that have been recognized by the appropriate receptor will be internalized via coated pits or coated vesicles. HDL transported through the cell by way of endosomes take up cholesterol and will then be secreted by the cell as cholesterol-laden particles. Normally, lysosomal HDL degradation would play but a minor role, but the mechanism is altered when there is increased cholesterol uptake, as may be gathered from our immunoelectron microscopic data.

On the basis of current data and our own findings, we may also postulate the synthesis of apo A by the intramural cells. In addition of HDL internalization, a cellular efflux of cholesterol seems to occur due to the binding of HDL merely to the cell surface, i.e. the socalled low affinity binding. This may lead to intracellular transfer of atherogenic lipids towards the cell membrane, as was observed in vitro in endothelial cells and myocytes. While the HDL receptor mechanism is of specific relevance to macrophages in vitro, this second mode of accumulation might also occur in situ in other cell populations.

Macrophage models have confirmed in vitro the synthesis and release of apo E under cholesterol overloading. This seems also to occur in vivo in the arterial wall, as shown by our in situ findings of apo E in histiocytic foam cells. Evidence of apo E was also seen in lipid-bearing smooth muscle cells. Accordingly, so-called reverse cholesterol transport must be of considerable importance even in vessels undergoing arteriosclerotic change, where it is involved in local metabolism and the conveyance of potentially atherogenic lipoproteins.

Despite the different etiology of CAS and RTA, their pathogenetic history obviously takes the same course with regard to intramural lipid distribution and metabolization. On account of the numerous functional and morphologic parallels between them, RTA may be regarded as a kind of human model of CAS that permits specific pathologic mechanisms and their complex interactions to be studied and understood much better than is possible during the slow development of CAS.

Acknowledgements. This work was supported by Deutsche Forschungsgemeinschaft grant V0 386/1.

References

Alexander K (1984) Krankheiten der Arterien. In: Siegenthaler W, Kaufmann W, Hornborstel H, Waller HD (ed) Lehrbuch der Inneren Medizin. Thieme, Stuttgart, pp 2.2–2.30

Amanuma K, Kanaseki T, Ikeuchi Y, Ohkuma S, Takano T (1986) Studies on fine structure and location of lipids in quick-freeze replicas of atherosclerotic aorta of WHHL rabbits. Virchows Arch [A] 410:231–238

Basu SK, Brown MS, Ho YK, Havel RJ, Goldstein JL (1981) Mouse macrophages synthesize and secrete a protein resembling apolipoprotein E. Proc Natl Acad Sci USA 78:7545–7549

Basu SK, Ho YK, Brown MS, Bilheimer DW, Anderson RGW, Goldstein JL (1982) Biochemical and genetic studies of the apoprotein E secreted by mouse macrophages and human monocytes. J Biol Chem 257:9788–9795

Bedossa P, Poynard T, Abella A, Paraf F, Lemaigre G, Martin E (1989) Localization of apolipoprotein A-I and apolipoprotein A-II in human atherosclerotic arteries. Arch Pathol Lab Med 113:777–780

Bondjers G, Wiklund O, Fager G, Camejo EH, Camejo G (1990) Transfer of lipoproteins from plasma to the cell populations of the normal and atherosclerotic tissue. Eur Heart J 11 [Suppl E]:158–163

Brown MS, Goldstein JL (1983) Lipoprotein metabolism in the macrophage: implications for cholesterol deposition in atherosclerosis. Annu Rev Biochem 52:223–261

Brown MS, Goldstein JL (1985) Arteriosklerose und Cholesterin: Die Rolle der LDL-Rezeptoren. Spektrum der Wissenschaft 1:96–106

Camejo G, Rosengren B, Olson U, Lopez F, Olofson SO, Westerlund C, Bondjers G (1990) Molecular basis of the association of arterial proteoglycans with low density lipoproteins: its effect on the structure of the lipoprotein particle. Eur Heart J 11 [Suppl E]:164–173

Carter RS, Siegel RJ, Chai AU, Fishbein MC (1987) Immunohistochemical localization of apolipoproteins A-I and B in human carotid arteries. J Pathol 153:31–36

Driscoll DM, Getz CS (1984) Extrahepatic synthesis of apolipoprotein E. J Lipid Res 25:1368

Feldman DL, Hoff HF, Gerrity RG (1984) Immunhistochemical localization of apoprotein B in aortas from hyperlipemic swine. Arch Pathol Lab Med 108:817–822

Francone OL, Fielding CJ (1990) Initial steps in reverse cholesterol transport: the role of short-lived cholesterol acceptors. Eur Heart J 11 [Suppl E]: 218–234

Gendre PMJ, Bounader-Bechennec FM (1989) Freeze-fracture study of the intramembrane particle density in the aortic smooth muscle cell plasmalemma of rabbits fed an atherogenic diet. Atherosclerosis 76:1–7

Gerrity RG (1981a) The role of the monocyte in atherogenesis. I. Transition of blood-borne monocytes into foam cells in fatty lesions. Am J Pathol 103:181–190

Gerrity RG (1981b) The role of the monocyte in atherogenesis. II. Migration of foam cells from atherosclerotic lesions. Am J Pathol 103:191–200

Getz GS, Mazzone T, Soltys P, Bates SR (1988) Atherosclerosis and apoprotein E. Arch Pathol Lab Med 112:1048–1055

Glenn KC, Ross R (1981) Human monocyte-derived growth factor(s) for mesenchymal cells activation of secretion of endotoxin and concavalin A. Cell 25:603–615

Goldstein JL, Brown MS (1977) The low-density lipoprotein pathway and its relation to atherosclerosis. Annu Rev Biochem 46:897–930

Haberland ME, Fong D, Cheng L (1990) Malondialdehyde, modified lipoproteins, and atherosclerosis. Eur Heart J 11 [Suppl E]:100–104

Harrach B, Robenek H (1990) Polyclonal antibodies against prefixed apolipoprotein A-I: an approach to circumventing fixation-induced loss of antigenicity in immunocytochemistry. Arteriosclerosis 10:564–578

Harrach B, Robenek H, Vollmer E, Roessner A, Bosse A, Drescher H, Böcker W (1989) Immunelektronenmikroskopische Lokalisation von Apolipoproteinen in Zellkulturen und dem arteriosklerotischen Plaque. Verh Dtsch Ges Pathol 73:675

Harris KPG, Russell GJ, Parvin SD, Veitch PS (1986) Alterations in lipid and carbohydrate metabolism attributable to cyclosporin A in renal transplant recipients. Br Med J 292:16

Hashimoto S, Wong H, Blissard D, Anderson D (1988) Cholesteryl ester accumulation in smooth muscle cells after uptake of necrotic products from atherosclerotic lesions. Exp Mol Pathol 49:196–205

Hegele RA (1989) Lipoprotein (a): an emerging risk factor for atherosclerosis. Can J Cardiol 5:263–267

Ho YK, Brown MS, Goldstein JL (1980) Hydrolysis and excretion of cytoplasmic cholesteryl esters by macrophages: stimulation by high density lipoproteins and other agents. J Lipid Res 21:391–398

Hoff HF, Gaubatz JW (1975) Ultrastructural localization of plasma lipoproteins in human intracranial arteries. Virchows Arch [A] 369:111–121

Hoff HF, Gaubatz JW (1977) Ultrastructural localization of apolipoprotein B in human aortic and coronary atherosclerotic plaques. Exp Mol Pathol 26:214–227

Hoff HF, Heideman CL, Jackson RL, Bayardo RJ, Kim HS, Gotto AM (1975a) Localization patterns of plasma apolipoproteins in human atherosclerotic lesions. Circ Res 37:72–79

Hoff HF, Lie JT, Titus JL, Byardo RJ, Jackson RL, De Bakey ME, Gotto AM (1975b) Lipoprotein in atherosclerotic lesions. Arch Pathol Lab Med 99:253–258

Hoff HF, O'Neil J, Pepin JM, Cole TB (1990) Macrophage uptake of cholesterol-containing particles derived from LDL and isolated from atherosclerotic lesions. Eur Heart J 11 [Suppl E]:105–113

Humbel B, Schwarz H (1989) Freeze substitution for immunochemistry. In: Verkleij AJ, Leunissen JLM (eds) Immunogold labeling in cell biology. CRC Press, Boca Raton, FL., pp 115–134

Kashyap ML (1989) Basic considerations in the reversal of atherosclerosis: significance of high-density lipoprotein in stimulating reverse cholesterol transport. Am J Cardiol 63:56H–59H

Kasiske BL (1988) Risk factors for accelerated atherosclerosis in renal transplant recipients. Am J Med 84:985–992

Kasiske BL, Umen AJ (1987) Persistent hyperlipidemia in renal transplant patients. Medicine 66:309–316

Kobayashi N, Okubo M, Marumo F, Uchida H (1983) De novo development of hypercholesterolemia and elevated high-density lipoprotein cholesterol: apoprotein A_1 ratio in patients with chronic renal failure following kidney transplantation. Nephron 35:239–240

Linden T, Wiklund O, Fager G, Olofsson SO, Bondjers G (1986) A new microimmunoassay for apolipoprotein B in arterial tissue. Atherosclerosis 62:227–237

Lowry RP, Soltys G, Peters L, Mangel R, Sniderman AD (1987) Type II hyperlipoproteinemia, hyperapobetalipoproteinemia, and hyperalphalipoproteinemia following renal transplantation: implications for atherogenic risk. Transplant Proc 19/4:3426–3430

Mawhinney TP, Augustyn JM, Fritz KE (1978) Glycosaminoglycan-lipoprotein complexes from aortas of hypercholesterolemic rabbits. I. Isolation and characterization. Atherosclerosis 31:155–167

Mitchinson MJ, Carpenter KLH, Ball RY (1990) The role of macrophages in human atherosclerosis. In: Glagov S, Newman WP, Schaffer AS (eds) Pathobiology of the human atherosclerotic plaque. Springer, Berlin Heidelberg New York, pp 121–128

Mora R, Lupu F, Simionescu N (1987) Prelesional events in atherogenesis. Atherosclerosis 67:143–154

Mora R, Lupu F, Simionescu N (1989) Cytochemical localization of β-lipoproteins and their components in successive stages of hyperlipidemic atherogenesis or rabbit aorta. Atherosclerosis 79:183–195

Munro JM, Cotran RS (1988) Biology of disease. The pathogenesis of atherosclerosis, atherogenesis and inflammation. Lab Invest 58:249–261

Nakashima Y, Matsushima T, Takahara K, Kuroiwa A, Nakamura M (1985) The analysis of lipids and glycosaminoglycans of low-density-lipoprotein-glycosaminoglycan complexes isolated from normal, fatty streaks, and fibrous plaque of human aortic intima. Int Angiol 4:487–493

Nicoll A, Duffield R, Lewis B (1981) Flux of plasma lipoproteins into human arterial intima. Atherosclerosis 39:229–242

Niendorf A, Rath M, Wolf K, Peters S, Arps H, Beisiegel U, Dietel M (1990a) Morphological

detection and quantification of lipoprotein (a) deposition in atheromatous lesions of human aorta and coronary arteries. Virchows Arch [A] 417:105 111
Niendorf A, Rath M, Wolf K, Arps H, Beisiegel U, Dietel M (1990b) Morphometrische Analyse der Ablagerungen des Lipoproteins (a) in atheromatösen Läsionen der Aorta und der Koronararterien. In: Assmann G, Betz E, Heinle H, Schulte H (eds) Neue Aspekte aus Zellbiologie und Molekulargenetik, Epidemiologie und Klinik. Vieweg, Braunschweig-Wiesbaden, pp 214–219
Palinski W, Rosenfeld ME, Ylä-Herttuala S, et al. (1989) Low density lipoprotein undergoes oxidative modification in vivo. Proc Natl Acad Sci USA 86:1372–1376
Palinski W, Ylä-Herttuala S, Rosenfeld ME, et al. (1990) Antisera and monoclonal antibodies specific for epitopes generated during oxidative modification of low density lipoprotein. Arteriosclerosis 10:325–335
Radhakrishnamurthy B, Srinivasan SR, Vijayagopal P, Berenson GS (1990) Arterial wall proteoglycans – biological properties related to pathogenesis of atherosclerosis. Eur Heart J 11 [Suppl E]:148–157
Rath M, Niendorf A, Reblin T, Dietel M, Krebber HJ, Beisiegel U (1989) Detection and quantification of lipoprotein(a) in the arterial wall of 107 coronary bypass patients. Arteriosclerosis 9:579–592
Rogers KA, Hoover RL, Castellot JJ, Robinson JM, Karnovsky MJ (1986) Dietary cholesterol-induced changes in macrophage characteristics. Relationship to atherosclerosis. Am J Pathol 125:284–291
Rosenfeld ME, Palinski W, Ylä-Herttuala S, Butler S, Witzum JL (1990) Distribution of oxidation-specific lipoprotein adducts and apolipoprotein B in atherosclerotic lesions of varying severity from WHHL rabbits. Arteriosclerosis 10:336–349
Ross R (1986) The pathogenesis of atherosclerosis—an update. N Engl J Med 314:488–500
Ross R (1990) Mechanisms of atherosclerosis—a review. Adv Nephrol 19:79–86
Salinas-Madrigal L, Pardo-Mindan FJ, Llausas-Magana E, Erro-Aguirre E (1988) Complications of renal transplant: a morphologic evaluation. Semin Diagn Pathol 5:80–103
Salisbury BGJ, Falcone DJ, Minick CR (1985) Insoluble low density lipoprotein-proteoglycan complexes enhance cholesteryl ester accumulation in macrophages. Am J Pathol 120:6–11
Schmitz G, Robenek H, Lohmann U, Assmann G (1985a) Interaction of high density lipoproteins with cholesteryl ester-laden macrophages: biochemical and morphological characterization of cell surface receptor binding, endocytosis and resecretion of high density lipoproteins by macrophages. EMBO J 4:613–622
Schmitz G, Niemann R, Brennhausen B, Krause R, Assmann G (1985b) Regulation of high density lipoprotein receptors in cultured macrophages. EMBO J 4:2773–2779
Schmitz G, Robenek H, Assmann G (1987) Role of high-density lipoprotein receptor cycle in macrophage cholesterol metabolism. Atherosclerosis Rev 16:95–107
Schmitz G, Brüning T, Williamson E, Nowicka G (1990) The role of HDL in reverse cholesterol transport and its disturbances in Tangier disease and HDL deficiency with xanthomas. Eur Heart J 11 [Suppl E]:197–211
Shekhonin B, Tararak EM, Samokhin GP, et al. (1990) Visualization of apo B, fibrinogen/fibrin, and fibronectin in the intima of normal human aorta and large arteries and during atherosclerosis. Atherosclerosis 82:213–226
Sjöstrand FS (1990) Common sense in electron microscopy. About cryofixation, freeze-substitution, low temperature embedding, and low denaturation embedding. J Struct Biol 103:135–139
Slotte JP (1990) HDL receptors and cholesterol efflux from parenchymal cells. Eur Heart J 11 [Suppl E]:212–217
Smith EB (1990) Transport, interactions and retention of plasma proteins in the intima: the barrier function of the internal elastic lamina. Eur Heart J 11 [Suppl E]:72–81
Smith EB, Staples EM (1980) Distribution of plasma proteins across the human aortic wall. Atherosclerosis 37:578–590
Srinivasan SR, Vijayagopal P, Dalfers ER, Abbate B, Radhakrishnamurthy B, Berenson GS (1986) Low density lipoprotein retention by aortic tissue. Atherosclerosis 62:201–208
Stary HC (1983) Macrophages in coronary artery, in aortic intima, and in atherosclerotic lesions of children and young adults up to age 29. In: Schettler FG, Gotto AM, Middelhoff G, Habenicht ARJ, Jurutka KR (eds) Sixth international symposium on atherosclerosis. Springer, New York Berlin Heidelberg, pp 462–466
Stary HC (1987a) Macrophages, macrophage foam cells, and eccentric intimal thickening in the coronary arteries of young children. Atherosclerosis 64:91–108

Stary HC (1987b) Evolution and progression of atherosclerosis in the coronary arteries of children and adults. In: Bates SR, Gangloff ED (eds) Atherosclerosis and aging. Springer, New York Berlin Heidelberg, pp 20–36

Stary HC (1990a) Changes in the cells of atherosclerotic lesions as advanced lesions evolve in coronary arteries of children and young adults. In: Glagov S, Newman WP, Schaffer SA (eds) Pathobiology of the human atherosclerotic plaque. Springer, Berlin Heidelberg New York, pp 93–106

Stary HC (1990b) The sequence of cell and matrix changes in atherosclerotic lesions in the first forty years of life. Eur Heart J 11 [Suppl E]:3–19

Steinberg D, Parthasarathy S, Carew TE, Khoo JC, Witzum JL (1989) Beyond cholesterol. Modifications of low-density lipoprotein that increase its atherogenicity. N Engl J Med 320:915–923

Steinmetz A, Kaffarnik H (1989) Lipoproteinrezeptoren und Apolipoprotein. Diagnose Labor 4:157–170

Tokuyasu KT (1984) Immuno-ultracryomicrotomy. In: Polak JM, Varndell JM (eds) Immunolabeling for electron microscopy. Elsevier, Amsterdam, pp 71–82

Vathsala A, Weinberg RB, Schoenberg L, et al. (1989) Lipid abnormalities in renal transplant recipients treated with cyclosporine. Transplant Proc 21:3670–3673

Vijayagopal P, Srinivasan SR, Radhakrishnamurthy B, Berenson GS (1981) Interaction of serum lipoproteins and a proteoglycan from bovine aorta. J Biol Chem 256:8234–8241

Vollmer E, Roessner A (1990) Neue Techniken für die feingewebliche Ultrastrukturanalyse. Arb. Gem. Rhein. Westf. Pathologen, Bochum, March 1990. Ber Pathol 111:372

Vollmer E, Roessner A, Wuisman P, Härle A, Grundmann E (1989a) The proliferation behavior of bone tumors investigated with the monoclonal antibody Ki-67. In: Roessner A (ed) biological characterization of bone tumors. Springer, Berlin Heidelberg New York (Current Topics in Pathology, vol 80:91–114)

Vollmer E, Brust J, Roessner A, et al. (1989b) Immunhistochemische Untersuchungen zur Verteilung von Apolipoproteinen in der arteriosklerotischen Gafäßwand menschlicher Arterien. Verh Dtsch Ges Pathol 73:445

Vollmer E, Roessner A, Bosse A, et al. (1991a) Immunohistochemical double labeling of macrophages, smooth muscle cells, and apolipoprotein E in the atherosclerotic Plaque. Path Res Pract 187:184–188

Vollmer E, Bosse A, Bögeholz J, et al. (1991b) Apolipoproteins and immunohistochemical differentiation of cells in the arterial wall of kidneys in transplant arteriopathy. Pathol Res Pract 187:957–962

Vollmer E, Brust J, Roessner A, et al. (1991c) Distribution patterns of apolipoproteins A_1, A_2 and B in the wall of atherosclerotic vessels. Virchows Arch [A] 419:79–88

Watanabe T, Hirata M, Yoshikawa Y, Nagafuchi Y, Toyoshima H, Watanabe T (1985) Role of macrophages in atherosclerosis. Lab Invest 53:80–90

Weisgraber KH, Mahley RW (1980) Subfractionation of human high density lipoproteins by heparin-sepharose affinity chromatography. J Lipid Res 21:316–325

Ylä-Herttuala S, Solakivi T, Hirvonen J, et al. (1987) Glycosaminoglycans and apolipoproteins B and A-I in human aortas. Arteriosclerosis 7:333–340

Yomantas S, Elner VM, Schaffner T, Wissler RW (1984) Immunhistochemical localisation of apolipoprotein B in human atherosclerotic lesions. Arch Pathol Lab Med 108:374–378

Yutani C, Go S, Imakita M, Ishibashi-Ueda H, Hatanaka K, Yamamoto A (1987) Autopsy findings in two patients with homozygous familial hypercholesterolemia. Special references to apolipoprotein B localization and internalization defect of low density lipoprotein. Acta Pathol Jpn 37:1489–1504

Collagens in Atherosclerotic Vessel Wall Lesions

J. RAUTERBERG, E. JAEGER, and M. ALTHAUS

1 Introduction

The proper function of the arterial wall depends decisively on its extracellular matrix, a highly complex structure of various proteins, glycoproteins, and proteoglycans. Morphologic and functional criteria permit a number of structural components to be defined, e.g., collagen fibrils, elastic fibers and membranes, microfibrils, and basement membranes, each of which consists of several different macromolecules. This matrix is synthesized and secreted mainly by smooth muscle cells in the medial and intimal layers and by fibroblasts and smooth

Current Topics in Pathology
Volume 87, Vollmer/Roessner (Eds.)

muscle cells in the adventitia. The structural components of the extracellular matrix are formed by specific interaction of the freshly synthesized macromolecules with other freshly synthesized or with already deposited macromolecules. Strict regulation of synthesis as well as of degradation of matrix components seem absolutely essential if the functional state of the arterial wall is to be maintained throughout the many years of an individual's life. The mechanisms of this regulation are poorly understood. They must include downregulation on a very low state over long periods of time, but also very rapid and effective enhancement of synthesis and degradation in tissue remodeling after injury as well as slight changes of metabolic rates in adaptive processes, e.g., if strengthening of the arterial wall becomes necessary during a prolonged increase in blood pressure.

One of the main characteristic features of the atherosclerotic vessel wall is a dysfunction of downregulation of the synthesis of extracellular matrix proteins, mainly in the intimal layer. In the intimal plaque the predominant cell type is a biosynthetic active phenotype, the so-called synthetic phenotype, of smooth muscle cells; high amount of a collagen-rich extracellular matrix are formed. Moreover, deposition of blood-derived lipoproteins, intensive invasion of the plaque area by blood monocytes, and differentiation of these monocytes into macrophages and lipid-laden foam cells take place. These cellular infiltrates certainly contribute considerably to the stimulation of vessel wall cells, intensifying their synthesis of matrix proteins.

One of the essential prerequisites for a better understanding of the processes leading from the well-controlled state of the normal artery to the apparent suspension of controlling mechanisms in the atherosclerotic vessel wall is a better knowledge of structural components of the matrix in the normal and diseased state. Though numerous data are available on the occurrence and local distribution of structural proteins, their role in the architecture of certain structural components and exact functional meaning are far from clear. In this review we will try to elucidate the situation, taking the protein family of collagens as an example. Whereas the function of some members of this family, e.g., the fibril-forming collagens, type I and type III, is relatively well known, the function of other types is more or less unclear, and it is not even known whether some of the recently discovered collagen types occur in the arterial wall or whether still undiscovered collagenous molecules may exist in this tissue.

The various collagen types play very different roles in the formation of supramolecular structures in the extracellular matrix of the vessel wall. Recent research has revealed interesting data on specific interactions between collagens and other proteins which are essential to the formation of structural matrix components, e.g., the interaction between type IV collagen, nidogen, and laminin in forming basement membranes. But overall, knowledge about specific affinities between macromolecules in the extracellular space is quite fragmentary.

Another field of interest which has emerged during recent years is the important role of matrix components in the regulation of cellular activities (NUISGENS et al. 1984). In this respect collagens seem to play an outstanding role, for instance in the downregulation of biosynthetic and proliferative activities of vessel wall cells (THIE et al. 1991). The basis of most kinds of cell–matrix interaction is specific affinities between distinct structural domains on the extracellular molecules and specific receptors on the cell surface; at present, great research efforts are being made to elucidate the molecular basis of cell–matrix interactions. This may be illustrated by the recent establishment of a new research program by the German Research Foundation named: "Molecular basis of cell–matrix interactions in biology and medicine." At present, the pathologic importance of disturbances of cell–matrix interactions can only be imagined and this subject will certainly be a major topic for research in the near future.

2 The Collagens of the Normal Vessel Wall and Their Participation in Structural Components of the Extracellular Matrix

The term "collagen," which initially described the protein which forms collagen fibers, is now used for a family of extracellular structural proteins which have in common a typical and exceptional kind of secondary and tertiary structure,

Table 1. Extracellular matrix of vessel walls: morphologically defined structures and the macromolecules from which they are formed

Morphologically defined structures	Macromolecules
Collagen fibrils	Type I collagen Type III collagen Type V collagen
Fibril-associated components	Type XII collagen Type XIV collagen Decorin Fibronectin
Microfibrils (beaded fibrils)	Type VI collagen
Linkage structures	Fibronectin Fibrillin Undulin Tenascin Thrombospondin and others
Elastin fibrils and membranes	Elastin Fibrillin
Basement membranes	Type IV collagen Laminin Nidogen BM 40 (SPARC) Type VIII collagen (?)
"Structureless ground substance"	Proteoglycans Hyaluronic acid

the triple helix. Nearly 30 different gene products have already been identified; they participate in at least 15 different molecules (for reviews see: KÜHN 1986a,b; BURGESON 1988; VAN DER REST and GARONE 1990; VUORIO and DE COMBRUGGHE 1990; LINSENMAYER 1991; KIELTY et al. 1993). Six of the collagen types have been detected so far in the arterial wall (Table 1). According to the structural components in which they are involved, they can be classified into three groups, following a suggestion made by MILLER (1985).

2.1 Fibril-Forming Collagens

As in most connective tissues, the quantitatively most outstanding group of arterial collagens are the fibril-forming collagens: These collagen molecules participate in the formation of fibers composed of bundles of fibrils which show a typical cross-striation pattern in the electron microscope after staining with heavy metal salts.

The collagen fibril represents the usual functional quaternary structure of type I collagen. It has recently become clear that collagen types III and V participate in the formation of the usual collagen fibrils in most tissues; at present it is not even known whether fibrillar or nonfibrillar structures formed solely by type III or type V collagen exist in vivo. Early reports based on immunohistologic studies (REMBERGER et al. 1975) claiming that the so-called reticulin occurring as small argyrophilic fibrils in the interstitium of several organs represents a tissue form of type III collagen could not be substantiated by later work. HENKEL and GLANVILLE (1982) provided chemical evidence that fibrils formed by type I and type III collagen are present in the arterial wall: They isolated from the insoluble collagen of the tunica media of bovine aorta after tryptic digestion a cross-link-containing peptide in which chains from type I and type III collagen are linked together. Evidence came from the work of FLEISCHMAJER et al. (1983) that type III collagen in skin is—at least partly—built as an incompletely processed molecule into the fibrils, in that they showed by immunohistologic electron microscopy, using gold labeling, fibrils which were decorated by outjutting N-terminal propeptides of type III collagen. As they found this phenomenon only in association with smaller fibrils, they suggested that type III collagen might perform a regulatory function in determining the diameter of collagen fibrils. ROMANIC et al. (1991) demonstrated the formation of composite fibrils from type I collagen and P(N) type III collagen (procollagen type III from which only the C-terminal propeptide has been cleaved) by treating a mixture of procollagen type III and pC collagen type I with procollagen-C-peptidase. In contrast, KEENE et al. (1987) reported for several tissues the presence of type III collagen on banded fibrils, regardless of fibril diameter.

Type V collagen was discovered in peptic extracts from placental tissue and fetal membranes. Since it has a similarly high degree of lysine hydroxylation and glycosylation as type IV collagen, it was initially believed to represent another type of basement membrane collagen. Its molecular structure, however, is more typical of a fibril-forming collagen: an uninterrupted triple helix of exactly the length of collagen types I, II, and III. Fibrils with a cross-striation pattern of 670 nm periodicity, however weak, can be precipitated; the formation of mixed fibrils with type I collagen has been reported (ADACHI and HAYASHI 1986). BIRK et al. (1990) found that, like type III collagen, type V collagen is able to reduce fibril diameter in this in vitro system.

It has been known for some time that the collagen of the corneal stroma, which is deposited in the form of fibrils with extremely uniform diameter, has a relatively high proportion of type V collagen. These fibrils were shown by BIRK et al. (1988) to contain type V collagen which can be visualized by electron microscopy after immunogold labeling only following partial solubilization, suggesting that type V collagen is present only in the internal region of the fibrils. Similar Observations have been made with type II collagen fibrils, in which type XI collagen—a fibril-forming cartilage-specific collagen homologous to type V collagen—can be demonstrated by immunoelectron microscopy only after partial digestion of the fibrils or at ends or breakage points of fibrils (MENDLER et al. 1989). In the normal vessel wall, type V collagen can be extracted from all layers (MURATA et al. 1986). Its occurrence in the arterial wall was also demonstrated by immunohistologic light microscopy (MCCULLAGH et al. 1980; SHEKKONIN et al. 1985, 1987; VOSS and RAUTERBERG 1986). Furthermore, a number of publications on other tissues showed type V collagen to occur in small blood vessels (SCHUPPAN et al. 1986). The reports correspond in describing a fine filamentous expression along smooth muscle cells, with a denser appearance in the subendothelium; they diverge, however, concerning the presence of such filamentous expression in the subendothelial basement membrane.

Until now no positive evidence has been provided to show that type V collagen is involved in the formation of cross-striated collagen fibrils in the vessel wall; so far its function remains more or less unclear. One interesting aspect should be mentioned: the extracellular matrix of the arterial wall contains considerable amounts of thrombospondin. This multidomain glycoprotein, which was first described among the proteins secreted by thrombin-activated platelets, has been shown to be synthesized and secreted in considerable amounts by cultivated endothelial cells and smooth muscle cells (for reviews see: LAWLER and HYNES 1986; SILVERSTEIN et al. 1986; FRAZIER 1987). Recently its presence in the extracellular matrix of vessel walls has been described by WIGHT et al. (1985), FAUVEL-LAFEVE and LEGRAND (1988), and ARBEILLE et al. (1991). A specific affinity of thrombospondin to type V collagen has been described by MUMBY et al. (1984) and it may well be that this interaction is important for the formation of certain structural elements in the vascular extracellular matrix.

Type V collagen occurs in two molecular forms $(\alpha 1(V))_2\ \alpha 2(V)$ (the "two-chain form") and $\alpha(V)\ \alpha 2(V)\ \alpha 3(V)$ (the "three-chain form") (NIYIBIZI et al. 1984). The two-chain form was found to be widespread throughout the organism in nearly all type I-containing matrices. While the occurrence of the three-chain form seems to be more restricted, it forms a relatively large proportion of type V molecules in the endometrial villi of the placenta and in the uterus (ABEDIN et al. 1981; RAUTERBERG and TROYER 1986). Type V collagen in the vessel wall is composed mainly of the two-chain form; the three-chain form has been shown to occur in small amounts in the intima (MURATA et al. 1986).

Conflicting data have been reported regarding the uniformity of vessel wall collagen fibrils. SHIRAISHI et al. (1980) described two populations of fibrils, both of which show increasing diameters up to the age of approximately 20 years, the smaller ones (70% of fibrils) reaching about 28 nm and the larger ones (30% of fibrils), 42 nm. The fibrils of both populations are relatively small as compared to tendon (> 100 nm) or skin fibrils (89.0 ± 12.9 for 20-year-old men). Other authors have described the existence of only one population of fibrils with relatively small diameter ranges in the aortic media of rats or cattle (RASPANTI et al. 1989). Comparison of electron micrographs of the surfaces of collagen fibrils from several tissues gained after freeze fracturing showed the existence of two morphologically different types of fibrils: one with strictly unidirectional packing of subfibrils or microfibrils, the other with a helical arrangement (RASPANTI et al. 1989). Those with straight packing occur in skeletal tissues bearing mainly unidirectional forces (tendon, ligament, bone) and seem to be characterized by two chemical peculiarities: they are virtually free of type III collagen and their main form of intermolecular cross-link, pyridinoline or hydroxypyridinoline, is solely derived from lysine or hydroxylysine. The "helical" form of fibrils occurs in all tissues having to provide tensile strength connected to a certain degree of compliance in more than one direction; they are reported to occur in skin, vessel walls, cornea, and the interstitial loose connective tissue of a number of organs. Histidine is involved in the main intermolecular cross-link in the collagen of these tissues, together with lysine and hydoxylysine. The content of collagen type III in tissues containing "helical" fibrils varies from virtually zero in adult cornea (TSENG et al. 1982) to about 40% in the medial layer of the adult aorta (MORTON and BARNES 1982) and up to 50% in fibrotic liver tissue (RAUTERBERG et al. 1982).

As already mentioned, cornea collagen contains, instead of type III collagen, an appreciable amount of type V. At present the question of whether either type III or type V collagen or both may participate in the regulation of fibril formation in the vessel wall remains open.

2.2 Fibril-Associated Collagens

In the course of recent years a new family of collagenous molecules has emerged which also participates in collagen fibril formation and for which the name FACIT collagen (fibril-associated collagen with interrupted triple helices) has been suggested (GORDON and OLSEN 1990). The first described was the cartilage-specific type IX collagen, which was localized on the surface of collagen fibrils by immunoelectron microscopy (VAUGHAN et al. 1988). Recently two further homologous collagens have been characterized (type XII and type XIV collagens) which are associated in a similar way with type I collagen fibrils; they have so far been detected in tendon and skin (GORDON et al. 1989; DUBLET and VAN DER REST 1991). FACIT collagen molecules consist of a shorter and a longer triple-helical region connected by a short nonhelical domain; both ends of the molecules have additional noncollagenous globular domains. The larger of the two triple helices aggregates binds specifically to type I or type II collagen fibrils. FACIT collagens seem to occur in a number of tissues; their occurrence in blood vessels, however, has not been reported to date.

2.3 Basement Membrane Collagens

Endothelial cells and smooth muscle cells in the arterial wall are associated with electron microscopically identifiable basement membranes. The endothelial monolayer is supported by a continuous basement membrane whereas the smooth muscle-associated basement membrane envelops each individual cell. The composition and architecture of basement membranes have been elucidated mainly for epithelial basement membranes. They contain type IV collagen beneath the noncollagenous glycoproteins laminin and nidogen, which together form a 1:1 molecular complex, and at least two proteoheparan sulfates (for reviews see: ABRAHAMSON 1986; TIMPL 1989; LEBLOND and INOUE 1989; INOUE 1989; PAULSSON 1992). There is immunohistologic evidence that the same components are present in both endothelial and smooth muscle cell-associated basement membranes (PALOTIE et al. 1983; SANES et al. 1990).

It was shown recently that, in addition to the well-described type IV collagen molecule, which is formed by two α1(IV) and one α2(IV) chains, there exist isoforms containing novel α(IV) chains, α3(IV), α4(IV), and α5(IV). Occurrence of these chains in arterial tissue has not been reported so far; SANES et al. (1990) noted absence of α3(IV) and α4(IV) from muscle arteries and capillaries. Isoforms have also been described for laminin. The so-called S-laminin replaces the B1 chain in the laminin molecule; S-laminin-containing molecules seem to represent the only form of laminin in muscle capillaries and arteries (SANES et al. 1990). Merosin represents an alternative laminin A chain. Merosin-containing laminin occurs in skeletal muscle basement membranes; it is absent, however, in arterial basement membranes.

Vessel-derived cultivated endothelial cells have been shown to produce another type of collagen, type VIII. This collagen type is also produced by cultivated cornea endothelial cells (SAGE et al. 1982), and it could be chemically (LABERMEYER and KENNEY 1983) and immunohistologically (KAPOOR et al. 1988) localized in Descemet's membrane, a specialized thick basement membrane separating the cornea from the underlying tissues. Whereas type IV collagen is secreted by all endothelial cells so far investigated, the production of type VIII collagen is not a common feature of cultivated endothelial cells, e.g., it is absent from the commonly used human umbilical vein endothelial cell (SAGE 1984) and its production may be linked to certain states of cell activation (IRUELA-ARISPE et al. 1991). Its presence has been demonstrated in extracts from fetal bovine aorta (JANDER et al. 1990). KITTELBERGER et al. (1989) reported immunohistologic evidence for its occurrence in the subendothelium of fetal and adult sheep aortas, whereas KAPOOR et al. (1988) failed to detect it in fetal bovine vessel walls using a monoclonal antibody which reacted with bovine Descemet's membranes. Thus the question remains open as to whether type VIII collagen is a regular or a transient component of the subendothelial basement membrane of blood vessels. In Descemet's membranes, type VIII collagen seems to participate in a special hexagonal framework (SAWADA et al. 1990). To date there has been no report of a similar structure within or associated with any other basement membrane. Consequently it is still unclear whether type VIII collagen is of any significance for the structure and function of vessel wall-specific basement membranes.

2.4 Microfibrillar Collagens: Type VI Collagen

Within the collagen family, type VI collagen represents a type of unique structural matrix molecule: a molecule which may best be described as a multidomain protein, possessing among these domains one with a collagenous triple-helical structure (for review see: RAUTERBERG et al. 1986; TIMPL and ENGEL 1987). It was initially characterized as a collagen ("intima collagen," "short-chain collagen") for methodological reasons, since solubilization by pepsin yields the triple-helical domain, representing approximately 30% of the total molecule. Nondegraded monomeric type VI collagen can be visualized electron microscopically as a dumbbell-like structure bearing two globular domains of approximately equal size on either side of the 100-nm triple-helical domain. The complete evaluation of the amino acid sequence of all three chains of type VI collagen, which has been achieved during recent years, suggests, however, a complicated domain structure for each of the "globules." A number of sequence motifs that also occur in other structural glycoproteins have been established. Each of the $\alpha1$ and $\alpha2$ chains has three motifs homologous to the A-domain of von-Willebrand protein, one in the N- and two in the C-terminal noncollagenous part (for review see COLOMBATTI and BONALDO 1991). The much longer $\alpha3$ chain even has nine von Willebrand A-like domains in the N-terminal and, like $\alpha1$ and $\alpha2$, two in the C-terminal region. In addition, there are three further domains with structural homology to other proteins in the C-terminus of the $\alpha3$ chain: the C3 domain, resembling proline-rich regions in some salivary proteins, the C4 domain homologous to the so-called type III domain of fibronectin, and the mostly C-terminal C5, which resembles some protease inhibitors, e.g., 50% identity to human urinary trypsin inhibitor.

The typical tissue form of type VI collagen, beaded fibrils with beads at a spacing of approximately 100 nm, has been demonstrated by immunogold electron microscopy in several tissues, lying between bundles of collagen fibrils (KEENE et al. 1988). The basic unit of these fibrils is a tetramer formed by parallel aggregation of two dimers which for their part are formed by an overlapping head-to-head aggregation of two monomers. Type VI collagen has unique adhesion properties to other macromolecules of the extracellular matrix (several collagen types and heparin) as well as to a number of cell types (AUMAILLEY et al. 1989). Since collagen affinity is located in the A domain in von-Willebrand protein, and heparin affinity in the III domain of fibronectin, the occurrence of homologous domains in type VI collagen may be linked to these affinities. The cell-binding motif RGD, typical of integrin-mediated cell adhesion, occurs several times within the triple-helical domain of type VI collagen.

Based on these structural and functional data, type VI collagen has been suggested to represent a kind of linkage protein which may be essential for tissue stability and integrity. This may be important especially for a vessel wall, in which the proportion of type VI collagen seems to be relatively high as compared to other tissues, though exact quantitative data are still not available, due mainly to the impossibility of complete solubilization into identifiable fragments.

3 Changes in Collagens in Atherosclerosis

Research on changes in arterial collagens in atherosclerosis has been directed mainly towards fibril-forming collagens. One of the most prominent events in atherosclerosis is indeed the deposition of huge amounts of fibrillar collagen during the formation of fibrous plaques. The development of the typical intimal plaque implies proliferation of smooth muscle cells and their enhanced synthesis of extracellular matrix; in addition, influx and deposition of blood-derived lipoproteins as well as infiltration of blood monocytes and lymphocytes determine the appearance of the atherosclerotic intima.

Characterization of collagens in the normal and atherosclerotic vessel wall has followed different routes. The quantitative ratio of collagen types in the tissue was determined after extraction of the collagens or collagen fragments and quantification after separation into the different types. In combination with determination of the total collagen content by measurement of hydroxyproline in the tissue hydrolysate, quantitative data for the tissue content of single collagen types became available. The local distribution of collagen types has been investigated by immunohistologic methods.

3.1 Quantitative Ratios of Collagen Types in Nonatherosclerotic and Atherosclerotic Human Vessel Walls

In spite of years of research in this field, knowledge of quantitative ratios of collagen types in the nonatherosclerotic and atherosclerotic vessel wall is still incomplete and in some respects controversial (for reviews see: Barnes 1985; Wagner 1990). The main reason is a highly cross-linked state of vessel wall collagen which makes quantitative extraction impossible.

3.1.1 Methods of Collagen Solubilization

Two methods of collagen extraction have been developed, both of which have limited applicability: extraction after limited pepsin digestion and solubilization by cyanogen bromide cleavage.

3.1.1.1 Solubilization by Limited Pepsin Digestion. Pepsin treatment at temperatures considerably below the denaturation point of the triple-helical structure digests the non-triple-helical terminal region of collagen molecules. Since intermolecular cross-links always involve these "telopeptides," their digestion leads to disruption of cross-links so that the collagen molecules become soluble. Peptic extraction is the only method allowing solubilization of appreciable amounts of collagens I, III, and V with intact triple helices from arterial tissues. Type IV collagen also becomes extractable by this method but due to interruptions in the triple helix, several fragments of different size are solubilized. Separation of the different collagen molecules and their constituent polypeptide chains can be achieved by electrophoretic or chromatographic methods; for separation and determination of their quantitative ratio, SDS-polyacrylamide gel electrophoresis (SDS-PAGE) has been the most widely applied method. The most serious disadvantage of peptic extraction is a different degree of solubilization, depending on the degree of cross-linking. Since solubility varies among the collagen types, the quantitative ratio of collagen types in the extract often does not correspond to the ratio in the whole tissue. Murata et al. (1986) showed that type V and type IV collagen were enriched in the first extracts. Type VI collagen is only poorly soluble after pepsin treatment, and it was shown by Trueb et al. (1987) that most published data on type VI collagen contents were underestimations due to this fact.

In the case of type I and type III collagen a considerable portion is solubilized not as monomers but as cross-link-containing oligomers which cannot be separated and identified by gel electrophoresis. The degree of solubilization achieved by sequential peptic extraction has been reported variously: whereas Murata and Motoyama (1990) report 25%–50% solubilization of collagens, Ooshima (1981) achieved 68%–76% and Hansson and Bentley (1983) up to 90% solubilization.

3.1.1.2 Solubilization by Cyanogen Bromide Cleavage. Cyanogen bromide digestion, which cleaves polypeptide chains at the C-terminal side of methionine residues, represents an alternative method yielding a mixture of peptides from which individual peptides can be separated, identified, and quantified. Since only a few sites within the amino acid sequence of collagen polypeptide chains are involved in cross-linking, the yield and electrophoretic mobility of most of the peptides are not influenced in cross-linked collagen. In the case of aortic tissue, collagens are solubilized completely by this method, leaving virtually pure elastin in the nonsolubilized residue. Most of the noncollagenous proteins can be removed prior to cyanogen bromide digestion by extraction with 8 *M* urea; these extracts contain only very small amounts of hydroxyproline. Subsequent cyanogen bromide digestion extracts mainly collagenous material, as is demonstrated by amino acid analysis, whereas elastin remains unsolubilized. The collagen-derived peptides can be further enriched by DEAE chromatography under conditions under which only noncollegenous peptides are retained on the column. The peptide mixture can be separated by PAGE and single bands quantified by densitometry (Weber et al. 1977; Morton and Barnes 1982). So far only ratios of type I to type III collagen have been calculated for cyanogen bromide digests of vessel wall collagen.

3.1.2 Comparison of Atherosclerosis-Related Changes in Type I and Type III Collagens in Arteries of the Elastic and Muscular Type (Aorta Abdominalis and Arteria Poplitea)

Both methods of collagen solubilization have been used for characterizing the quantitative differences between collagen types in normal and atherosclerotic vessels. Nearly all data reported on human vessels refer to the aorta. Recently reviewed results (Wagner 1990; Rauterberg and Jaeger 1992) show two tendencies: (a) in the thickened intima of atherosclerotic vessels, the type I/type III ratio is shifted towards more type I collagen; (b) the occurrence of type V collagen in the intima of the atherosclerotic vessel is enhanced as compared with normal intima (Ooshima 1981; Morton and Barnes 1982; Murata et al. 1986).

As an example of the application of cyanogen bromide digestion for the determination of type I to type III ratios, a comparison between an elastic and a muscular type of artery (aorta abdominalis and arteria poplitea) is described below.

Tissue samples were obtained from autopsies: the upper part of the aorta abdominalis (between the hiatus aorticus diaphragma and the arteria renalis) and the complete arteria poplitea dextra from the same individuals. The tunica intima, media, and adventitia were separated and an aliquot of each used for hydroxyproline determination. The residual material was frozen in liquid nitrogen, homogenized in a freezer mill, and extracted according to the scheme shown in Fig. 1. This procedure essentially follows the method described by

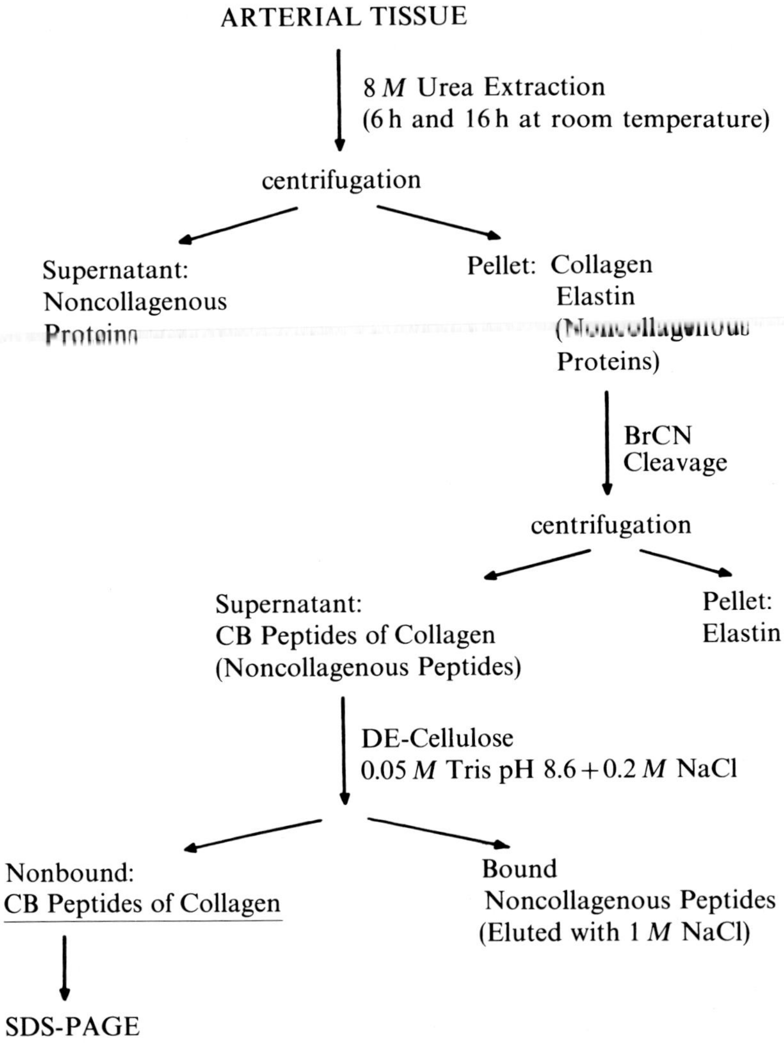

Fig. 1. Scheme of sequential tissue extraction by urea and by cyanogen bromide digestion

WEBER et al. (1979) and by MORTON and BARNES (1982). To eliminate noncollagenous cleavage products, the cyanogen bromide-extracted material—after desalting and lyophilization—was applied to chromatography on a short column of DEAE-cellulose. Nearly all the noncollagenous peptides were bound to the column whereas the collagen-derived peptides were not retained.

The amount of the three fractions obtained (8 *M* urea extract, cyanogen bromide extract, and cyanogen bromide residue) served as a gauge of noncollagenous protein, collagen, and elastin, respectively.

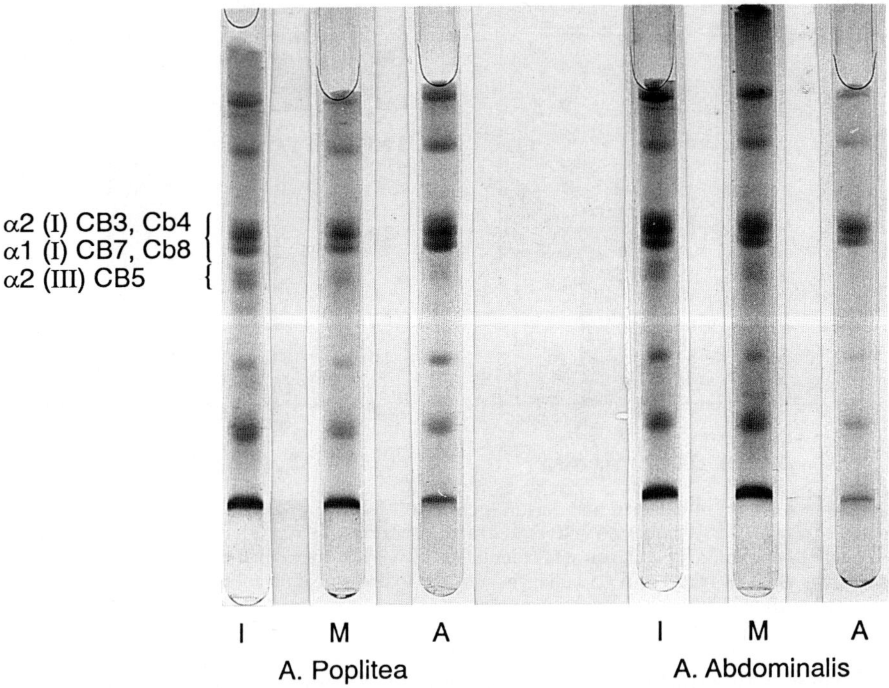

Fig. 2. SDS-polyacrylamide gel electrophoresis of collagen-derived cyanogen bromide peptides from the tunica intima (*I*), tunica media (*M*), and tunica adventitia (*A*) of nonatherosclerotic arteria poplitea and aorta abdominalis. Cyanogen bromide digestion was performed on the urea-extracted tissues; the extract was purified by DEAE-cellulose chromatography prior to electrophoresis as described in the text

The DEAE-cellulose-purified cyanogen bromide extracts were applied to SDS-PAGE and the gels were subjected to densitometry after staining with Coomassie blue. Figure 2 shows as an example the stained gels of the cyanogen bromide digests of the tunica intima, media, and adventitia from the nonatherosclerotic arteria poplitea and aorta of a 19-year-old male. The peak areas belonging to the type III-derived peptide α1(III) CB5 and the type I peptides α1(I) CB7 and CB8 and α2(I) CB3 and CB4 were determined and the portion of type III collagen as a percentage of total type III plus I was calculated using the formula:

$$\%\ \text{type III collegen} = \frac{A(III) \times 100}{0{,}3564 \times A(I) + A(III)}$$

A(III): peak area type III—derived peptide α1(III) CB5
A(I): peak area type I—derived peptides α1(I) CB7, CB8 and α2(I) CB3

Figure 3 shows the amounts of elastin and collagen. In the aorta the proportion of elastin, which in the normal vessel exceeds that of collagen, is

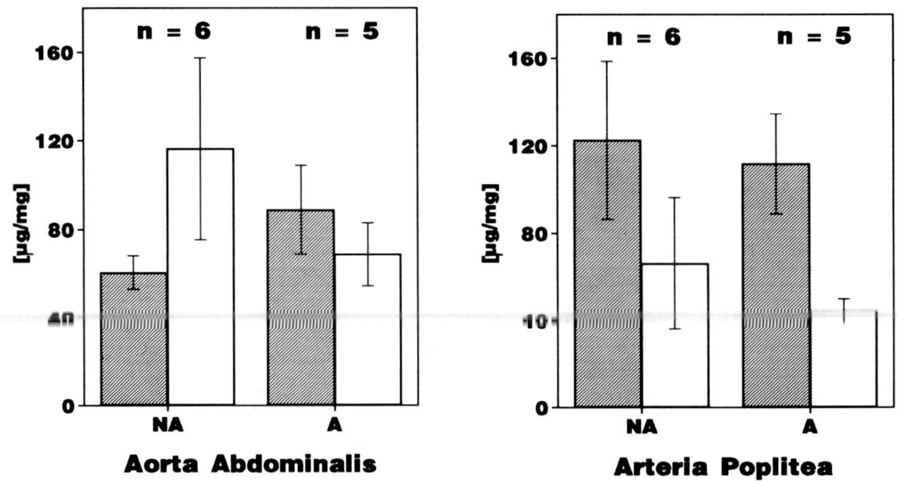

Fig. 3. The amounts of collagen and elastin (µg/mg wet tissue) in the intimal plus medial layer of nonatherosclerotic (*NA*) and atherosclerotic (*A*) aorta abdominalis and arteria poplitea. As described in the text, the amount of collagen was calculated from hydroxyproline measurement taking into account the ratio of type I and III collagens and the hydroxyproline content of elastin

diminished, while that of collagen dramatically enhanced. In the arteria poplitea only the proportion of elastin is diminished; that of collagen does not change.

Figure 4 shows the ratios of type III to type I collagen for the three layers of normal and atherosclerotic vessels (aorta abdominalis and arteria poplitea).

In the nonatherosclerotic vessels the proportions of type I collagen and type III collagen are quite similar in the tunica media and the tunica adventitia of both vessels. There is a difference, however, in the tunica intima: in the arteria poplitea the proportion of type III collagen is higher than in the media, whereas in the aorta the proportions in the intima and media are similar. The situation in the arteria poplitea corresponds more to that in aortas of young individuals (15 years and younger), where the intimal layer is considerably thinner than in nonatherosclerotic aortas of individuals aged 20 and older (J. RAUTERBERG, unpublished results); indeed, the youngest individuals in this study (10 and 15 years of age) also had a higher proportion of type III collagen in their intima than in the media.

In the atherosclerotic group, a shift towards a higher proportion of type I collagen can be observed in the tunica intima of both vessels; this shift is more prominent in the arteria poplitea than in the aorta.

In the media the situation is quite different: a considerable shift to more type III collagen in the media of the atherosclerotic aorta can be observed, whereas in the arteria poplitea there is virtually the same type I–type III ratio in the media of both groups. For both vessels it can be stated, however, that the proportion of type III collagen in the intima as compared to that in the media is considerably lower in the atherosclerotic than in the normal vessels.

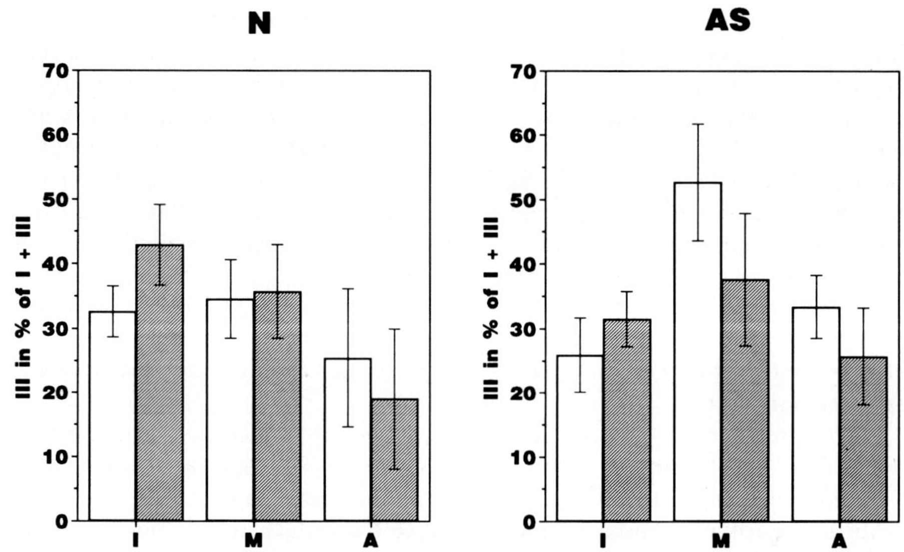

Fig. 4. Quantitative ratios of type I and type III collagen (type III in % of type I plus type III collagen) in the intima (*I*), media (*M*), and adventitia (*A*) of the nonatherosclerotic (*N*) and atherosclerotic (*AS*) aorta abdominalis (*white columns*) and arteria poplitea (*shaded columns*)

These results suggest that the increased proportion of type I collagen is characteristic not only of the atherosclerotic intimal plaque in the aorta but also of the thickened intima of an atherosclerotic artery of the muscular type, the arteria poplitea.

In neither vessel is this development in the intima paralleled by a change in the proportion of media collagens; whereas in the arteria poplitea the proportion remains unchanged, there is an increase in type III collagen in the media of the atherosclerotic aorta compared to the normal aorta. This increase probably reflects a merely age-dependent change, since in earlier work we found an increase in the relative amount of type III collagen in aortic media independent of atherosclerosis (J. RAUTERBERG, unpublished results).

3.2 Immunohistologic Characterization of Collagen Deposition in Normal and Atherosclerotic Vessels

The distribution of the different collagen types in the normal and atherosclerotic vessel wall has been investigated by a number of authors using immunohistologic methods, in most cases indirect immunofluorescence. The human aorta has been most intensively studied, and the results of several publications (SHEKKONIN et al. 1985; VOSS and RAUTERBERG 1986; MCCULLAGH et al. 1980; LABAT-ROBERT et al. 1985; SHEKKONIN et al. 1987) may be summarized as follows:

Only small differences can be detected in the distribution of type I and III collagens. Both occur in mostly identical patterns in the normal, fibrillar structures parallel to elastic membranes and smooth muscle cells. GAY et al. (1975) described a closer association of type III fibrils to elastin; this finding has not been confirmed by other authors. Both collagen types co-localize with fibronectin (SHEKKONIN et al. 1987). Both collagens stain more intensively in the adventitia than in the media. Type V collagen, too, shows fibrillar expression, however faint, in the media; most authors emphasize a close association with smooth muscle cells (GAY et al. 1981). More intensive type V-specific staining is observed in the subendothelial layer and in close association with subendothelial basement membrane of the vasa vasorum in the deep media and adventitia. In contrast to types I and III, type V is virtually absent from the adventitial extracellular matrix.

The presence of type VI collagen has been demonstrated in a pattern resembling fibronectin in all layers of the aorta (RAUTERBERG et al. 1986). Type IV collagen, co-localizing with laminin, has been shown to be restricted to the subendothelial basement membrane, to the surface area of smoth muscle cells and to the basement membrane of the vasa vasorum.

There are only a few reports on the distribution of collagens in arteries of the muscular type. Due to the dense packing of smooth muscle cells in the media, the distribution of all extracellular matrix components occurring in the media appears to be very similar (VOSS and RAUTERBERG 1986).

In the atherosclerotic aorta, the extracellular matrix of fibrous plaques stains intensively for type I as well as for type III collagen. In diffuse intimal thickenings as well as in small and presumably young plaques both collagens co-localize with fibronectin, whereas in larger fibrous plaques the amount of fibronectin seems to be greatly reduced in favor of type I and III collagens (SHEKKONIN et al. 1987).

Type V collagen seems to be restricted to fine fibrillar expression in the vicinity of the subendothelial basement membrane and to a more focal-like occurrence in fibrous plaques. Thus the immunohistologic appearance of type V collagen does not correspond to the results obtained by chemical methods, which show increased deposition of type V collagen in fibrous plaques.

Type IV collagen is very poorly stained within the area of atherosclerotic plaques and is practically limited to the basement membranes of the endothelium covering the plaque area.

Type VI collagen can be found throughout the atherosclerotic plaque in a distribution resembling that of type I and type III collagen.

4 Synthesis of the Different Collagen Types by Vessel Wall Cells

Only two cell types represent the resident cells in the tunica intima and media of the arterial wall: the smooth muscle cell (SMC) and the endothelial cell (EC). In normal vessels, ECs are restricted to a monolayer covering the inner side of all blood vessels, thus forming the virtual blood–tissue barrier. Only in the aorta do ECs occur within the deeper media as an element of the vasa vasorum. In all other arteries the tunica media is formed exclusively by SMCs, while the occurrence of the usual connective tissue-forming cell, the fibroblast, is restricted to the tunica adventitia (Ross and Glomset 1976). Therefore SMCs must be responsible for the synthesis of all the components participating in the formation of the medial extracellular matrix. SMCs also occur in the intima in the usually small layer between the subendothelial basement membrane and the elastica interna. In most larger human arteries this subendothelial layer becomes thickened even during infancy, especially at sites exposed to enhanced hydrodynamic stress, e.g., at the outlet of branching vessels. The intimal extracellular matrix is probably a product of SMCs and ECs; in intimal thickening with increasing numbers of SMCs, the portion formed by this cell type should be correspondingly enhanced.

4.1 Collagen Synthesis by Smooth Muscle Cells

Smooth muscle cells are known to change their phenotype profoundly when taken into culture. During the first 2 days after enzymatic liberation from the tissue, they show a similar appearance to that in the arterial wall: their cytoplasm contains mainly myofilaments and electrophoretic analysis of actins shows a high proportion of α-actin. After a few days of culture, however, they begin to change from this "contractile" state into a "synthetic" one: the contractile apparatus is reduced whereas the cytoplasm is filled more and more by the rough endoplasmic reticulum (Campbell et al. 1989). Most investigations on collagen synthesis have been done on cells which have already reached the synthetic state. These cells synthesize collagen actively; the proportion of collagens among secreted proteins is similar to that found in fibroblast cultures. The mainly produced collagen type is type I; the proportion of type III varies between 25% and <10%. Synthesis of collagen types IV, V, and VI has also been detected but few quantitative data are available. For SMCs from rabbit aortas, Okada et al. (1989) found, by densitometry of SDS gels of the pepsin-treated labeled collagens, proportions of 82.7%, 14.9%, 0.8%, and 1.6% for collagen types I, III, IV, and V, respectively.

Only a few reports have described changes in collagen synthesis parallel to the change of phenotype. Ang et al. (1990) characterized the newly synthesized collagen during phenotype change of cultivated rabbit aortic SMCs. They found a 25- to 30-fold increase in general collagen synthesis. The proportion of collagen type I increased from 78.1% to 90.3% from the contractile to the synthetic phenotype, and a similar shift was found in the proportion of corresponding mRNAs. Ang et al. found no change in the portion of type V collagen (ca. 3%–5% of total collagen). Okada et al. (1989) described a return to a contractile state if cultivated rabbit aortic SMCs were kept in a medium containing dimethylsulfoxide (DMSO). After 8 days culturing in 1% DMSO they found a remarkable relative increase in type IV collagen, from 0.8% to 9.2% of total collagens.

Characterization of SMCs in vivo by morphologic, immunohistologic, and biochemical criteria (actin isoforms) demonstrates a similar change in the phenotype of SMCs during the development of atherosclerotic plaques (CAMPBELL and CAMPBELL 1985; CAMPBELL et al. 1989). This corresponds well to the general enhancement of collagen synthesis and to the shift towards more type I collagen among the synthesized collagens.

Another mechanism of regulation of collagen synthesis in SMCs was recently demonstrated by THIE et al. (1991). Similar to fibroblasts (NUISGENS et al. 1984), SMCs which are seeded into a gel of collagen I fibrils are dramatically inhibited in their collagen synthesis; their total protein synthesis is reduced as well, but to a lesser extent.

4.2 Synthesis of Extracellular Structural Proteins by Endothelial Cells

As already mentioned, it is unknown which proportion of the subendothelial matrix is synthesized by ECs. Probably the basement membrane, which is associated with the endothelial layer, is produced by them; it can be shown that ECs cultured on a collagen gel produce a continuous basement membrane in the absence of SMCs (TÜMMERS et al. 1987). In addition, it may well be that a certain amount of matrix components deposited between the endothelial basement membrane and the elastica interna is derived from ECs.

Characterization of collagens secreted by cultivated ECs has not been very helpful in investigating the in vivo situation. The pattern of collagens synthesized by cultivated ECs varies profoundly according to species and tissue of origin as well as culture conditions (SAGE et al. 1981). The main product of bovine aortic ECs, for instance, is type III collagen, whereas pig aortic ECs under identical conditions synthesize type III and type I collagen in comparable amounts (LEVENE et al. 1984; SANKEY and BARNES 1984) and ECs from human umbilical veins secrete mainly type IV collagen. So far the mechanisms regulating in vivo expression of the different collagen types remain unknown. Changes in the secretion of collagen and other matrix proteins may well play an important role in the initiation of atherogenesis. It is known that basement membrane production in diabetic patients is increased in the microvasculature as well as in larger vessels, leading to thickened subendothelial basement membranes (OSTERBY 1990). The highly increased atherosclerotic risk of diabetes patients is well documented.

5 Localization of Active Synthesis of Collagens in Human Arteries by Detection of mRNA-Containing Cells Using the Method of In Situ Hybridization

In addition to the investigation of collagen synthesis in vessel wall cells at the level of protein synthesis in experimental model systems (cell culture, experimental animals), it is possible to localize cells expressing collagen mRNA using the method of in situ hybridization and thus to obtain evidence about an earlier stage of biosynthetic activation of vascular cells. In contrast to both model systems, this method can be applied to human vessels, since small tissue samples which can be obtained from certain kinds of surgery can be investigated.

5.1 Occurrence of Type I and Type III mRNA in Cells of Atherosclerotic Human Renal and Iliac Arteries

In a recent study (JAEGER et al. 1991) we used ^{35}S-UTP-labeled RNA probes complementary to type I and type III collagen mRNA to localize cells actively expressing collagen mRNA in frozen sections of normal and atherosclerotic arteries. Specimens were obtained from surgery (renal arteries from resections of kidneys, and iliac arteries from organ transplantation). The patients' ages ranged from 14 to 75 years; arteries included two unaffected and nine atherosclerotic samples with lesions of different stages, presenting as fatty streaks, locally restricted fibrous plaques, and complicated lesions. The cellular environment of collagen mRNA-expressing cells was investigated by immunohistochemistry using antibodies to cell-specific antigens. Serial sections made in parallel to these sections investigated by in situ hybridization were immunohistochemically stained with antibody HHF35 (TSUKADA et al. 1987a, b) reacting with SMC-specific α-actin in order to identify cells with enhanced mRNA content.

Detection of monocytes and macrophages was achieved using monoclonal antibodies 27E10 (ZWADLO et al. 1986), which recognizes blood-borne monocytes, and 25F9 (ZWADLO et al. 1985), specific for mature macrophages. A polyclonal antibody (Fa. Dako, Hamburg) specific for von Willebrand protein was used to visualize the endothelial layer and to detect possible involvement of capillarization processes in intimal plaque formation, which have been suggested as contributory factors to local accumulation of growth factors in human atherosclerotic plaques (WILCOX et al. 1988). The state of proliferating activity was determined using the monoclonal antibody Ki67, which is specific for a nuclear proliferation-associated antigen occurring in rapidly dividing cells.

5.1.1 Methodology of In Situ Hybridization

Five-micrometer cryostat sections were cut from all arteries, placed onto poly-L-lysine coated slides, fixed in 4% paraformaldehyde solution for 1 min, and stored in 70% ethanol at 4°C. cDNAs coding for the α1(I) (CHU et al. 1982) and for the α1(III) collagen chains (MISCULIN et al. 1986) were transcribed with the help of gemini vectors pGem3 and pGem4 (Promega Biotec, Madison, USA). ^{35}S labeled complementary "antisense" probes were used for hybridization. "Sense" transscripts of α1(III) cDNA were used as negative control. Pretreatment of tissue sections, hybridization and stringency conditions, washing procedures, and posthybridization RNase digestion of surplus template have already been described in detail (JAEGER et al. 1990).

5.1.2 Enhanced Collagen mRNA Synthesis in Human Atherosclerotic Arteries

In situ hybridization with probes for type I and type III collagen revealed the normal human artery wall with an intima of two or three cell layers to be virtually free of collagen mRNA-expressing cells. In contrast, renal and iliac arteries with intimal fibrous plaque formation showed the presence of type I and type III mRNA containing smooth muscle cells throughout intimal plaque regions. Activated cells were located in close vicinity to immigrated monocytes and macrophages (Fig. 5). Fibrous plaques in the early stages of development contained merely monocytes, whereas advanced atherosclerotic lesions showed immigration of both monocytes and mature macrophages.

Three of the renal arteries with severe fibrous plaque formation were virtually free of collagen mRNA-expressing smooth muscle cells within the fibrous intima. In atherosclerotic intimal plaques of serial sections, no immigration of monocytic cells was detectable in any of the three samples.

Summarizing, we found a very low level of collagen gene expression connected with virtual absence of monocytic cells in normal human arteries. In atherosclerotic sample, in contrast, immigrated monocytes in the early stages of plaque formation, and both monocytes and macrophages in advanced intimal fibrous plaques, were always accompanied by smooth muscle cells expressing enhanced levels of type I and type III collagen mRNA. Intimal smooth muscle cells in atherosclerotic plaques devoid of cells of the monocyte/macrophage system always expressed undetectable levels of collagen mRNA similar to those in normal arteries.

5.2 Human Aortic Coarctation as an Example of High Blood Pressure-Induced Enhancement of Collagen Gene Expression

The thoracic aorta from patients with aortic coarctation develops myoproliferative hyperplasia in the proximal part of the vessel due to the influence of locally enhanced blood pressure. In a previous study (JAEGER et al. 1990), nine samples of human aortic coarctation were investigated using the same methodology. They permit collagen mRNA expression in the high blood pressure-exposed thickened proximal aortic segment to be compared to mRNA expression in the normal distal aortic segment. Using this model system, the influence of enhanced blood pressure on mRNA expression for different collagen types can be studied.

Fig. 5a–d. Renal artery with fibrous plaque formation showing type I collagen mRNA expressing intimal smooth muscle cells visualized by in situ hybridization of serial sections (**a, c**) and located in close vicinity to immigrated macrophages identified by immunocytochemical staining of further serial sections (**b, d**; *arrows*); 67-year-old male patient. **a, b**: × 150; **c, d**: × 200

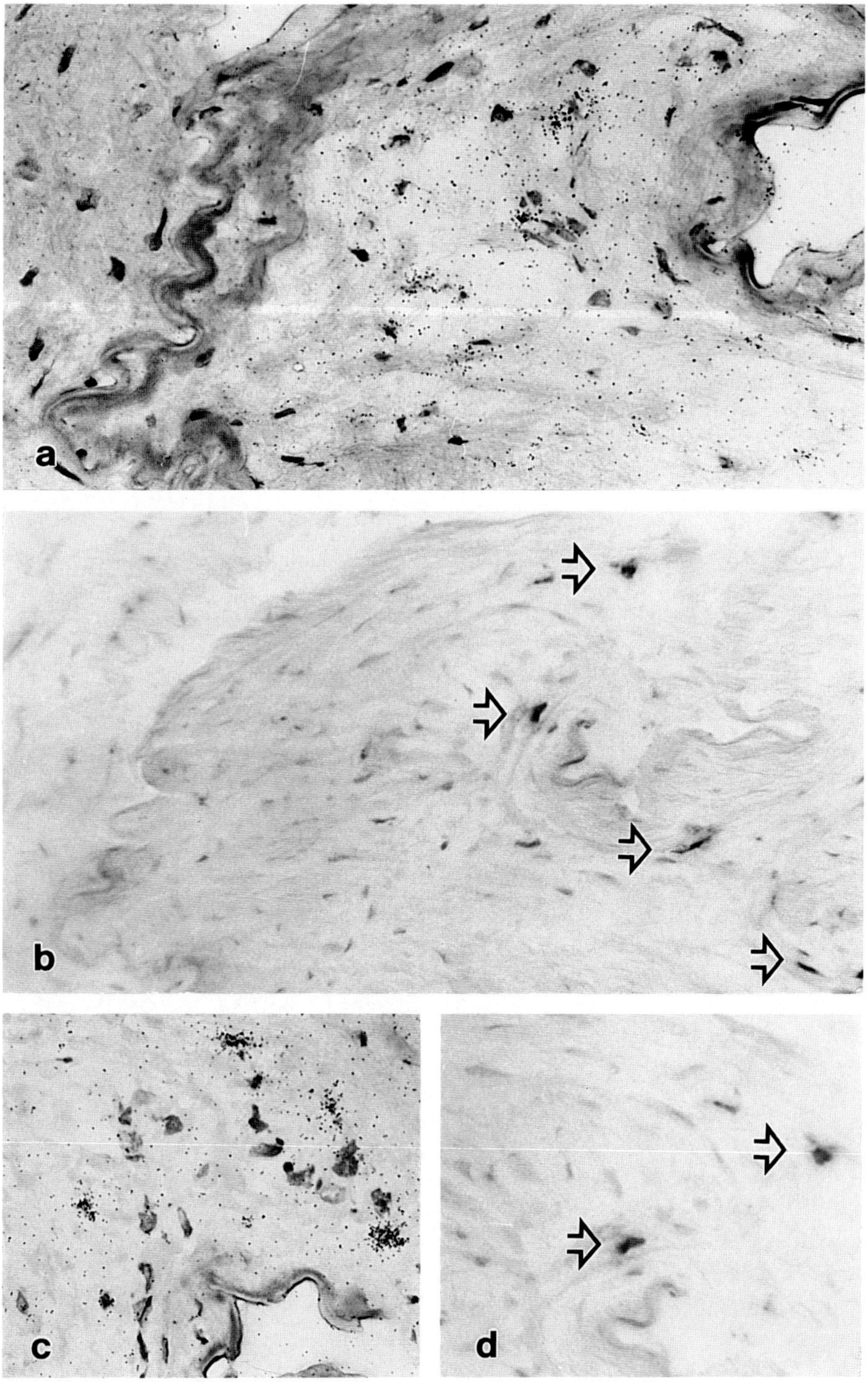
a
b
c
d

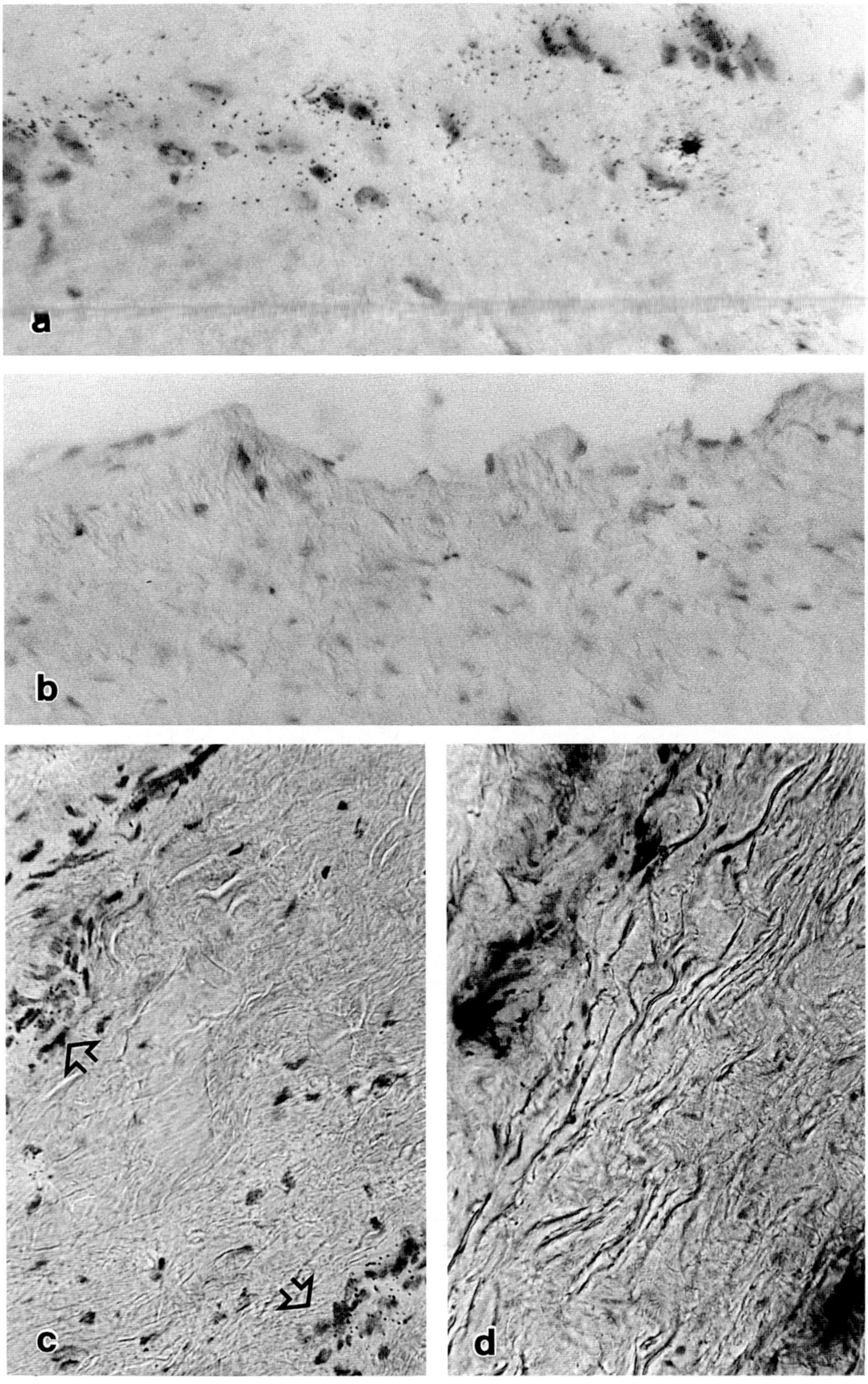
a
b
c
d

The hyperplastic intima and media appeared rich in extracellular matrix, with fewer cells than are found in the normal vessel wall. Smooth muscle cells within the thickened intimal and medial layers in the prestenotic segment expressed enhanced amounts of both type I and type III collagen mRNA when compared to the poststenotic aortic part. In arteries from patients younger than 14 years, intimal as well as medial smooth muscle cells were responsible for enhanced expression of collagen mRNA, whereas in older patients the signal was mostly restricted to the subendothelial layer of the vessel (Fig. 6A). In the distal vessel wall segment, intimal and medial collagen RNA expression was found to be as low as in the normal non-atherosclerotic vessel wall. Also histologically, the vessel wall structure appeared to be unaltered. In the stenotic segment of aortic coarctations, collagen mRNA expression in intimal and medial smooth muscle cells is also enhanced when compared to the distal segment. Whereas expression of type I mRNA surpasses expression of type III mRNA in the atherosclerotic vessel wall and in the proximal segment of aortic coarctations, the expression of both collagen mRNAs similar is in the region of stenosis. This finding has also been confirmed on the level of protein synthesis in cultured smooth muscle cells from human aortic coarctations where cells of the stenotic part synthesized more type III collagen than did proximal smooth muscle cells (RAUTERBERG and ALLAM, unpublished).

In the proximal as well as in the stenotic segment of aortic coarctations, immuno-histochemistry of serial sections demonstrated a virtual absence of invaded monocytes and macrophages within the intimal and medial areas of proliferation (Fig. 6b). Monocytic cells were detected neither in the vicinity of collagen mRNA containing smooth muscle cells nor at other sites within the hyperplastic areas except the highly capillarized deep media and adventitia mainly in the stenotic part of the vessel. Monocytic cells were found near capillaries in this region and enhanced collagen mRNA expression in neighbouring smooth muscle cells was observed (Fig. 6c, d).

6 Collagen Gene Expression in Atherosclerotic Plaques and in Nonatherosclerotic Intimal Thickening

A recent report by the Committee on Vascular Lesions of the Council of Arteriosclerosis of the American Heart Association emphasizes that arteriosclerotic lesions and atherosclerotic plaque formation can be clearly distinguished from intimal thickenings occurring as "physiological adaptions to

Fig. 6a–d. Stenotic segment of aortic coarctation, showing intimal smooth muscle cells expressing enhanced amounts of type I collagen mRNA (**a**) in the virtual absence of monocytic cells in corresponding regions of a serial section (**b**). In the highly capillarized deep media of the stenotic part, we found close co-localization of type I collagen mRNA-expressing smooth muscle cells surrounding the capillaries (**c**, *arrows*) and macrophages (**d**); 16-year-old male patient. **a, b**: × 500; **c, d**: × 400

mechanical stresses secondary to variations in flow, wall tension or both" (STARY et al. 1992). The authors differentiate two forms of adaptive intimal thickening: a diffuse thickening and an excentric thickening. Excentric thickening occurs mainly at branches and may, in the case of an arterial bifurcation, involve half the circumference of the parent and daughter vessels. Morphologically these "physiological intimal thickenings" are divided into the lumen-directed proteoglycan-rich layer and the elastin-rich "mucoelastic" layer. Both contain smooth muscle cells as the clearly dominating cell type, with low density in the proteoglycan-rich layer and higher density in the mucoelastic layer. Invading cells, mainly monocytes, may occur sporadically and in relatively low numbers.

Taking this definition as a basis for classification, the intimal vessel wall thickening occurring in the aorta proximal to aortic coarctations certainly represents a nonatherosclerotic adaptive type of lesion. The results on localization of collagen I and III mRNA-containing cells suggest different mechanisms of activation of collagen synthesis in this adaptive type of lesion and in the atherosclerotic plaques of renal and iliac arteries: In atherosclerotic intimal plaques of renal and iliac arteries, collagen mRNA-producing cells were closely co-localized with cells of the monocyte/macrophage system that had invaded and were focally distributed throughout the plaque region. In no sample among the investigated atherosclerotic vessels were message-containing cells detected without neighboring monocytic cells, suggesting the induction of transcriptional activity in intimal smooth muscle cells by secretory products of the monocytes or macrophages.

A number of cytokines and growth factors produced and secreted by macrophages have been described as being involved in the process of atherosclerotic plaque formation, in part by altering the rate of collagen synthesis. For example, transforming growth factor β (TGF-β) has been reported to stimulate the synthesis of extracellular matrix components in a number of mesenchymal cells (for review see ROBERTS et al. 1988) as well as type I and III collagen synthesis in cultured fibroblasts (VARGA et al. 1987). The macrophage-derived monokine interleukin-1 (IL-1) may have a stimulatory (KÄHARI et al. 1987; POSTLETHWAITE et al. 1988) as well as an inhibitory effect (BHATNAGAR et al. 1986) on collagen gene transcription and translation. Tumor necrosis factor (TNF), which is likewise secreted by macrophages, has been shown to inhibit collagen gene transcription and collagen synthesis in cultured human fibroblasts (SOLIS-HERRUZO et al. 1988). Platelet-derived growth factor, also secreted by macrophages, has been found in normal arteries with low cell turnover (BARRETT and BENDITT 1988), but in addition is an active contributor to atherosclerotic lesion formation and a potent stimulator of monocyte and smooth muscle cell migration and proliferation (NILSSON 1986; ROSS 1987).

Thus, enhancement of the rate of collagen mRNA transcription in smooth muscle cells in the local vicinity of immigrated monocytes or macrophages may be the consequence of a stimulating effect exerted by macrophage secretory products on cells in their local environment within the atherosclerotic intimal plaque.

In inborn aortic coarctations, also, enhancement of collagen synthesis contributes essentially to reactive vessel wall thickening of the proximal segment. In contrast to atherosclerotic plaque formation, hypertension-induced intimal and medial vessel wall thickening in the investigated aortic coarctations was observed without the involvement of immigrated monocytic cells. In the proximal as well as in the stenotic part of the aorta, focally distributed intimal and medial smooth muscle cells in younger patients and subendothelial smooth muscle cells in older patients showed expression of type I and type III collagen mRNA without immunohistochemically detectable monocytes or macrophages in their vicinity. These results suggest that smooth muscle cell growth and synthetic activity in high blood pressure-induced vessel wall thickening are controlled by mechanisms other than activation by macrophage-derived cytokines. Smooth muscle cells are known to be active producers of several growth factors, e.g., fibroblast growth factor (FGF), PDGF, and IL-1, and may undergo an autocrine stimulation process during proliferation. CROUCH et al. (1989) showed a stimulatory effect on collagen mRNA production in pulmonary artery smooth muscle cells when these cells were exposed to conditioned calf serum harvested from cultured medial smooth muscle cells from hypertensive calves. They suggest the existence of a soluble factor that is generated from medial smooth muscle cells, leading to enhanced production of collagen in hypertensive arteries at a pretranslational level.

It has to be borne in mind that the general co-localization of mRNA-containing smooth muscle cells with monocytic cells in atherosclerotic plaques does not exclude the existence of additional control mechanisms as have been discussed for hypertensive vessels, probably also mediating synthetic activation of vessel wall cells during atherosclerotic plaque formation. Further in situ and immunocytochemical investigations with probes and antibodies for cytokines and growth factors involved in biosynthetic activation of vascular cells will provide valuable insights into cellular activation processes in vessel wall proliferation.

So far no reports are available on similar studies on activation of cells to synthesize collagens other than types I and III. In an animal model involving the induction of myointimal thickening by removal of the endothelium by balloon catheterization, BARNES (1983) investigated the activity of collagen biosynthesis by incubating tissue samples in a medium containing radioactively labeled amino acids. By determination of labeled collagens using peptic extraction and gel electrophoretic separation, he showed that type I collagen synthesis was more enhanced than type III and type IV in comparison with uninjured vessels. Similar results were reported by RYAN et al. (1988) using a different model. These authors induced atherosclerosis in external jugular veins of sheep which were linked in vivo by anastomosis with the common carotid artery. McGUIRE et al. (1989) extracted RNA from samples of aortic tissue of spontaneously hypertensive rats and found that the thickened aortic walls of the animals contained enhanced levels of mRNAs of the beasement membrane components laminin and type IV collagen. In the same animal model, SARZANI et al. (1989) found that, of several growth factor mRNAs, only TGF-β mRNA was enhanced in the vessel wall of hypertensive animals. As already stated, TGF-β has a pronounced stimulating effect on the synthesis of several extracellular matrix proteins by mesenchymal cells (ROBERTS et al. 1988), among them smooth muscle cells (SCHLUMBERGER et al. 1991).

Research into the effect of cytokines and combinations of cytokines on collagen synthesis by vessel wall cells is at a very early stage. With better knowledge in this field, and after more extensive studies on in situ activation of collagen synthesis in the different states of atherosclerosis and on the role of cell–cell interactions in this activation, the mechanisms of dysregulation of collagen synthesis in atherosclerotic vessel walls will be better understood. This knowledge is an important prerequisite to finding new ways of intervening in the atherosclerotic process.

References

Abedin MZ, Ayad S, Weiss JB (1981) Type V collagen: the presence of appreciable amounts of α3(V) chain in uterus. Biochem Biophys Res Commun 102:1237–1245

Abrahamson DR (1986) Recent studies on the structure and pathology of basement membranes. J Pathol 149:257–278

Adachi E, Hayashi T (1986) In vitro formation of hybrid fibrils of type V collagen and type I collagen—limited growth of type I collagen into thick fibrils by type V collagen. Connect Tiss Res 14:257–266

Ang AH, Tachas G, Campbell JH, Bateman JF, Campbell GR (1990) Collagen synthesis by cultures of rabbit aortic smooth muscle cells—alteration with phenotype. Biochem J 265:461–469

Arbeille BB, Fauvel FMJ, Lemesle MB, Tenza D, Legrand YJ (1991) Thrombospondin: a component of microfibrils in various tissues. J Histochem Cytochem 39:1367–1375

Aumailley M, Mann K, von der Mark K, Timpl R (1989) Cell attachment properties of collagen type VI and Arg-Gly-Asp dependent binding to its α2(VI) and α3(VI) chains. Exp Cell Res 181:463–474

Barnes MJ (1983) Collagen polymorphism in the normal and diseased blood vessel wall. Atherosclerosis 46:249–251

Barnes MJ (1985) Collagens in atherosclerosis. Collagen Rel Res 5:65–97

Barnes MJ, Morton LF, Levene CI (1976) Synthesis of collagen types I and III by pig medial smooth muscle cells in culture. Biochem Biophys Res Commun 70:339–347

Barrett TB, Benditt EP (1988) Platelet-derived growth factor gene expression in human atherosclerotic plaques and normal artery wall. Proc Natl Acad Sci USA 85:2810–2814

Bhatnagar R, Penfornis H, Mauviel A, Loyau G, Saklatvala J, Pujol J-P (1986) Interleukin-1 inhibits the synthesis of collagen in fibroblasts. Biochem Int 13:709–720

Birk DE, Fitch JM, Babiarz JP, Linsenmayer TF (1988) Collagen type I and type V are present in the same fibril in avian corneal stroma. J Cell Biol 106:999–1008

Birk DE, Fitch JM, Babiarz JP, Doane KJ, Linsenmayer TF (1990) Collagen fibrillogenesis in vitro—interaction of type-I and type-V collagen regulates fibril diameter. J Cell Science 95:649–657

Burgeson RE (1987) The collagens of skin. In: Wuepper KD, Geddedahl T (eds) Biology of heritable skin diseases. Curr Probl Dermatol 17:61

Campbell GR, Campbell JH (1985) Smooth muscle phenotypic changes in arterial wall homeostasis. Implications for the pathogenesis of atherosclerosis. Exp Mol Pathol 42:139–162

Campbell JH, Kocher O, Skalli O, Gabbiani G, Campbell GR (1989) Cytodifferentiation and expression of α-smooth muscle actin messenger RNA and protein during primary culture of aortic smooth muscle cells—correlation with cell density and proliferative state. Arteriosclerosis 9:633–643

Chu M-L, Myers JC, Bernard MP, Ding J-F, Ramirez F (1982) Cloning and characterization of five overlapping cDNAs specific for the human pro α3(I) collagen chain. Nucl Acids Res 10:5925–5934
Chu ML, Zhang R-Z, Pan T, Stokes D, Conway D, Kao H-J, Glanville R, Mayer U, Mann K-H, Dentzmann R, Timpl R (1990) Mosaic structure of globular domains in the human type VI collagen α3 chain: similarity to von Willebrand factor, fibronectin, actin, salivary proteins, and aprotein type protease inhibitors. EMBO J 9:385–393
Colombatti A, Bonaldo P (1991) The superfamily of proteins with von-Willebrand factor type-A-like domains—one theme common to components of extracellular matrix, hemostasis, cellular adhesion, and defense mechanisms. Blood 77:2305–2315
Crouch EC, Parks WC, Rosenbaum JL, et al. (1989) Regulation of collagen production by medial smooth muscle cells in hypoxic pulmonary hypertension. Am Rev Respir Dis 140:1045–1051
Dublet B, van der Rest M (1991) Type XIV collagen, a new trimeric molecule extracted from fetal bovine skin and tendon with a triple helical disulfide-bonded domain homologous to type IX and type XII collagen. J Biol Chem 266:6853–6858
Fauvel-Lafeve F, Legrand YJ (1988) Immunochemical identification of a thrombospondin-like structure in an arterial microfibrillar extract. Thromb Res 50:305–316
Fleischmajer R, Olsen BR, Timpl R, Perlish JS, Lovelace O (1983) Collagen fibril formation during embryogenesis. Proc Natl Acad Sci USA 80:3354–3358
Frazier WA (1987) Thrombospondin, a modular adhesive glycoprotein of platelets and nucleated cells. J Cell Biol 105:625–632
Gay S, Balleisen L, Remberger K, Fietzek PP, Adelmann BC (1975) Immunohistochemical evidence for the presence of collagen type III in human arterial walls, arterial thrombi and in leukocytes, incubated with collagen in vitro. Klin Wochenschr 53:899–902
Gay S, Martineshernandes A, Rhodes RK, Miller EJ (1981) The collagenous exocytoskeleton of smooth muscle cells. Collagen Rel Res 1:377–384
Gordon MK, Olsen BR (1990) The contribution of collagenous proteins to tissue-specific matrix assemblies. Curr Opin Cell Biol 2:833–838
Gordon MK, Gerecke DR, Dublet R, van der Rest M, Olsen BR (1989) Type XII collagen; a large multidomain molecule with partial homology to type IX collagen. J Biol Chem 264:19772–19778
Hanson AN, Bentley JP (1983) Quantitation of type I to type III collagen ratios in small samples of human tendon, blood vessels and atherosclerotic plaque. Anal Biochem 130:32–40
Henkel W, Glanville RW (1982) Covalent crosslinking between molecules of type I and type III collagen. The involvement of the N-terminal, non-helical regions of the α1(I) and α1(III) chains in the formation of intermolecular crosslinks. Eur J Biochem 122:205–213
Inoue S (1989) Ultrastructure of basement membranes. Int Rev Cytol 117:57–98
Iruela-Arispe ML, Diglio CA, Sage EH (1991) Modulation of extracellular matrix proteins by endothelial cells undergoing angiogenesis in vitro. Arteriosclerosis Thrombosis 11:805–815
Jaeger E, Rust S, Scharffetter K, et al. (1990) Localization of cytoplasmic collagen mRNA in human aortic coarctation: mRNA enhancement in high blood pressure-induced intimal and medial thickening. J Histochem Cytochem 38:1365–1375
Jaeger E, Rust S, Roessner A, et al. (1991) Joint occurrence of collagen mRNA containing cells and macrophages in human atherosclerotic vessels. Atherosclerosis 31:55–68
Jander R, Korsching E, Rauterberg J (1990) Characteristics and in vivo occurrence of type-VIII collagen. Eur J Biochem 189:601–607
Kähari V-M, Jyrki H, Eero V (1987) Interleukin-1 increases collagen production and mRNA levels in cultured skin fibroblasts. Biochim Biophys Acta 929:142–147
Kapoor R, Sakai LY, Funk S, Roux E, Bornstein P, Sage EH (1988) Type VIII collagen has a restricted distribution in specialized extracellular matrix. J Cell Biol 107:721–730
Keene DR, Sakai LY, Bächinger HP, Burgeson RE (1987) Type III collagen can be present on banded collagen fibrils regardless of fibril diameter. J Cell Biol 115:2393–2402
Keene DR, Engvall E, Glanville RW (1988) Ultrastructure of type VI collagen in human skin and cartilage suggests an anchoring function for this filamentous network. J Cell Biol 107:1995–2006
Kielty CM, Hopkinson I, Grant ME (1993) The collagen family: structure, assembly and organization in the extracellular matrix. In: Royce PM, Steinmann B (eds) Connective tissue and its heritable disorders. Alan R. Liss, New York, pp 103–147
Kittelberger R, Davis PF, Greenhill NS (1989) Immunolocalization of type VIII collagen in vascular tissue. Biochem Biophys Res Commun 159:414–419
Kühn K (1986a) The collagen family—variation in the molecular and supermolecular structure. Rheumatology 10:29–69

Kühn K (1986b) The collagens—molecular and macromolecular structures. In: Tschesche H (ed) Proteinases in inflammation and tumor invasion. Walter de Gruyter, Berlin, pp 107–143

Labat-Robert J, Szendroi M, Godeau G, Robert L (1985) Comparative distribution patterns of type I and type III collagens and fibronectin in human arteriosclerotic aorta. Pathol Biol 33:261–265

Labermeyer U, Kenney MC (1983) The presence of EC collagen and type IV collagen in bovine Descemet's membranes. Biochem Biophys Res Commun 116:619–625

Lawler J, Hynes R-O (1986) The structure of human thrombospondin, an adhesive glycoprotein with multiple calcium-binding sites and homologies with several different proteins. J Cell Biol 103:1635–1648

Leblond CP, Inoue S (1989) Structure, composition, and assembly of basement membrane. Am J Anat 185:367–390

Levene CI, Bartlet C, Heale G (1984) Phenotypic changes in morphology and collagen polymorphism of cultured bovine and porcine aortic endothelium. Arteriosclerosis 52:59–71

Linsenmayer TF (1991) Collagen. In: Hay ED (ed) Cell biology of extracellular matrix, 2nd ed. Plenum, New York, pp 7–44

McCullagh KG, Duance VC, Bishop KA (1980) The distribution of collagen types I, III and V (AB) in normal and atherosclerotic aorta. J Pathol 130:45–65

McGuire PG, Brocks DG, Killen PD, Orkin RW (1989) Increased deposition of basement membrane macromolecules in specific vessels of the spontaneously hypertensive rat. Am J Pathol 135:291–299

Mendler M, Eich-Bender SG, Vaughan L, Winter KH, Bruckner P (1989) Cartilage contains mixed fibrils of collagen types II, IX and XI. J Cell Biol 108:191–197

Miller EJ (1985) Recent information on the chemistry of the collagens. In: Butler WT (ed) Chemistry and biology of mineralized tissues. Ebsco Media, Birmingham, pp 80

Misculin M, Dalgleish R, Kluve-Beckermann B, Rennard SI, Tolstoshev P, Brantly M, Crystal RG (1986) Human type III collagen gene expression is coordinatively modulated with the type I collagen genes during fibroblast growth. Biochemistry 25:1408–1413

Morton LF, Barnes MJ (1982) Collagen polymorphism in the normal and diseased blood vessel wall—investigation of collagen types I, III and V. Atherosclerosis 42:41–51

Mumby SM, Raugi GJ, Bornstein P (1984) Interaction of thrombospondin with extracellular matrix proteins: selective binding to type V collagen. J Cell Biol 98:646–652

Murata K, Motoyama T (1990) Collagen species in various sized human arteries and their changes with intimal proliferation. Artery 17:96–106

Murata K, Motoyama T, Kotake C (1986) Collagen types in various layers of the human aorta and their changes with the atherosclerotic process. Atherosclerosis 60:251–262

Nilsson J (1986) Growth factors and the pathogenesis of atherosclerosis. 62:185–199

Niyibizi C, Fietzek PP, van der Rest M (1984) Human placenta type V collagens. Evidence for the existence of an $\alpha 1(V)$ $\alpha 2(V)$ $\alpha 3(V)$ collagen molecule. J Biol Chem 259:14170–14174

Nuisgens B, Merill C, Lapiere C, Bell E (1984) Collagen biosynthesis by cells in a tissue equivalent matrix in vitro. Collagen Rel Res 4:351–364

Okada Y, Katsuda S, Matsui Y, Minamoto T, Nakanishi I (1989) Altered synthesis of collagen types in cultured arterial smooth muscle cells during phenotypic modulation by dimethyl sulfoxide. Acta Pathol Jpn 39:15–22

Ooshima A (1981) Collagen αB chains: increased proportion in human atherosclerosis. Science 213:660–668

Osterby R (1990) Basement membrane morphology in diabetes mellitus. In: Rifkin H, Poste D (eds) Diabetes mellitus, theory and practice. Elsevier, New York, pp 220–233

Palotie A, Tryggvason K, Peltonen L (1983) Components of subendothelial aorta basement membrane: immunohistochemical localization and role in cell attachment. Lab Invest 49:362–370

Paulsson M (1992) Basement membrane proteins: structure, assembly, and cellular interactions. Crit Rev Biochem Mol Biol 27:93–127

Postlethwaite AE, Raghow R, Stricklin GP, Poppleton H, Seyer JM, Kang AH (1988) Modulation of fibroblast functions by interleukin 1: increased steady-state accumulation of type I procollagen messenger RNAs and stimulation of other functions but not chemotaxis by human recombinant interleukin 1 α and β. J Cell Biol 106:311–318

Raspanti M, Ottani V, Ruggeri A (1989) Different architectures of the collagen fibril: morphological aspects and functional implications. Int J Macromol 11:367–371

Rauterberg J, Jaeger E (1992) Collagen and collagen synthesis in the atherosclerotic vessel wall. In: Robenek H, Sievers N (eds) Cell interactions in atherosclerosis. CRC, Boca Raton, Fl. (in press)

Rauterberg J, Troyer D (1986) Type V collagen: heterogeneity in different tissues. In: Laurent P, Grimaud JA, Bienvenue J (eds) Marker proteins in inflammation, vol. 3. Walter de Gruyter, Berlin, pp 343–356

Rauterberg J, Schlief H-E, Pott G (1982) The collagen of the normal and fibrotic liver. In: Gerlach U, Pott G, Rauterberg J, Voss B (eds) Connective tissue of the normal and fibrotic human liver. Thieme, Stuttgart, pp 36–37

Rauterberg J, Jander R, Troyer D (1986) Type VI collagen—a structural glycoprotein with a collagenous domain. Front Matrix Biol 11:90–109

Remberger J, Gay S, Fietzek PP (1975) Immunhistochemische Untersuchungen zur Kollagencharakterisierung in Leberzirrhosen. Virchows Arch [A] 367:231–240

Roberts AB, Flanders KC, Kondajah P, et al. (1988) Transforming growth factor β: biochemistry and roles in embryogenesis, tissue repair and remodeling, and carcinogenesis. Recent Prog Horm Res 44:157–197

Romanic AM, Adachi E, Kadler KE, Hojima Y, Prockop DJ (1991) Co-polymerization of pNcollagen III and collagen I. pNcollagen III decreases the rate of incorporation of collagen I into fibrils, the amount of collagen I incorporated, and the diameter of the fibrils formed. J Biol Chem 266:12703–12705

Ross R (1987) Growth factors in the pathogenesis of atherosclerosis. Acta Med Scand [Suppl] 715:33–38

Ross R, Glomset JA (1976) The pathogenesis of atherosclerosis I. N Engl J Med 295:369–375

Ryan PA, Davis PF, Stehbens WE (1988) The biochemical composition of haemodynamically stressed vascular tissue. III. The collagen composition of experimental arteriovenous fistulae. Atherosclerosis 71:157–163

Sage H (1984) Collagen synthesis by endothelial cells in culture. In: Jaffe EA (ed) Biology of endothelial cells. Martinus Nijhoff, Boston, pp 161–171

Sage H, Bornstein P (1982) Endothelial cells from umbilical vein and a hemangioendothelioma secrete basement membrane largely to the exclusion of interstitial procollagens. Arteriosclerosis 2:27–36

Sage H, Pritzl P, Bornstein P (1981) Secretory phenotype of endothelial cells in culture: comparison of aortic, venous, capillary, and corneal endothelium. Arteriosclerosis 1:427–442

Sage H, Pritzl P, Bornstein P (1982) Endothelial cells secrete a novel collagen type in vitro independently of prolyl hydroxylation. Collagen Rel Res 2:465–479

Sanes JR, Engwall E, Butkowski R, Hunter DD (1990) Molecular heterogeneity of basal lamina: isoforms of laminin and collagen IV at the neuromuscular junction and elsewhere. J Cell Biol 111:1685–1699

Sankey E, Barnes MJ (1984) Comparison of the collagenous products synthesised in culture by pig aortic endothelial and smooth-muscle cells. J Biochem 218:11–18

Sarzani R, Brecher P, Chobanian AV (1989) Growth factor expression in aorta of normotensive and hypertensive rats. J Clin Invest 83:1404–1408

Sawada H, Konomi H, Hirosawa K (1990) Characterization of the collagen in the hexagonal lattice of Descemet's membrane—relation of type VIII collagen. J Cell Biol 110:219–227

Schlumberger W, Thie M, Rauterberg J, Robenek H (1991) Collagen synthesis in cultured aortic smooth muscle cells—modulation by collagen lattice culture, transforming growth factor β1, and epidermal growth factor. Arteriosclerosis Thromb 11:1660–1666

Schuppan D, Becker J, Boehm H, Hahn EC (1986) Immunofluorescent localization of type-V collagen as a fibrillar component of the interstitial connective tissue of human oral mucosa, artery and liver. Cell Tissue Res 243:535–543

Shekkonin BV, Domogatsky AP, Muzykantov VR, Idelson GL, Rukosuev VS (1985) Distribution of type-1, type-3, type-4 and type-5 collagen in normal and atherosclerotic human arterial wall—immunological characteristics. Collagen Rel Res 5:355–368

Shekkonin BV, Domogatsky AP, Idelson GL, Koteliansky VE, Rukosuev VS (1987) Relative distribution of fibronectin and type I, III, IV, V collagens in normal and atherosclerotic intima of human arteries. Atherosclerosis 67:9–16

Shiraishi M, Segewa M, Takebayashi S (1980) An electron-microscopic study on aging of collagenous fiibrils in the larger blood vessels of humans. J Electron Microsc 29:139–143

Silverstein RL, Leung LLK, Nachman RL (1986) Thrombospondin: a versatile multifunctional glycoprotein. Arteriosclerosis 6:245–254

Solis-Herruzo JA, Brenner DA, Chojkier M (1988) Tumor necrosis factor-α inhibits collagen gene transcription and collagen synthesis in cultured human fibroblasts. J Biol Chem 263:5841–5845

Stary HC, Blankenhorn DH, Chandler AB, et al. (1992) A definition of the intima of human arteries and of its atherosclerosis-prone regions—a report from the Committe on Vascular Lesions of the Council on Arteriosclerosis, American Heart Association—special report. Arteriosclerosis Thromb 12:120–134

Thie M, Schlumberger W, Semich R, Rauterberg J, Robenek H (1991) Aortic smooth muscle cells in collagen lattice culture—effects on ultrastructure, proliferation and collagen synthesis. Eur J Cell Biol 55:295–304

Timpl R (1989) Structure and biological activity of basement membrane proteins. Eur J Biochem 180:487

Timpl R, Engel J (1987) Type VI collagen. In: Mayne R, Burgeson RE (eds) Structure and function of collagen types. Academic, Orlando, pp 105–143

Trüeb B, Schreier T, Bruckner P, Winterhalter K (19870 Type VI collagen represents a major fraction of connective tissue collagens. Eur J Biochem 166:699–703

Tseng SCG, Smuckler D, Stern R (1982) Comparison of collagen types in adult and fetal bovine corneas. J Biol Chem 256:2627–2633

Tsukada T, Tippens D, Gordon D, Ross R, Gown AM (1987a) HHF35, a muscle-actin-specific monoclonal antibody. 1. Immunocytochemical and biochemical characterization. Am J Pathol 126:51–60

Tsukada T, McNutt MA, Ross R, Gown AM (1987b) HHF35, a muscle-actin-specific monoclonal antibody. 2. Reactivity in normal, reactive, and neoplastic human tissues. Am J Pathol 127:389–402

van der Rest M, Garrone R (1990) Collagens as multidomain proteins. Biochimie 72:473

Tümmers M, Troyer D, Banch HJ, Rauterberg J (1987) Endothelial cells on fibrillar collagen gels and plastics substrate dependent morphology, synthesis, and secretion. Eur J Cell Biol 46, Suppl 22:75

Varga J, Rosenbloom J, Jimenez SA (1987) Transforming growth factor β (TGF β) causes a persistent increase in steady-state amounts of type I and III collagen and fibronectin mRNAs in normal human dermal fibroblasts. Biochem J 247:597–604

Vaughan L, Mendler M, Huber S, Bruckner P, Winterhalter KH, Irwin MI, Mayne R (1988) D-periodic distribution of collagen type IV along cartilage fibrils. J Cell Biol 106:991

Voss B, Rauterberg J (1986) Localization of collagen types I, III, IV and V, fibronectin and laminin in human arteries by the indirect immunofluorescence method. Pathol Res Pract 181:568

Vuorio E, de Combrugghe B (1990) The family of collagen genes. Ann Rev Biochem 59:837–872

Wagner WD (1990) Modification of collagen and elastin in the human atherosclerotic plaque. In: Glagov S, Neumann WP, Schaffer SA (eds) Pathobiology of the human atherosclerotic plaque. Springer, New York, pp 167–188

Weber L, Meigel WN, Rauterberg J (1977) SDS-polyacrylamide gel electrophoretic determination of type I and type III in small skin samples. Arch Dermatol Res 258:251–257

Wight TN, Raugi GJ, Mumby SM, Bornstein P (1985) Light microscopic immunolocation of thrombospondin in human tissues. J Histochem Cytochem 33:295–302

Wilcox JN, Smith KM, Williams LT, Schwartz SM, Gordon D (1988) Platelet-derived growth factor mRNA detection in human atherosclerotic plaque by in situ hybridization. J Clin Invest 82:1134–1143

Zwadlo G, Bröcker E-B, von Bassewitz D-B, Feige U, Sorg C (1985) Monoclonal antibody to a differentiation antigen present on mature macrophages and absent from monocytes. J Immunol 134:1487–1492

Zwadlo G, Schlegel R, Sorg C (1986) A monoclonal antibody to a subset of human macophages found only in the peripheral blood and inflammatory tissue. J Immunol 137:512–518

Metabolism of Fibromuscular and Atheromatous Plaques in an Experimental Model: Causal Mechanisms for the Development of Intimal Necrosis

H. HEINLE, D. KLING, and E. BETZ

1 Introduction

Hallmarks in the development of atherosclerosis are intimal accumulation of leukocytes, especially monocytes/macrophages, proliferation of cells characterized as modified smooth muscle cells, formation of extracellular matrix, and incorporation of lipids either within intimal cells or associated with extracellular material (for reviews see: HAUSS 1973; GEER and WEBSTER 1974; ROSS and GLOMSET 1976; CAMEJO 1982; GOTLIEB 1982; KLURFELD 1983; THOMAS and KIM 1983; ROSS 1986; MUNRO and COTRAN 1988; STARY 1990).

Of the different types of arteriosclerotic lesions (for classification see: GEER and WEBSTER 1974; ROSS and GLOMSET 1976; DOERR 1978; MUNRO and COTRAN 1988; STARY 1990), the advanced or atheromatous lesion as characterized by

Current Topics in Pathology
Volume 87, Vollmer/Roessner (Eds.)

necrotic intimal areas seems to be the most important in causing further stenosing processes which are responsible for the clinical symptoms of atherosclerosis. For example, in myocardial infarction, thrombus formation occluding the artery is often found in association with atheromas (HORT et al. 1982; HORT 1985). In relation to public health it is important to note that this type of lesion is very common in the coronary arteries of people in Western countries (SOLBERG and STRONG 1983). In a recent study, STARY (1990) found that advanced atheromatous plaques were present in the left anterior descending branch in nearly 70% of persons who died at between the ages of 35 and 39 years (in most cases due to accidents, homicide or suicide).

Knowledge of the pathophysiologic mechanisms leading to the formation of atheromatous lesions is still rather scanty. The final development of necrosis is often discussed in relation to the increased diffusion distances within the intimal thickening, which are held to impair the nutritional supply to deeper areas of the vessel wall. This will be a major topic of this chapter and will be dealt with later.

In recent years great emphasis has been placed on exploring the initial steps of atherogenesis. However, information on the dynamics of the cellular processes evoked by the different noxes or risk factors and leading to plaque formation, as well as on their underlying molecular interactions and mechanisms, cannot be obtained from humans. Studies on experimental models or cell culture systems are therefore necessary, despite their limitations when applied to the interpretation of human disease. The results obtained to date indicate that a large variety of substances acting as growth factors, chemoattractants, or other signaling molecules participate in the regulation of the normal cellular functions of the arterial wall and may be disturbed in atherosclerosis. These factors may derive from the cells of the vessel wall itself, from blood cells, from the nervous system, or from hormones, lipoproteins, etc. which are supplied from the blood (GUTSTEIN et al. 1978; ROSS et al. 1982; BOWEN-POPE et al. 1985; DAVIES 1986; NILSSON 1986; ROSS 1986; HANSSON et al. 1988; MUNRO and COTRAN 1988). The mechanisms by which the target cells, i.e., mainly smooth muscle cells, leukocytes (monocytes/macrophages), and endothelial cells, recognize these factors have been well investigated only in certain special cases, e.g., for platelet-derived growth factor (ROSS et al. 1986; FERNS et al. 1991) or for low-density lipoprotein and its oxidatively modified forms (STEINBERG et al. 1989; NIENDORF and BEISIEGEL 1991). Nevertheless, the resulting changes in the behavior of these cells which lead to atherogenesis are strictly dependent on intact cellular intermediary and energy metabolism. For example, recently it was shown in rat aorta that proliferation of intimal smooth muscle cells as induced by endothelial denudation is strongly decreased when the glucose supply is impaired by fasting (RIDRAY et al. 1991). This finding illustrates that the initial steps in atherogenesis, too, depend on the availability of energy-providing substrates, reflecting the importance of the cellular energy metabolism.

Although the enzymatic and biochemical properties of the arterial wall and metabolic alterations in atherosclerosis were investigated and reviewed some time ago (KIRK 1963; ADAMS 1967; ZEMPLENYI 1974; ST. CLAIR 1976; WISSLER et al. 1976), the view that the physiologic and pathophysiologic cellular events in the vessel wall are closely related to and dependent on the metabolism has been somewhat neglected in the last few years. In this chapter we would like to focus again on problems of energy metabolism in atherosclerosis and concentrate on two questions:

1. Are there alterations in cellular energy metabolism in the proliferative phase of atherogenesis and how can they be characterized?
2. Can the development of necrosis in the advanced phase of the lesion be ascribed to alterations in energy metabolism, and to what extent is hypercholesterolmia involved?

Since many of the results which will be presented were obtained from an experimental model, we will first—in order to permit comparisons—summarize some morphologic findings on human atherosclerotic plaques of the coronary arteries as well as those characterizing the animal model. Thereafter, a description of the metabolic properties will be given.

2 Morphologic Characteristics of Human Atherosclerotic Lesions

No attempt will be made here to provide a comprehensive morphologic description of human atherosclerotic plaques; rather only some characteristic features of lesions of coronary arteries (GEER and WEBSTER 1974; HORT 1985; CLIFF et al. 1988; DAVIES et al. 1988; STARY 1990) will be summarized. STARY studied normal and atherosclerotic segments of the left coronary anterior descending branch in persons who died before the age of 40 from causes other than myocardial infarction. Therefore, one can assume that the lesions which were found were mostly at a nonocclusive stage, causing no clinical symptoms. In contrast to this are the findings of HORT (1985), CLIFF et al. (1988), and DAVIES et al. (1988), who investigated coronary vessels of patients who died from myocardial infarction or of hearts removed for transplantation. In these cases, final stages of very advanced lesions can be expected to occur.

In normal coronary arteries the thickness of the intima increases with age. In the subendothelial space a small number of macrophages, smooth muscle cells rich in intracellular organelles, and sometimes mast cells are found. The extracellular matrix consists of proteoglycans, elastin, and collagen.

Lesion development is characterized by increasing numbers of intimal macrophages, which in the initial phase seem to invade as monocytes from the arterial lumen. In advanced, neovascularized lesions, monocyte emigration from the medial and intimal capillaries is also found (BAYLISS HIGH and ADAMS 1980). The number of smooth muscle cells increases, too. This may be caused by (a) migration of cells from the media into the intima, a process seen in many experimental models and also described in human coronary atherosclerosis (SCHLOTE et al. 1980), (b) proliferation, or (c) a combination of both processes. Findings from many experimental models allow the conclusion that proliferation of initimal smooth muscle cells is the dominant mechanism responsible for the increase in cell content of the lesion (SCHWARTZ et al. 1986; KLING et al. 1992).

Intracellular lipid vacuoles are found in very early stages of lesion formation, whereas later on typical foam cells appear, derived either from macrophages or from smooth muscle cells. In fatty streaks which are found even in the arteries of children (STARY 1990), foam cells are locally concentrated in the intima. More advanced lesions grow thicker and additionally contain different types of lymphocytes, abundant extracellular material, and even more lipids. When the lipids form massive extracellular deposits, very often associated with cellular necrosis, the lesion is called atheroma. In fibroatheroma a cap is found covering the uppermost part of the plaque. The cap consists of smooth muscle cells and collagen-rich extracellular material. In this type of human lesion, very often macrophages and T-lymphocytes are found to be concentrated in the shoulder regions of the plaques (JONASSON et al. 1986; HANSSON et al. 1989). Granulocytes are not very frequent in human plaques (JONASSON et al. 1986; STARY 1990); however, many experimental studies show that in acute injuries, granulocytes can enter the vessel wall (KLING et al. 1987a). It is important to note that there is no evidence for endothelial destruction in the normal human coronary artery or in initial lesions (STARY 1990), yet it seems that the endothelium is injured as the plaques become larger (DAVIES et al. 1988). Further signs of advanced lesions are mineralization with calcium, neovascularization, hemorrhage, and often thrombus formation.

3 The Animal Model of Atherosclerosis Used in the Present Studies

3.1 Experimental Protocol for Induction of the Lesions

The animal model of atherosclerosis which was used for the studies reported here is based on the transmural electrical stimulation of the arterial wall and has been described in detail previously (BETZ and SCHLOTE 1979; BETZ et al. 1980; BETZ and HÄMMERLE 1984). In short: in male New Zealand rabbits with a body weight of 2.5–3.5 kg a Teflon cuff bearing two graphite-coated gold electrodes was loosely implanted around the right common carotid artery so that pulsatile wall movements were not hindered. The two electrodes were placed diametrically opposed and close to the adventitia of the vessel. The electrodes were subcutaneously connected with a small socket fixed in the skull which allowed the repeated application of DC impulses, so that the same polarization of the electrodes was always applied. The stimulation was achieved in the freely moving animals in two daily sessions, 30 min in the morning and 15 min in the afternoon. The DC impulses (15 ms/imp., 0.1 mA, 10 Hz) were regulated to constant current. The contralateral arterial segment remained electrically unstimulated, although in some cases sham operated, and always served as an intra-individual control. According to their diet, the animals were categorized into two groups: group 1 received a normal rabbit standard chow (Altromin, Lage, FRG), while group 2 received the same chow enriched with 1% cholesterol.

For morphologic studies, animals were stimulated for periods lasting between several days and 4 weeks. Subsequently the carotid arteries were exposed and either excised and fixed by immersion in paraformaldehyde for light microscopy or perfusion-fixed in situ under physiologic pressure using glutaraldehyde/cacodylate as a fixative for electron microscopy (KLING et al. 1987a). For the metabolic investigations, the stimulation was applied for 4–5 weeks. The procedure employed to obtain the tissue samples for these studies is described in Sects. 4.1 and 4.2.

3.2 Morphologic Alterations Induced by Electrical Stimulation; Definition of the Experimental Lesions

The responses of the arterial wall evoked by the DC stimulation, also with respect to the influence of hypercholesterolemia, are very well characterized by morphologic studies (BETZ and SCHLOTE 1979; BETZ et al. 1980; EITEL et al. 1980; BETZ and HÄMMERLE 1984; KLING et al. 1987a; BETZ 1991; KLING et al. 1991). The results obtained from these investigations show that at the anodic region of the stimulated vessel wall, the site where plaque development will occur, extravasation of granulocytes, monocytes, and lymphocytes can be observed as the initial cellular event. The cells penetrate the endothelial lining and invade the intima. Although the endothelium shows some structural irregularities during this phase, it is continuously present as a morphologically complete cell layer. After the first day of stimulation, smooth muscle cells which now reveal signs of an intermediate phenotype appear in pores of the lamina elastica interna as well as in the intima. Since in the normal carotid artery of rabbits the intima is void of cells, one can assume that these cells have migrated from the media into the intima. Thereafter plaque thickness increases, mainly due to proliferation of the intimal smooth muscle cells and their production of extracellular matrix. The number of leukocytes slowly decreases. Thus, after 4 weeks of stimulation, plaques are formed which contain 10–18 intimal cell layers.

The cellular dynamics of these initial steps were qualitatively similar in the animals of groups 1 and 2, with the thickness of the proliferates after 4 weeks not significantly different between the two groups. Figure 1 shows cross-sections of the intimal lesions of both groups corresponding to the 1-week stage. The obvious difference in this stage is the presence of intracellular lipid vacuoles under hypercholesterolemia. Yet, accurate analysis of the cell kinetics showed that mononuclear cells contributed to a higher degree to the intimal constituents in the plaques of group 2 than in those of group 1 (KLING et al. 1991). After 4

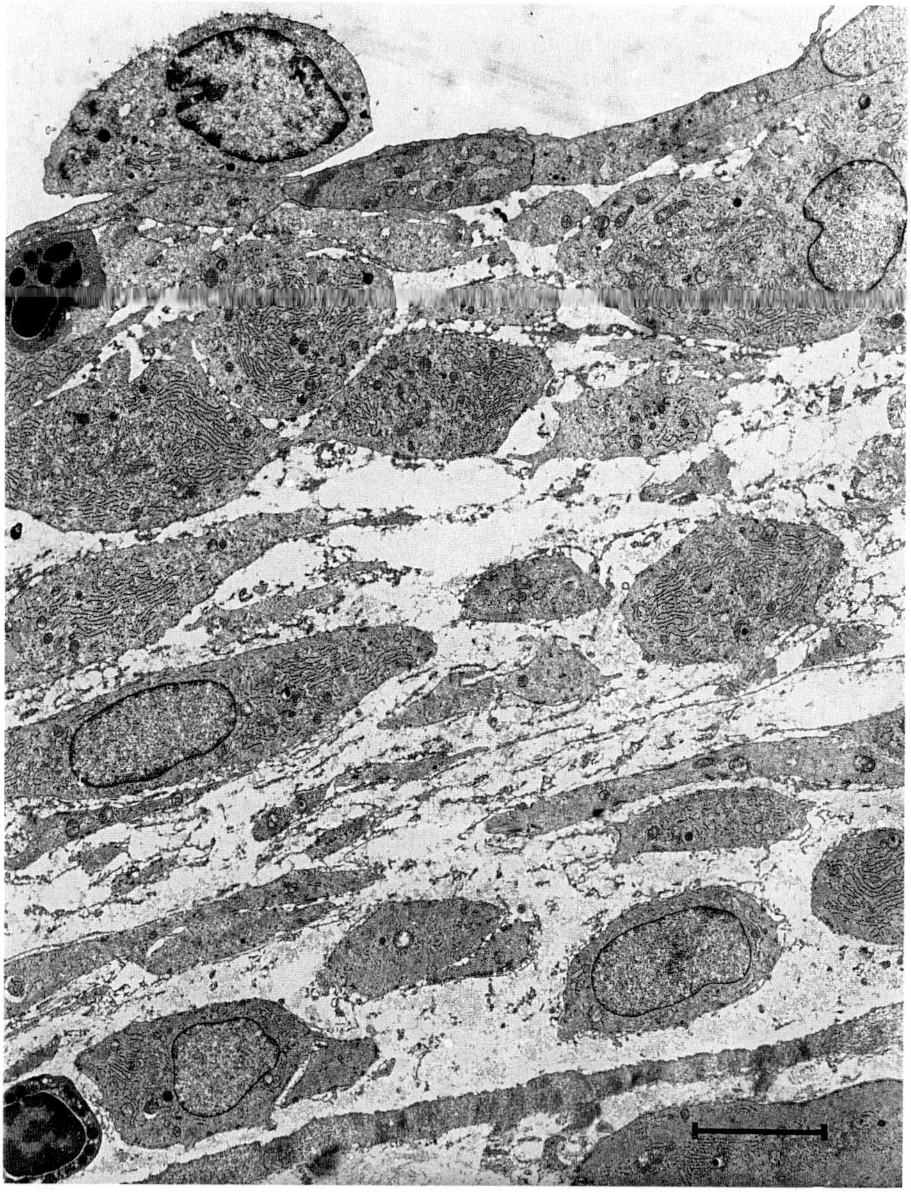

Fig. 1a, b. Electron microscopic pictures of cross-sections through intimal plaques in an initial proliferative stage, induced by DC stimulation of rabbit carotid artery under either **a** normocholesterolemia or **b** hypercholesterolemia. The endothelial lining (*top*) and the internal lamina (*bottom*) are easily recognized. The dominant intimal cell type is smooth muscle of the activated phenotype. In **a** a mononuclear cell is adhering to the endothelium; in **b** the intimal lipid vacuoles are visible. The *bars* represent 4 μm

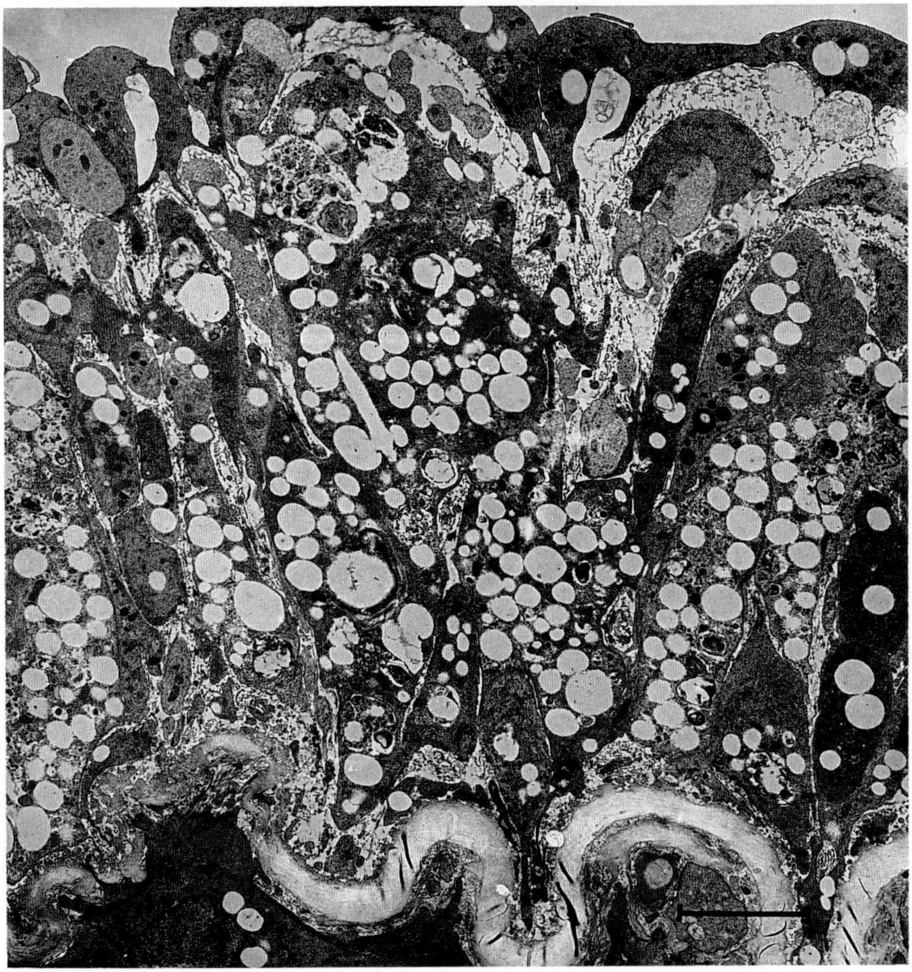

b

weeks, in group 1 only 5% of the intimal cells were macrophages, while in group 2 the figure was about 20%. Furthermore, lipid incorporation, foam cells, and signs of intimal necrosis at later stages were only or predominantly found in group 2.

This morphologic description provides the rationale for the nomenclature we use for the lesions induced by DC stimulation: Since the plaques formed under normocholesterolemia are dominated by smooth muscle cells and fibrous extracellular matrix, we call them *fibromuscular lesions*; under hypercholesterolemia the lipid incorporation, the higher content of macrophages, and the tendency to develop necrosis are very characteristic so that these lesions are called *atheromatous*. Additionally, by comparison with human lesions it is evident that this model closely resembles—on a morphologic level—the fibrofatty lesion of the coronary arteries. Since, as in man, the intimal necrosis is closely associated with lipid incorporation, this model seems suitable for the investigation of basic metabolic mechanisms which might be responsible for necrosis.

3.3 Functional Alterations Induced by DC Stimulation

In order to complete the characterization already provided for the model of transmural DC stimulation, some further results of functional studies will be briefly summarized (HEINLE et al. 1980b, 1987; TARCZY et al. 1981; BETZ and WIEGEL 1982; WIEGEL 1985; APFEL and BETZ 1985; KLING et al. 1987b).

In vivo studies during the initial phase of lesion development revealed a transiently increased permeability of the endothelium for macromolecules, e.g., albumin or horseradish peroxidase, and an altered electrical resistance of the stimulated arterial wall. The increase in permeability became manifest parallel to plaque growth.

In vitro investigations on the passive and active mechanical properties of the vessel segments stimulated for 4 weeks showed increased wall stiffness and increased contractility in comparison to the unstimulated controls. For example, application of the contraction-inducing agonists norepinephrine or serotonin to isolated arteriosclerotic segments of animals of group 2 revealed a shift of the dose–response relation to lower agonist concentrations as well as an increase in the maximal force response. In arteriosclerotic segments of group 1 contractility was not augmented so clearly; in fact, depolarization-induced contractions evoked diminished maximal forces in these cases.

4 Metabolic Characterization of Fibromuscular and Atheromatous Plaques

4.1 Determination of Turnover Rates for Glucose, Oxygen, and Lactate

In order to characterize metabolic fluxes in the lesions, in vitro turnover rates of glucose, oxygen, and lactate were determined using plaques induced in animals of both groups according to the protocol outlined in Sect. 3.1. After 4 weeks of stimulation, the corresponding segments of the stimulated and control carotid arteries were excised and further dissected in a physiologic saline solution at 37°C (KNEHR et al. 1980; HEINLE et al. 1982). When glucose uptake and lactate production were to be measured, the plaques were isolated as an intima–media preparation and incubated for 90 min in 50 µl of oxygenated, HEPES-buffered Tyrode solution (complete composition in HEINLE et al. 1982). Thereafter, glucose and lactate were determined in the incubation medium, and the rates of consumption and production, respectively, were calculated from the concentration

Table 1. In vitro uptake of glucose and oxygen, production of lactate, and ATP turnover in fibromuscular and atheromatous plaques of rabbit carotid arteries

		J_{Glu}	J_{Lac}	J_{O_2}	J_{O_2}/J_{Lac}	J_{ATP}
Group 1 ($n = 5$)	Fibromuscular plaques	55.8 ± 24.5	29.4 ± 12.8	42.6 ± 15.8	1.45	312
	Unstimulated controls	43.9 ± 16.8	18.0 ± 9.5	21.6 ± 4.3	1.20	174
Group 2 ($n = 8$)	Atheromatous plaques	85.7 ± 28.8	45.4 ± 16.9	65.5 ± 8.4	1.44	480
	Unstimulated controls	52.9 ± 16.2	24.2 ± 8.5	40.9 ± 4.9	1.69	294

The turnover rates J are given in $\mu mol\, h^{-1} g^{-1}$ dry weight. J_{ATP} was calculated from $J_{ATP} = 1.25 \cdot J_{LAC} + 6.42 \cdot J_{O_2}$ according to PETERSON and PAUL (1974)

changes and related to the dry weight or DNA content of the corresponding samples. In order to measure oxygen consumption a special chamber was used with an incubation volume of about 250 µl and a polarographic measuring device for continuous registration of the oxygen partial pressure. From the decrease in oxygen pressure over a period of time, its consumption could be calculated and related to dry weight or DNA content of the samples (KNEHR et al. 1980; ENGEL et al. 1984).

The results of these determinations are summarized in Table 1. It is obvious that in both groups all measured turnover rates are increased in the arteriosclerotic plaques when compared to those of the unstimulated controls. This indicates, under the incubation conditions used, an increased energy turnover in the cells of the intimal lesions. Since the ATP turnover can be calculated from oxygen uptake and lactate production under assumptions discussed by PETERSON and PAUL (1974), these calculated values are included in the table. These results show that the lowest value is obtained for the controls of group 1. Hypercholesterolemia also seems to influence the basic energy metabolism of the "normal" arterial wall by increasing its ATP turnover. The highest value is found in the plaques of the hypercholesterolemic animals (group 2). This finding also holds true when the turnover rates are related to the DNA contents of the corresponding tissue samples (HEINLE 1985).

However, these data have to be considered in comparison to results obtained from other models which are summarized in Table 2. Furthermore, they must be discussed critically in relation to methodologic problems that limit the interpretation of such measurements. Beginning with the latter point it is clear that the homeostatic situation during in vitro incubation is quite different from the in vivo situation of the intact vessel wall (for a comprehensive discussion see HEINLE 1985). For example, there are differences in the composition of the surrounding medium, in the pressure and transport gradients across the vessel wall, and in the neuronal supply of the tissue, etc. Therefore, the turnover rates determined in vitro reflect only metabolic capacities corresponding to the incubation conditions applied and cannot be regarded as identical with in vivo fluxes.

Table 2. In vitro uptake of glucose and oxygen, lactate production, and ATP turnover in atherosclerotic plaques. Data from literature

		J_{Glu}	J_{Lac}	J_{O_2}	J_{O_2}/J_{Lac}	J_{ATP}	Reference
Rabbit	aorta						
	Intact	54.4	13.6	35.0	2.58	242	
	Injured	23.2	20.8	23.0	1.11	175	MORRISON et al. (1976)
Rabbit	aorta						
	Atherosclerotic	19.0	36.4	29.3	0.81	235	
	Normal	7.4	13.6	17.0	1.25	127	MORRISON et al. (1972)
Rabbit	aorta						
	Atherosclerotic	54.4	20.4	15.5	0.76	125	
	Normal	60.4	21.2	6.5	0.31	71	STANGE and PAPENBERG (1978)
Rhesus	monkey						
	Atheorosclerotic	–	48.4	30.0	0.62	255	
	Normal	–	19.6	19.6	1.0	151	ST. CLAIR (1976)

The values are calculated from the data in the corresponding references and are given in $\mu mol\,h^{-1}\,g^{-1}$ dry weight. (In relating wet weight to dry weight, a factor of 0.25 was used)

Another problem arising from the artificial handling of the tissue samples is the possibility of severe alterations in metabolic networks, which have been observed especially in smooth muscle after cooling, or injuries to the endothelium (SCOTT et al. 1970; MORRISON et al. 1976). These alterations lead to changes in the metabolic fluxes, i.e., increased lactate production under aerobic conditions. This provides an explanation for the formerly frequent observation of high aerobic glycolysis in arterial tissue. Under optimal tissue protection, low lactate production is found in the presence of oxygen, and a Pasteur effect can be induced under anaerobic conditions (ARNQVIST and LUNDHOLM 1976). As shown by MORRISON et al. (1976), the ratio of fluxes of oxygen and lactate is an appropriate indicator of tissue preservation and undisturbed metabolic properties. Therefore, this calculated value is included in both Tables 1 and 2. The value $J_{O_2}/J_{Lac} = 2.58$ given in Table 2 for intact arterial tissue was never reported by groups studying atherosclerotic vessels, yet the ratio calculated from the fluxes measured in our experiments (Table 1) are closer to this value than the comparable ones of Table 2.

Quantitative calculations with the turnover rates reveal further discrepancies (HEINLE 1985): Assuming that the consumed glucose is mainly used for ATP regeneration under steady-state conditions and that the oxygen consumption is not uncoupled from ATP production, the fluxes of glucose, oxygen, and lactate must be in a strong stoichiometric relation. However, calculations show that this clear relationship does not exist. Instead, either an overshoot consumption of oxygen is found or further substrates must be oxidized in order to explain the high oxygen consumption. Candidates for substrates providing energy by oxidative degradation are glutamate and free fatty acids (ODESSY and CHACE 1982). The latter, at least, might be more readily available in tissues obtained from hyperlipidemic animals. Additionally, it was shown in short-term in vitro experiments that carbohydrate-related energy metabolism in cells of the arterial wall is compartmentalized so that energy derived from lactate production is used for sodium-potassium pumping whereas energy from oxidative phosphorylation is used for the contractile apparatus (PAUL 1983; LYNCH and PAUL 1983). Both might be differently stimulated in the different types of lesions.

A last point has to be borne in mind when explaining the turnover rates of arteriosclerotic lesions: Since the intimal lesions also contain cells other than smooth muscle cells, e.g., macrophages, which have a much higher oxygen consumption than the smooth muscle (BJÖRNHEDEN and BONDJERS 1987), the overall consumption could be increased due to their activity.

Despite these numerous objections and limitations which might be responsible for the large quantitative difference in the results summarized in Tables 1 and 2, the qualitative differences between normal and arteriosclerotic specimens are documented in all cited studies i.e., in arteriosclerotic tissue increased oxygen consumption and lactate production were found under in vitro conditions [this was also the case in studies not included in Tables 1 and 2, in which only oxygen and not lactate was measured, e.g. MUNRO et al. (1961), HAJJAR et al. (1988) or, for review, CRAWFORD and BLANKENHORN (1991)]. Although not necessarily identical to the in vivo situation, these results demonstrate increased metabolic capacities of the cells within the lesion and an increased ATP turnover. Explanations for this phenomenon are still hypothetical and may be seen, for example, in an increased energy demand for synthetic processes, for contraction, or for active transport of potassium, sodium, or calcium due to increased passive membrane permeabilities. These points will be discussed later. Nevertheless, the results presented here (Table 1) show that the enhanced energy turnover within the lesions is due on the one hand to the lesion formation "per se" (as found in the fibromuscular plaque) and on the other to the modulatory effect of hypercholesterolemia. Since in the other experimental models of atherosclerosis referred to in Table 2, hypercholesterolemia is an essential part of the method to induce the atherosclerotic lesion, the model of DC stimulation offers a unique possibility to discriminate this effect.

The increased energy turnover of the plaque cells can only be balanced by an improved supply of substrates, also within the vessel wall. Therefore the question arises as to whether alterations in the arterial wall can be detected under in vivo conditions reflecting, perhaps, a limited cellular supply of substrates. Since hypercholesterolemia contributes to the increased energy turnover, again the model of DC stimulation is very suitable for the study of this question. In the next section experiments will be described in which metabolite contents in fibromuscular and atheromatous lesions were determined in freeze-stopped tissues.

4.2 Determination of Tissue Contents of Substrates and Metabolites

The approach involving characterization of the metabolism of atherosclerotic tissue by the measurement of turnover rates can be extended by determining the tissue content of selected substrates or metabolites. Since the supply of the arterial wall with substrates, e.g., glucose or oxygen, is provided either from the lumen or from the adventitial vasa vasorum, it would be most interesting to ascertain their spatial distribution from the intima to the adventitia. Therefore, we developed a new technique by which we were able to measure the content of glucose, lactate, glycogen, ATP, and ADP so that metabolite concentration gradients across the vessel wall could be established (HEINLE 1987). The gradient of oxygen partial pressure throughout the vessel wall was only provisionally determined in our model; in order to provide this information, some results obtained from other systems will be discussed in a separate section (4.2.3).

4.2.1 Determination of Tissue Gradients of Glucose, Lactate, Glycogen, ATP, and ADP

For these measurements, intimal plaques induced by DC stimulation in rabbits of groups 1 and 2 (with a stimulation time of 4–5 weeks; see sect. 3.1) were used, together with corresponding unstimulated vessel wall segments as controls. In order to maintain conditions within the tissue samples which closely resemble those in the in vivo situation, the specimens were quick-frozen after in situ preparation, as previously described (HEINLE 1987). Shortly after removal of the cuff with the electrodes, the area below the anode (approx. $1 \times 5\,mm^2$) which could be expected to contain the intimal plaque (see Sect. 3.2) was quickly excised and frozen on a cover slide cooled in liquid nitrogen. The endothelial surface was directed toward the glass surface so that after embedding, freezing on the tissue holder of the microtome, and removal of the cover glass, 10-μm-thick slices parallel to the endothelial layer could be obtained with a cryomicrotome (frigocut 2700, Reichert Jung, Heidelberg, FRG). The tissue samples, including those obtained from unstimulated segments, were sliced from the endothelium to the adventitia so that consecutive slice numbers could be assigned to definite distances from the luminal surface. The slices were lyophilized in tissue holders as described by LOWRY and PASSONNEAU (1972) and stored in a desiccator at −40°C. After further preparation of the dried slices and weighing (10–25 μg dry weight per slice; larger samples were divided), glucose, glycogen, and lactate were determined by fluorimetric methods originally described by LOWRY and PASSONNEAU (1972) and modified by HEINLE (1987). ATP was assayed by chemiluminescence using the luciferine–luciferase reaction kit of Boehringer (Mannheim, FRG). Light emission was measured in a Biolumat LB 9500 (Berthold, Wildbad, FRG). The same test system was used for the determination of ADP; however, prior to the chemiluminescence reaction this metabolite was phosphorylated to ATP with phosphoenolpyruvate and pyruvate kinase (in principle according to BERGMEYER 1974). In this way the sum of ATP and ADP is obtained. In order to discriminate the ATP content of the slice used for the ADP reaction, the ATP/DNA ratio of a neighboring tissue specimen was calculated, and based on this ratio, the ATP content of the "ADP slice" was

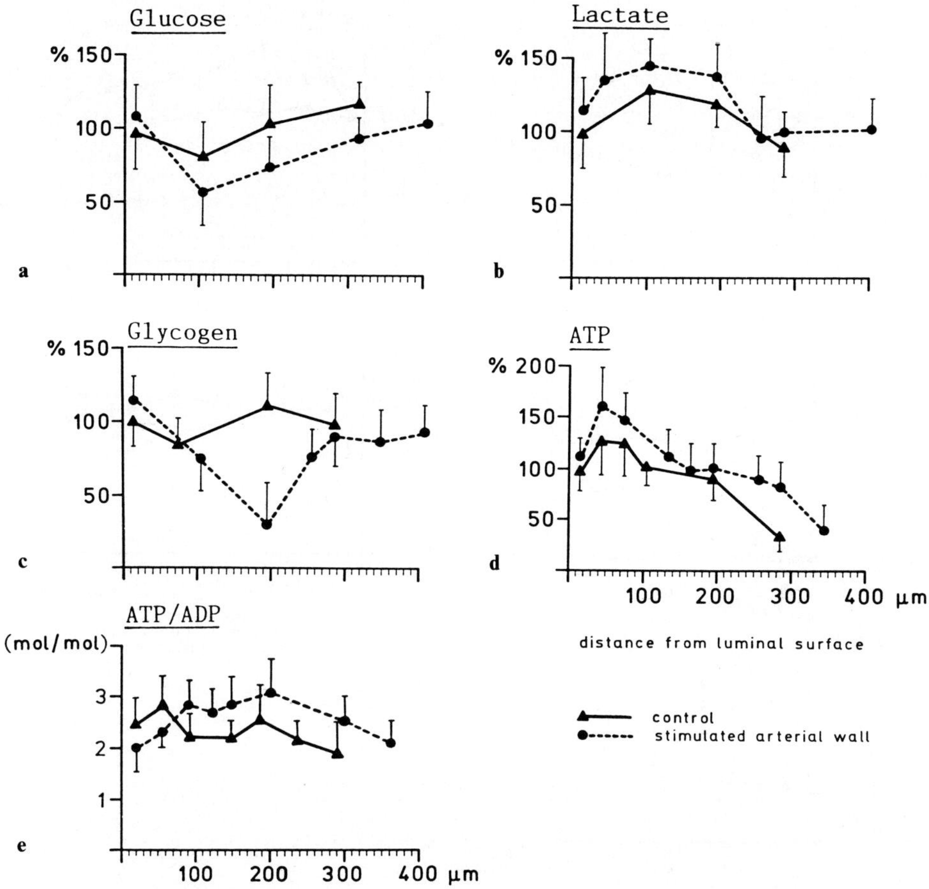

Fig. 2a–e. Gradients of tissue contents of glucose, lactate glycogen, and ATP, and the ratio of ATP/ADP across rabbit carotid artery stimulated by DC impulses under normocholesterolemia. "Control" corresponds to unstimulated vessel wall of the contralateral artery. The signs represent mean values ± SD ($n = 6$), calculated for ranges each corresponding to a thickness of 30 µm. The absolute values (corresponding to 100%) are 580 (glucose), 750 (lactate), 1300 (glycogen), and 140 (ATP), all indicated in nmol/mg DNA

determined. Thereafter the content of ADP alone was obtained by subtraction. All measurements were calibrated with corresponding standards; the results were related to the dry weight as well as to the DNA content of the corresponding slices.

The results of these measurements are given in Fig. 2 for group 1 and in Fig. 3 for group 2. In these diagrams the normalized contents of glucose, glycogen, lactate, and ATP as well as the ATP/ADP ratio are plotted with respect to the distance from the endothelium. Since in rabbits there are no subendothelial cells in the normal carotid artery, the intima of the segments used as controls is less than 10 µm and cannot be separated by the applied

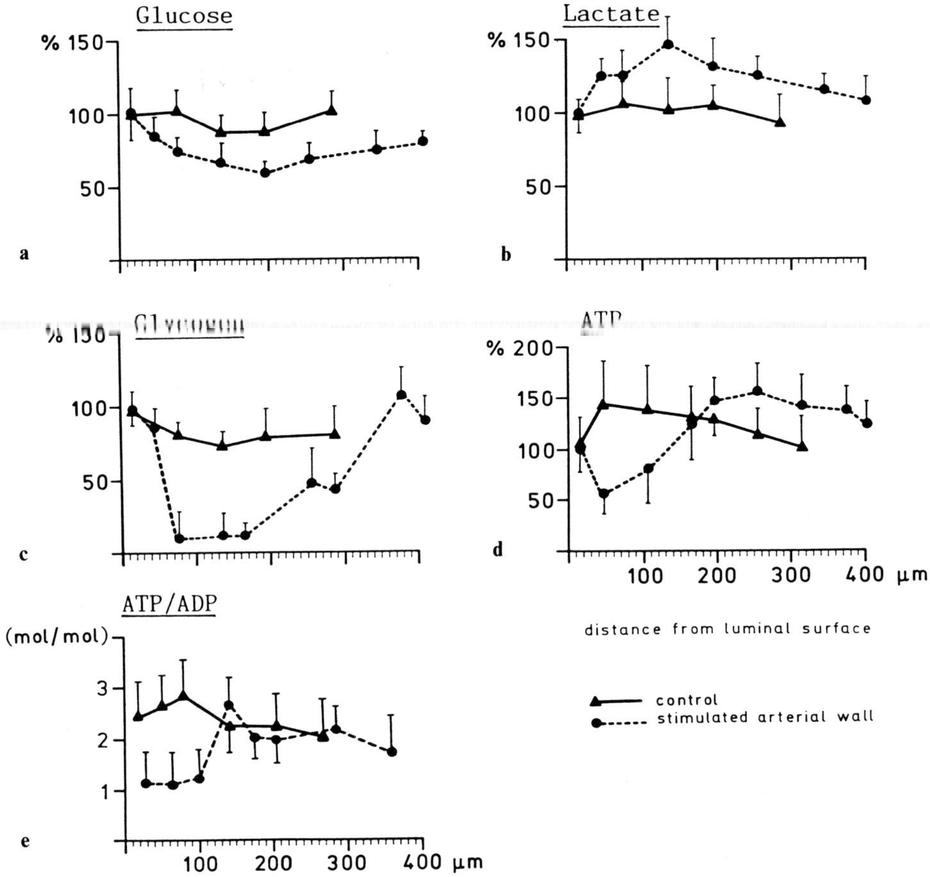

Fig. 3a–e. Gradients of tissue contents of glucose, lactate, glycogen, and ATP, and the ratio of ATP/ADP across rabbit carotid artery stimulated by DC impulses under hypercholesterolemia. For further explanation, see Fig. 2. The absolute values (based on measurements on nine animals and corresponding to 100%) are 420 (glucose), 630 (lactate), 820 (glycogen), and 142 (ATP), again given in nmol/mg DNA

technique. The media corresponds to about 15–20 slice (150–200 µm), and the slices up to 300 µm belong to the adventitia. In the stimulated arterial walls with the atherosclerotic lesion, the intima has thickened to about 150–200 µm, whereas the media is practically unaltered. Due to the electrodes and the dissection of the cuff, the thickness of the adventitia is usually somewhat decreased in the stimulated segment (findings from the morphologic studies mentioned in Sect. 3.2). For these reasons, the wall thickness of the normal carotid artery corresponds to about 300 µm, and that of the atherosclerotic one to about 400 µm.

Regarding the results obtained from group 1 (Fig. 2), it is obvious that in fibromuscular plaques glycogen is greatly decreased in the layers 100–200 µm

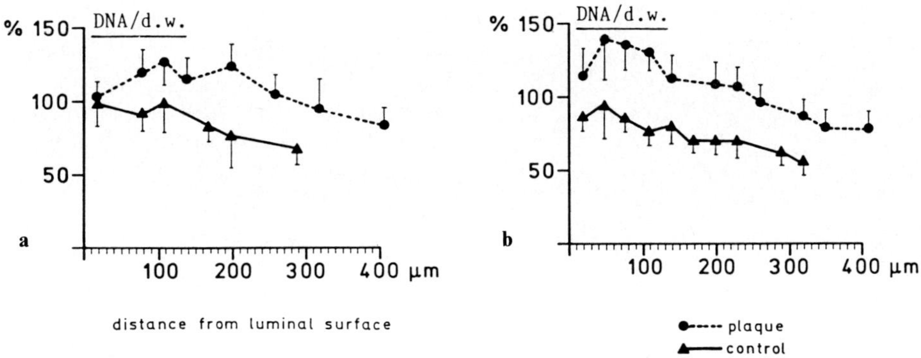

Fig. 4a, b. Gradients of the ratio of DNA/dry weight (*d.w.*) across rabbit carotid artery stimulated by DC impulses under **a** normocholesterolemia or **b** hypercholesterolemia. For further explanation, see Fig. 2. The absolute values (Corresponding to 100%) are **a** 9.9 μg DNA/mg d.w.

below the endothelium. In comparison to the control values, the content of glucose is slighly decreased in these layers, whereas there is a small increase in lactate and ATP. There are no significant differences in the ATP/ADP ratio between the fibromuscular plaque and normal media. Figure 3 clearly reveals the deviations from the results just mentioned. In the atheromatous plaque it is most impressive to see the low content sometimes even the absence of glycogen in the layers between 50 and 150 μm. Also, ATP and the ATP/ADP ratio are greatly decreased in these layers. Lactate is slightly more increased in the intima than under normocholesterolemia, and the decrease of glucose seems to be shifted to deeper layers. In the adventitia of all tissue sample investigated, comparable contents of the metabolites were found.

Determination of the DNA content in the slices revealed that in all intimal slices of fibromuscular and atheromatous plaques, the ratio of DNA to dry weight was similar to (or even higher than) that in normal media (Fig. 4). These DNA gradients indicate that the cells of the analyzed tissues were stopped under vital conditions and that also in group 2 the lesions were still prior to the stage of manifestation of large necrotic centers, which of course could not be evaluated in these experiments with histologic methods.

The intimal alterations of the tissue contents of lactate, glycogen and ATP are illustrated in Fig. 5, which shows the respective gradients drawn into a morphological picture of a corresponding cross section of a typical atheromatous plaque (group 2).

Results obtained with this technique from plaques which were found in the thoracic aorta of the hypercholesterolemic rabbits after the experimental period of 4–5 weeks (HEINLE 1987) showed a morphologic situation very similar to that in lesions of the carotid artery, i.e., there was clear discrimination between intima and media, with intimal myocytes and macrophages. In both cell types lipid incorporation was found and the thickness of the subendothelial space ranged from 150 to 200 μm. In addition, the concentration profiles of glucose,

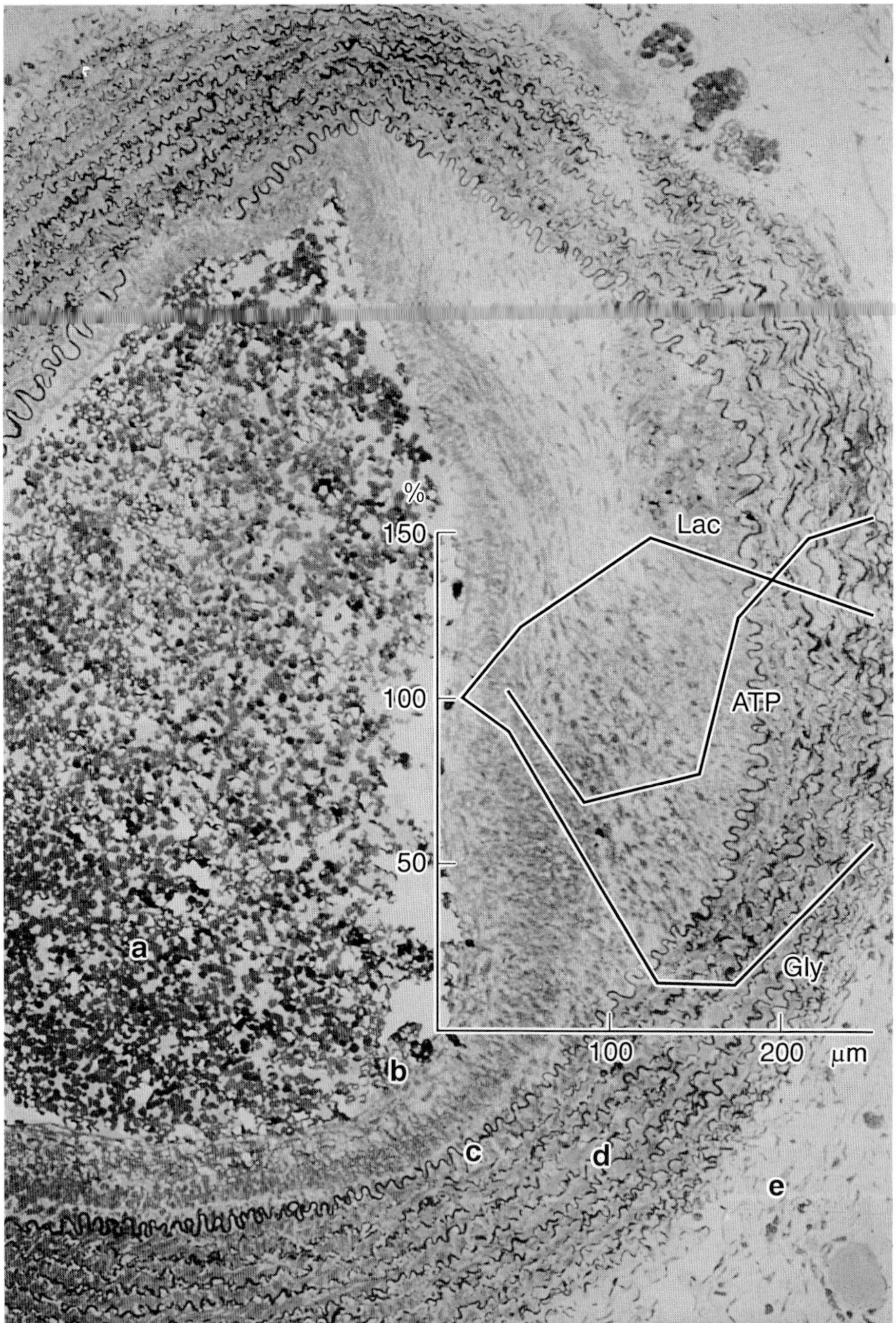
%
150
100
50
Lac
ATP
Gly
100
200
μm
a
b
c
d
e

glycogen, lactate, and ATP closely resembled those of the carotid artery lesions of group 2. This means that in the intimal layers, glycogen and ATP were greatly reduced. This finding allows the more general statement that plaque development under hypercholesterolemia, irrespective of its initial causal mechanism, is associated with metabolic alterations leading to an impairment of the energy metabolism, with decreased stores of the energy-providing glycogen and decreased ATP content.

4.2.2 Discussion of the Results

As in the case of the results outlined in Sect. 4.1, when discussing these data one first has to consider certain methodologic problems. As regards the construction of the metabolite concentration gradients across the vessel wall, it is evident that the excision of the tissue sample alters its geometry. In situ, the vessel wall is stretched by the blood pressure, which is released after dissection. This means that primarily the distribution of the extracellularly occurring substances such as glucose and lactate becomes diffuse; the dislocation of the intracellular compounds such as the adenine nucleotides or glycogen should be less pronounced. This might be one reason why the profiles across the vessel wall are more differentiated for glycogen and ATP than for glucose and lactate. Furthermore, one must be aware that even if the tissues are quick-frozen, there might be alterations in the metabolite contents due to narcosis, anoxia, or the freezing technique (Faupel et al. 1972). This problem especially concerns the contents of ATP and ADP, which are very sensitive to hypoxia (Faupel et al. 1972). Therefore, it is possible that the values for ATP and the ATP/ADP ratio reported here are lower than those in vivo. However, since all specimens were handled identically, the decreased values in the atheromatous plaques show either the pathophysiologic fact of decreased cellular levels of ATP or, at least, altered metabolic properties in these areas with a reduced ability to maintain ATP during preparation of the tissue until the freeze-stop. This could be caused by increased ATP breakdown or impaired rephosphorylation. Irrespective of the exact mechanism, this impairment of the energy metabolism seems to be important for the development of necrosis.

Comparison with results reported by others shows that no data are available for the atherosclerotic carotid artery of the rabbit. However, measurements on homogenates obtained from either complete vessel walls or intima media preparations from different types of normal arteries resulted in concentrations similar to the mean values that can be calculated from the control profiles given here

Fig. 5. Gradients of lactate (Lac), glycogen (Gly) and ATP calculated as relative values from the data of Fig. 4 and superimposed onto a cross section (H&E staining) of a typical atheromatous plaque obtained from group 2. In this case, the stimulation period was 5 weeks; in the upper third of the intimal lesion, beginning necrosis at the base of the plaque is visible. *a*, lumen; *b*, intima; *c*, lamina elastica interna; *d*, media; *e*, adventitia

(MORRISON et al. 1976; ZEMPLENYI 1977; KIRSCH et al. 1978; PAUL 1981). With respect to atherosclerotic tissue, in particular the contents of ATP and ADP were determined by NUMANO et al. (1979) in the intima and media of aorta of rabbits fed a cholesterol-enriched diet for 15 weeks. They analyzed the tissues after microdissecting lyophilized cross-sections of aorta and found that in the thickened intima the contents of both ATP and ADP were reduced to about 40%–60% of levels in the normal media. However, ATP/ADP ratio values in the intima were not significantly changed and amounted to approximately 1. Other information on atherosclerotic tissue is rather scanty. According to KIRK (1963) the glycogen content is decreased by 50% in human atherosclerotic lesions of the femoral artery, and it was postulated by SMITH (1982) that the lactate content should be increased in intimal lesions.

This information confirms the view already derived from our results that the metabolic alterations within a growing plaque lead to a situation in which the increased energy demand causes a depletion of energy-providing substrates, i.e., glucose and, especially, glycogen. Such depletion was found in fibromuscular plaques (group 1) as well as in the atheromatous plaques of group 2—even in those which developed in the aorta under the influence of hypercholesterolemia. However, the ability to maintain both the level of ATP and the ATP/ADP ratio seemed to be particularly impaired in the arteries of the cholesterol-fed rabbits. Since the plaques of the carotid artery in such animals are prone to develop necrotic centers, it is tempting to speculate that the ATP depletion or the deterioration of ATP regeneration is responsible for cellular injury ultimately leading to necrosis. Possible mechanisms by which hypercholesterolemia might contribute to the impairment of ATP metabolism will be discussed in Sect. 6.3.

4.2.3 Gradients of Oxygen Partial Pressure in Atherosclerotic Plaques

As described in Sect. 4.1, oxygen consumption was measured in fibromuscular and atheromatous plaques induced by DC stimulation in the rabbit carotid artery. Since in both cases increased uptake was found, it would be interesting to know whether or not altered concentration profiles are also found for oxygen within the thickened arterial wall. Orientating measurements performed in our laboratory provided a profile of oxygen partial pressure with a minimum (but not anoxia) in the inner third of the vessel wall. In order to provide an overview, some published data from other investigations will be discussed (see also the review of CRAWFORD and BLANKENHORN 1991).

Means of measuring oxygen partial pressure profiles within the arterial wall have long been a topic of discussion. One problem in obtaining accurate results used to be the sensitivity of the platinum electrodes to the mechanical pressure exerted by the tissue when the electrode penetrated the arterial wall. With this technical limitation, profiles of oxygen partial pressure were registered in normal arterial wall, which showed values close to zero near the lamina elastica interna and a sharp increase to levels of normal arterial oxygenation after penetration of this boundary (MOSS et al. 1968).

After the development of recessive electrodes in which the surface of the platinum wire was protected from the pressure generated by the tissue, the registered gradients were revealed to decrease continuously within the arterial wall, with a minimum at the inner third of the media. Thus, the formerly found diffusion barrier at the lamina elastica interna could be declared to be an artifact. Towards the adventitia the oxygen partial pressure increased again. Measurements in atherosclerotic vessels showed that the minimum values in the oxygen profile are even lower below an intimal atherosclerotic thickening (HEUGHAN et al. 1973; JURRUS and WEISS 1977; SCHNEIDERMAN and GOLDSTICK 1978; HAJJAR et al. 1988). These findings further extend the view, that the cells within the intimal atherosclerotic lesions develop an increase in their energy metabolism which exhausts their stores of energy-providing substrates and also leads to lower levels of oxygen pressure within the tissue. These alterations may be enhanced by the prolonged diffusion distance from the lumen or vasa vasorum into the intima or by impaired diffusional transport due to changes in the extracellular space. Nevertheless, these changes seem to be relevant to the increased tendency toward development of intimal necrosis. However, if necrotic areas are present, the acellular regions decrease their oxygen demand, so that anoxic spots are not a characteristic sign of necrotic regions.

5 Intimal Plaques and Intimal Necrosis

The discrepancy between the energy consumption of the cells and their supply of required substrates might provide an explanation for the development of the necrotic centers frequently found at the base of intimal plaques in the vicinity of a fragmentated internal lamina. For example, SCOTT et al. (1966) reported that in human atherosclerotic plaques, necrosis is always found when their thickness increases to more than 0.6–0.8 mm. On the other hand, it was shown by VELICAN and VELICAN (1982) that in human arteries, intimal necrosis very often occurs at distances from the endothelium that are clearly shorter than the above-mentioned critical distance, so that insufficiency of diffusional transport cannot be the reason for the necrosis.

Further insights into the different pathophysiologic mechanisms of necrosis are provided by our results obtained with the DC stimulation model. As described in Sect. 3.2, this model offers the possibility of inducing intimal plaques of either the fibromuscular or the atheromatous type which grow during the stimulation time of 4 weeks to a similar thickness of approximately 15 cell layers (BETZ and SCHLOTE 1979; BETZ and HÄMMERLE 1984). However, development of intimal necrosis is mainly seen in the presence of hypercholesterolemia and is associated with the impairment of ATP metabolism of the cells within the atheroma. Therefore, one can postulate that there is a mechanism leading to intimal necrosis that is probably due to insufficiency of diffusional transport of substrates or metabolites. Another mechanism seems to be dependent on altered plasma lipoprotein levels induced by dietary cholesterol administration. In the final section some mechanisms will be discussed by which hypercholesterolemia can impair cellular energy metabolism and contribute to intimal necrosis.

6 Hypercholesterolemia-Related Mechanisms Which Could Support Intimal Necrosis

Since the increase of plasma cholesterol induced by dietary cholesterol supplementation in rabbits is mainly due to an increase in the concentrations of low-density lipoproteins (LDL), which also represent an important risk factor for human coronary artery disease, we would like to discuss some interactions of this plasma constituent and its oxidatively modified forms with components of the arterial wall. These mechanisms might contribute essentially and causally to the development of intimal necrosis.

6.1 Influence of Hypercholesterolemia on the Monocyte/Macrophage System

The results obtained from the morphologic studies using the DC stimulation model show that in the initial phase of plaque development, macrophages are an important component of the intima (Sect. 3.2). Yet, during the first 2 weeks, no significant difference could be found in the intimal content of macrophages between the hypercholesterolemic and the normocholesterolemic group. Thereafter, the number of mononuclear cells in the intima decreased in both groups, though the decline was significantly slower in the hypercholesterolemic group. This means that after a stimulation period of 4 weeks, atheromatous plaques contain 3-4 times more mononuclear cells than the fibromuscular lesions. The question of how LDL-related hypercholesterolemia may contribute to this effect can be discussed in light of the hypothesis mainly elaborated by Steinberg and co-workers (for review see, e.g. STEINBERG et al. 1989; STEINBRECHER et al. 1990; ROSENFELD 1991), according to which LDL is active chiefly after its oxidative modification. The mechanism underlying this chemical reaction is a peroxidative attack by the polyunsaturated fatty acids present in LDL and a concomitant modification of the apoproteins by aldehydic degradation products of the fatty acids. This reaction is assumed to take place within the intima in contact with endothelial or smooth muscle cells or macrophages. Although the reaction products formed might not in all cases be uniformly due to differences in either the LDL or the mechanism of oxidation, they have numerous effects on different cellular systems. Among them are chemoattraction of monocytes, as well as inhibition of migration of mononuclear cells after incorporation into monocytes or macrophages (QUINN et al. 1987). Under the assumption that LDL oxidation also occurs in the intima after DC stimulation of the arterial wall, at least the last-mentioned effect may contribute to the increased macrophage content in the atheromatous plaques. In the human lesion, too, these mechanisms could contribute to the increased macrophage content in the intima.

The role of macrophages in atherosclerosis is still only partially understood. Besides beneficial effects (e.g., removal of lipids, induction of wound-healing processes after injury), they also exert cytotoxic effects that probably increase the danger of developing necrosis. One of these, as already mentioned, is enhanced uptake of various substrates (e.g., oxygen), causing an insufficiency in the supply to the other intimal cells (BJÖRNHEDEN and BONDJERS 1987; see Sect. 4.1). Additionally, more direct cytotoxic effects are ascribed to activated macrophages which secrete a great variety of products with very different physiologic functions and pathophysiologic importance (NATHAN 1987). Those most responsible for cytotoxicity are reactive oxygen species such as superoxide anion, hydroxyl radicals or hydrogen peroxide (BADWEY and KARNOWSKY 1980), nitric oxide in combination with superoxide (RADI et al. 1991), and various hydrolytic enzymes which can influence and attack surrounding cells and extracellular material by different mechanisms (NATHAN 1987).

With respect to the effects of reactive oxygen metabolities, such as hydrogen peroxides, on the arterial wall, we performed investigations the results of which will be included in Sect. 6.3.

6.2 Influence of Hypercholesterolemia on Lipid Peroxidation Reactions

The peroxidation of polyunsaturated fatty acids in lipoproteins or membranes is regarded as a widespread pathophysiologic mechanism responsible for cellular damage in very different pathologic situations. The quantification of this reaction is very often based on the test with thiobarbituric acid, although it has been demonstrated that this test is not very specific and therefore only of limited value. Nevertheless, it has been shown by this and other methods that in various animal models with hypercholesterolemia (TSAI and CHEN 1975; HEINLE and LIEBICH 1980; HEINLE et al. 1991a), and in patients with coronary artery disease or diabetes mellitus (LOEPER et al. 1983; NISHIGAKI et al. 1981), increased plasma levels of degradation products of lipid peroxidation occur. The origin of these substances is not clear and could be based on (a) the increased peroxidation of the polyunsaturated fatty acids needed for cholesterol esterification, (b) the augmented concentration of oxidized LDL, or (c) decreased detoxification by reduction of lipid hydroperoxides in blood or in tissues. Nevertheless, these findings confirm that under conditions of hypercholesterolemia the vessel wall is exposed to peroxidative stress (HEINLE and LIEBICH 1980). Furthermore, it was reported long ago and recently confirmed (GLAVIND et al. 1952; MOWRI et al. 1986) that atheromas contain peroxides of polyunsaturated fatty acids and their degradation products. Again, their origin is not clear. They could be derived either from oxidized LDL formed in the intima or from lipids oxidized, for example, by the reactive oxygen metabolites secreted by macrophages.

Since our experiments with low-molecular-weight hydroperoxides and oxidized LDL showed that both severely impair the energy metabolism of the normal arterial wall, these results will be discussed in the next section.

6.3 Influence of Low-Molecular-Weight Hydroperoxides and Oxidized LDL on Energy Metabolism of Normal Arterial Wall

In order to induce oxidative stress on the arterial wall in vitro, we administered the low-molecular-weight hydroperoxides hydrogen peroxide and *tert*-butylhydroperoxide, the hydroperoxides of linolenic acid and oxidized LDL, respectively, to excised segments of the aorta and the common carotic artery of normally fed rabbits. Effects on the tissue contents of glycogen and ATP on the activity of glycogen phosphorylase *a* and—as an indication of alterations of intracellular calcium—on contractility were determined. The details of the experiments and the incubation conditions of the tissue samples have already been reported elsewhere (Heinle 1984, 1989; Heinle et al. 1991b).

6.3.1 Influence of Low-Molecular-Weight Hydroperoxides

These studies showed that at concentrations above 0.2 m*M*, hydrogen peroxide and *tert*-butylhydroperoxide induce a strong activation of glycogen breakdown which can be explained by the simultaneously observed five fold increase in the ratio of active glycogen phosphorylase *a* to inactive phosphorylase *b* (Heinle 1982, 1989). Concomitantly, ATP is decreased by about 50% whereas the ATP/ADP ratio is decreased from about 2.3 (as found in fresh arterial tissue) to approximately 1.2. With respect to alterations of contractility, it was found that at concentrations of about 0.3 m*M* the peroxides were able to induce contraction in relaxed arterial rings (Heinle 1984). This indicates that cytosolic levels of calcium ions are increased under these conditions. Lower peroxide concentrations did not cause contraction. However, even at concentrations of 10 μ*M*, potentiated contraction enhancement was found when the contractile apparatus was simultaneously activated, e.g., by depolarization. This finding can be interpreted as a facilitative effect of the hydroperoxides on cytosolic calcium release. The linolenic acid hydroperoxide as synthesized in the reaction with soy been lipoxidase revealed similar effects on contractility in concentrations up to 20 μ*M*.

6.3.2 Influence of Oxidized LDL

In experiments similar to those just described, we studied the effects of oxidized LDL on arterial segments of normally fed rabbits (Heinle et al. 1991b). LDL

Table 3. Influence of oxidized LDL and *tert*-butylhydroperoxide (tBHP) on glycogen and ATP content of aortic preparations from normally fed rabbits

	Fresh tissue	Incubation in PSS	Incubation with native LDL	Incubation with oxidized LDL	Incubation with tBHP
Glycogen	12.9 ± 3.6	10.3 ± 2.5	9.5 ± 2.4	2.6 ± 1.9*	5.0 ± 3.1
ATP	2.2 ± 0.5	1.9 ± 0.6	1.6 ± 0.8	0.4 ± 0.3*	1.1 ± 0.4

PSS, physiologic salt solution
* Difference from incubation with native LDL was significant, with $P < 0.05$ (Student's *t*-test)
All values are given in μmol/g dry weight (and represent mean values ± SD, $n = 5$). Concentration of LDL (native and oxidized) was 2 mg/ml in each case; that of tBHP was 1 m*M*

was oxidized in vitro according to ESTERBAUER et al. (1987) and added to the incubation medium in concentrations up to 2 mg/ml. The alterations in the tissue contents of glycogen and ATP and the effects on contractility were measured.

The results of the metabolic determinations are summerized in Table 3. They show that oxidized LDL has effects similar to those of low-molecular-weight hydroperoxides on these parameters of energy metabolism, with a great decrease in glycogen and ATP. For the sake of comparison, the ATP-decreasing effect of incubation in the presence of *tert*-butylhydroperoxide is also documented in the table.

The parallelism in the effects is also seen in relation to the influence on contractility. Here again, contraction was induced when high concentrations of oxidized LDL (> 1 mg/ml) were applied to relaxed arterial segments, whereas low concentrations (below 0.5 mg/ml) had a contraction-enhancing effect only under the condition of simultaneous stimulation by depolarization.

This very strong similarity in the effects evoked by low-molecular-weight hydroperoxides and oxidized LDL suggests that the responses are due to the same mechanisms. This seems possible since it has been shown that oxidized LDL contains a wide variety of different peroxidative reaction products of polyunsaturated fatty acids (ESTERBAUER et al. 1987) which might mimic the influence of the separately applied low-molecular-weight hydroperoxides. However, additional effects of other components of oxidized LDL or the whole lipoprotein cannot be excluded (TANNER et al. 1991).

The concentration ranges of the peroxides and oxidized LDL used for these experiments might exceed those expected to be present in the arterial wall, yet they are able to induce in a short time alterations in the normal arterial wall which are similar to those found in atherosclerotic plaques under the long-term influence of hypercholesterolemia. These findings suggest that hypercholesterolemia can contribute to the development of intimal necrosis by generating oxidative stress. The underlying mechanisms seem to be related, on the one hand, to increased calcium release from intracellular stores which are sensitive to thiol oxidation (TRIMM et al. 1986) and which can be blocked by thiol alkylation (TRIES 1990). Since many metabolic systems and energy-consuming intracellular pathways (e.g., synthetic processes, contraction, active ion transport) are regulated by cytosolic calcium, its increase causes a stimulation of the ATP turnover, which in turn needs an increased substrate supply (see Sect. 4.1).

On the other hand, it is known that hydroperoxides are detoxified intracellularly by the glutathione peroxidase–glutathione disulfide reductase system, which needs $NADPH_2$ to be completely effective. The latter is mainly provided by the pentose phosphate pathway, which also needs glucose or glycogen as a substrate. Therefore, it is conceivable that under conditions of oxidative challenge there are limitations to the glucose/glycogen metabolism, which cannot simultaneously maintain the supply for the energy-providing reactions and for the production of the reducing equivalents. This provides an explanation for the discussed energy insufficiency of the atheromatous plaques.

7 Concluding Remarks and Clinical Implications

The investigations presented here on the experimental model of atherosclerosis produced by transmural DC stimulation of the arterial wall reveal that development of intimal necrosis is to a great extent dependent on hypercholesterolemia and seems to be related to alterations in energy metabolism. In atheromatous plaques as induced under hypercholesterolemia, increased turnover rates of glucose, oxygen, and ATP and decreases in the contents of glycogen and ATP and in the ATP/ADP ratio were found to reflect an insufficient energy balance. In fibromuscular lesions the alterations were less pronounced. The underlying mechanisms causing necrosis within atheromas seem to be mainly dependent on peroxidative reactions which can be induced by oxidized LDL or by reactive oxygen metabolites released from activated macrophages.

With respect to human atheromatosis it is important to note that the development of clinical symptoms in atherosclerotic subjects is closely related to the occurrence of atheromatous plaques and that many risk factors cause augmented lipid peroxidation or increased generation of reactive oxygen metabolites. This has been shown for hypercholesterolemia (LOEPER et al. 1983; AVOGARO et al. 1988), diabetes mellitus (WOLFF et al. 1991), and smoking (HARATS et al. 1990). Therefore, one can assume that oxidative stress is a generally occurring mechanism probably responsible for aggravation of atherosclerosis.

Occlusive thrombosis causing ischemic complications is very often found in areas with intimal ruptures due to intimal necrotic centers (HORT 1985). However, activation of thrombocytes could also be stimulated in areas still morphologically intact when the cellular ADP level is increased due to impaired energy metabolism. It is known that degradation products of the adenine nucleotides can be released from the cells in order to maintain a high ATP/ADP ratio, thus stimulating luminal thrombosis. These results suggest that peroxidative stress is a very important factor aggravating atherosclerotic reactions of the vessel wall, and it seems worthwhile to improve the corresponding antioxidant capacities by suitable dietary or therapeutic precautions.

Acknowledgements The experiments of our group presented in this work were in part supported by grants from the Deutsche Forschungsgemeinschaft, from the Erwin Riesch-Stiftung, the Karl

Kuhn-Stiftung, and the Alfred Teufel-Stiftung. The excellent technical assistance of Ms. H. Ableiter, Ms. S. Dreher, and Ms. R. Weidler is gratefully acknowledged.

References

Adams CWM (1967) Vascular histochemistry in relation to the chemical and structural pathology of cardiovascular disease. Lloyd-Luke, London

Apfel H, Betz E (1985) Der elektrische Widerstand von Arterienwänden bei Atheromentwicklung. Angio Arch 7:91–93

Arnqvist HJ, Lundholm L (1976) Influence of oxygen tension on the metabolism of vascular smooth muscle: demonstration of a Pasteur effect. Atherosclerosis 25:245–252

Avogaro P, Bittolo Bon G, Cazzolato G (1988) Presence of a modified low density lipoprotein in humans. Arteriosclerosis 8:79–87

Badwey JA, Karnowsky M (1980) Active oxygen species and the function of phagocytotic leukocytes. Annu Rev Biochem 49:695–726

Bayliss High OB, Adams CWM (1980) The role of macrophages and giant cells in advanced human atherosclerosis. Atherosclerosis 36:441–447

Bergmeyer HU (ed) (1974) Methoden der enzymatischen Analyse. Verlag Chemie, Weinheim, pp 2178–2182

Betz E (1991) Animal models and cultures of vessel wall cells in atherosclerosis research. Z Kardiol 80 [Suppl 9]:7–13

Betz E Hämmerle H (1984) The action of antiatherogenic drugs on the development of atheroma and on cultures of smooth muscle cells and fibroblasts. Funkt Biol Med 3:46–55

Betz E, Schlote W (1979) Responses of vessel walls to chronically applied electrical stimuli. Basic Res Cardiol 74:10–20

Betz E, Wiegel W (1982) Smooth muscle hypersensitivity to norepinephrine of atheromatous proliferates in carotid arteries. In: Heisted DD, Marcus MC (eds) Cerebral blood flow. Effects of nerves and neurotransmitters. Elsevier/North-Holland, Amsterdam, pp 177–182

Betz E, Roth J, Schlote W (1980) Proliferation of smooth muscle cells in long-term local stimulation of carotid arteries. Folia Angiol 28:28–31

Björnheden T, Bondjers G (1987) Oxygen consumption in aortic tissue from rabbits with diet induced atherosclerosis. Arteriosclerosis 7:238–247

Bowen-Pope DF, Ross R, Seifert RA (1985) Locally acting growth factors for vascular smooth muscle cells: endogenous synthesis and release from platelets. Circulation 72:735–740

Camejo G (1982) The interactions of lipids and lipoproteins with the extracellular matrix of arterial tissue: its possible role in atherogenesis. Adv Lipid Res 19:1–53

Cliff WJ, Heathcote CR, Moss NS, Reichenbach DD (1988) The coronary arteries in cases of cardiac and noncardiac sudden death. Am J Pathol 132:319–329

Crawford DW, Blankenhorn DH (1991) Arterial wall oxygenation, oxyradicals, and atherosclerosis. Atherosclerosis 89:97–108

Davies MJ, Woolf N, Rowlews PM, Pepper J (1988) Morphology of the endothelium over atherosclerotic plaques in human coronary arteries. Br Heart J 60:459–464

Davies PF (1986) Vascular cell interactions with special reference to the pathogenesis of atherosclerosis. Lab Invest 55:5–21

Doerr W (1978) Arteriosclerosis without end. Principles of pathogenesis and an attempt at a nosologic classification. Virchows Arch [A] 380:91–106

Drake TA, Hannani K, Fei HH, Lavi S, Berliner JA (1991) Minimally oxidized low density lipoprotein induces tissue factor expression in cultured human endothelial cells. Am J Pathol 138:601–607

Eitel W, Schmid G, Schlote W, Betz E (1980) Early arteriosclerotic changes of the carotid artery wall induced by electrostimulation. A study by scanning and transmission electron microscopy. Pathol Res Pract 170:211–229

Engel E, Knehr HE, Betz E (1984) Messungen des Sauerstoffverbrauchs von Arterienwandelementen. Funktionsanalyse biologischer Systeme 12:83–89

Esterbauer H, Jürgens G, Quehenberger O, Koller E (1987) Autoxidation of human low density lipoprotein: loss of polyunsaturated fatty acids and vitamin E on generation of aldehydes. J Lipid Res 28:495–509

Faupel RP, Seitz HJ, Tarnowsky W, Thiemann V, Weiß CH (1972) The problem of tissue sampling from experimental animals with respect to freezing technique, anoxia, stress, and narcosis. Arch Biochem Biophys 148:509–522

Ferns GAA, Raines EW, Sprugel KH, Motani AS, Reidy MA, Ross R (1991) Inhibition of smooth muscle accumulation after angioplasty by an antibody to PDGF. Science 253:1129–1132

Geer JC, Webster WS (1974) Morphology of mesenchymal elements of normal artery, fatty streaks and plaques. Adv Exp Med Biol 43:9–33

Glavind J, Hartmann S, Clemmesen J, Jessen KE, Dam H (1952) Studies of the role of lipoperoxides in human pathology. Acta Pathol Microbiol Scand 30:1–6

Gotlieb AJ (1982) Smooth muscle and endothelial cell function in the pathogensis of atherosclerosis. Can Med Assoc J 126:903–908

Gutstein WH, Harrison J, Parl F, Kin G, Avitable M (1978) Neuronal factors contribute to atherogenesis. Science 199:449–451

Hajjar DP, Farber IC, Smith SC (1988) Oxygen tension within the arterial wall: relationship to altered bioenergetic metabolism and lipid accumulation. Arch Biochem Biophys 262:375–380

Hansson GK, Jonasson L, Holm J, Clowes MM, Clowes AW (1988) Gamma-interferon regulates vascular smooth muscle proliferation and Ia antigen expression in vivo and in vitro. Circ Res 63:712–719

Hansson GK, Holm J, Jonasson L (1989) Detection of activated T-lymphocytes in the human atherosclerotic plaque. Am J Pathol 135:169–175

Harats D, Bennaim M, Dabach Y, Hollander G, Havivi E, Stein O, Stein Y (1990) Effects of vitamin C and vitamin E supplementation on susceptibility of plasma lipoproteins to peroxidation induced by acute smoking. Atherosclerosis 85:47–54

Hauss WH (1973) Über die Rolle des Mesenchyms in der Genese der Arteriosklerose. Virchows Arch [A] 359:135–156

Haust MD (1974) Light and electron microscopy of human atherosclerotic lesions. Adv Exp Med Biol 104:33–59

Heinle H (1982) Peroxide induced activation of glycogen phosphorylase a activity in vascular smooth muscle. Biochem Biophys Res Commun 107:597–601

Heinle H (1984) Vasoconstriction of carotid artery induced by hydroperoxides. Arch Int Physiol Biochem 92:267–271

Heinle H (1985) Stoffwechseländerungen der Gefäßwand bei experimenteller Arteriosklerose. Habilitations schrift, University of Tübingen

Heinle H (1987) Metabolite concentration gradients in the arterial wall of experimental atherosclerosis. Exp Mol Pathol 46:312–320

Heinle H (1989) Influence of oxidative stress on metabolic and contractile functions of arterial smooth muscle. In: Acker H (ed) Oxygen sensing in tissues. Springer, Berlin Heidelberg New York, pp 151–164

Heinle H, Liebich H (1980) The influence of diet-induced hypercholesterolemia on the degree of oxidation of glutathione in rabbit aorta Atherosclerosis 37:637–640

Heinle H, Knehr H, Schmid G, Eitel W Betz E (1980a) Biochemical variations in electrically induced intimal smooth muscle cell proliferates of the rabbit carotid artery. Artery 8:393–397

Heinle H, Tarozy M, Schmid G, Betz E (1980b) Morphological and functional alterations in the arterial wall after local electrical stimulation. Bibl Anat 20:79–82

Heinle H, Stowasser F, Betz. E (1982) Metabolic changes in modified smooth muscle cells of rabbit carotid arteries. Basic Res Cardiol 77:82–92

Heinle H, Kling D, Lindner V (1987) Increased contractile responses of isolated arteriosclerotic rabbit carotid arteries to various vasoactive stimuli. Int Angiol 6:53–58

Heinle H, Tries S, Esterbauer H (1988) Effects of H_2O_2, arachidonic acid hydroperoxide and 4-hydroxynonenal on arterial smooth muscle contraction. Pflügers Arch 412 [Suppl]:R85

Heinle H, Ableiter H, Betz E (1991a) Diet-induced hypercholesterolemia decreases osmotic resistance of rabbit erythrocytes: possible involvement of the thiol-protecting system. Nutr Metab Cardiovasc Dis 1:125–129

Heinle H, Veigel C, Tries S (1991b) The influence of oxidatively modified low density lipoprotein on parameters of energy metabolism and contractile function of arterial smooth muscle. Free Radic Res Commun 11:281–286

Heughan C, Niinikoshi J, Hunt TK (1973) Oxygen tension in lesions of experimental atherosclerosis of rabbits. Atherosclerosis 17:361–367

Hort W (1985) Morphologie der koronaren Herzerkrankung. In: Schettler G, Gross R (eds) Arteriosklerose: Grundlagen, Diagnostik, Therapie. Deutscher Ärzte Verlag, Cologne, pp 35–44

Hort W, Kalbfleisch H, Frenzel H (1982) Coronary atherosclerosis and its relation to myocardial infarction. Verh Dtsch Ges Inn Med 88:1298–1301

Hunt JV, Wolff SP (1991) Oxidative glycation and free radical production—a causal mechanism of diabetic complication. Free Radic Res Commun 12:115–123

Jonasson L, Holm J, Skalli O, Bondjers G, Hansson GK (1986) Regional accumulations of T cells, macrophages, and smooth muscle cells in human atherosclerotic plaque. Arteriosclerosis 6:131–138

Jurrus ER, Weiss HS (1977) In vitro oxygen tensions in the rabbit aortic arch. Atherosclerosis 28:223–232

Kirk JE (1963) Intermediary metabolism of human arterial tissue and its change with age and atherosclerosis. In: Sandler M, Bourne GH (eds) Atherosclerosis and its origin. Academic Press, New York, pp 67–117

Kirsch WM, Ferguson JF, Ignelzi R (1978) Regional differences in arterial metabolic rates: its significance in relation to cerebral vasospasm. Adv Neurol 20:47–57

Kling D, Holzschuh T, Betz E (1987a) Temporal sequence of morphological alterations in artery walls during experimental atherogenesis. Occurrence of leukocytes. Res Exp Med 187:237–250

Kling D, Holzschuh T, Strohschneider T, Betz E (1987b) Enhanced endothelial permeability and invasion of leukocytes into the artery wall as inital events in experimental atherosclerosis. Int Angiol 6:21–28

Kling D, Heinle H, Harlan JM (1991) Participation of leukocytes in the development of experimentally induced arteriosclerosis. Morphological and functional aspects. In: Hauss WH, Wissler RW, Bauch HJ (eds) Abhandlungen der Rhein. Westf. Akademie der Wissenschaften, Westdeutscher Verlag, pp 105–115

Klurfeld DM (1983) Interactions of immune function with lipids and atherosclerosis. CRC Crit Rev Toxicol 11:333–365

Knehr HE, Heinle H, Betz E (1980) Enhanced oxygen uptake and lactate production of smooth mucsle cell proliferates of rabbit carotid arteries. Pflügers Arch 387:73–77

Loeper J, Emerit J, Goy J, Bedu O, Loeper J (1983) Lipid peroxidation during human atherosclerosis. IRCS Med Sci 11:1034–1035

Lowry DH, Passonneau JV (1972) A flexible system of enzymatic analysis. Academic, New York

Lynch RM, Paul RJ (1983) Compartmentation of glycolytic and glycogenolytic metabolism in vascular smooth muscle. Science 222:1344–1346

Morrison AD, Berwick L, Orci L, Winegrad AI (1976) Morphology and metabolism of an aortic intima-media preparation in which an intact endothelium is preserved. J Clin Invest 57:650–660

Morrison ES, Scott RF, Kroms M, Frick J (1972) Glucose degradation in normal and atherosclerotic aortic intima-media. Atherosclerosis 16:175–184

Moss AJ, Samuelson P, Angell C, Minken SL (1968) Polarographic evaluation of transmural oxygen availability in intact muscular arteries. J Atheroscler Res 8:803–810

Mowri H, Chinen K, Ohkuma S, Takano T (1986) Peroxidized lipids isolated by HPLC from atherosclerotic aorta. Biochem Int 12:347–352

Munro MJ, Cotran RS (1988) The pathogenesis of atherogenesis: atherogenesis and inflammation. Lab Invest 58:249–261

Munro AF, Rifkind BM, Leibescheutz HJ, Campbell RSF, Howard BR (1961) Effect of cholesterol feeding on the oxygen consumption of aortic tissue from the cockerel and the rat. J Atheroscler Res 1:296–304

Nathan CF (1987) Secretory products of macrophages. J Clin Invest 79:319–326

Niendorf A, Beisiegel U (1991) Low-density lipoprotein receptors. Curr Top Pathol 83:187–218

Niinikoshi J, Heughan C, Hunt TK (1973) Oxygen tension in the aortic wall of normal rabbits. Atherosclerosis 17:353–359

Nilsson J (1986) Growth factors and the pathogenesis of atherosclerosis. Atherosclerosis 62:185–199

Nishigaki I, Hagihara M, Tsunekawa H, Maseki M, Yagi K (1981) Lipid peroxides levels of serum lipoprotein fractions of diabetic patients. Biochem Med 25:373–378

Numano F, Yamaguchi S, Jaima M, Watabiki S, Sakurada S, Mashimo N, Maezawa H (1979) Microassay of adenine nucleotides in intima and media of the aortic wall. Exp Mol Pathol 31:468–478

Odessy R, Chace KV (1982) Utilization of endogenous lipid, glycogen, and protein by rabbit aorta. Am J Physiol 243:H128–H132

Paul RJ (1981) Chemical energetics of vascular smooth muscle. In: Bohr DF, Somlyo AP, Sparks H (eds) Handbook of physiology, Sect 2. The cardiovascular system, vol 2. Vascular smooth muscle. Williams & Wilkins, Baltimore, pp 201–235

Paul RJ (1983) Functional compartmentalization of oxidative and glycolytic metabolism in vascular smooth muscle. Am J Physiol 244:C399–C409

Peterson JW, Paul RJ (1974) Aerobic glycolysis in vascular smooth muscle: relation to isometric tension. Biochem Biophys Acta 357:167–176

Quinn MT, Parthasarathy S, Fong LG, Steinberg D (1987) Oxidatively modified low density lipoproteins: a potential role in recruitment and retention of monocytes/macrophages during atherogenesis. Proc Natl Acad Sci USA 84:2995–2998

Radi R, Beckmann JS, Bush KM, Freeman BA (1991) Peroxynitrite oxidation of sulfhydryls. The cytotoxic potential of superoxide and nitric oxide. J biol Chem 266:4244–4250

Ridray S, Capron L, Hendes D, Picon L, Ktorza A (1991) Effects of fasting and refeeding on the proliferative response of rat aorta to injury. Am J Physiol 261:H190–H195

Rosenfeld ME (1991) Oxidized LDL affects multiple atherogenic cellular responses. Circulation 83:2137–2140

Ross R (1986) The pathogenesis of atherosclerosis—an update. N Engl J Med 314:488–500

Ross R, Glomset JA (1976) The pathogenesis of atherosclerosis. N Engl J Med 295:369–377, 420–425

Ross R, Raines E, Bowen Pope DF (1982) Growth factors from platelets, monocytes, and endothelium: their role in the cell proliferation. Ann NY Acad Sci 397:18–24

Ross R, Raines EW, Bowen Pope DF (1986) The biology of platelet derived growth factor. Cell 46:155–158

Schlote W, Boellard JW, Betz E (1980) Experimental atherosclerosis—the animal model and its relation to the human disease. Folia Angiol 28:76–79

Schneiderman G, Goldstick TK (1978) Carbon monoxide-induced arterial wall hypoxia and arteriosclerosis. Atherosclerosis 30:1–15

Schwartz SM, Campbell GR, Campbell JH (1986) Replication of smooth muscle cells in vascular disease. Circ Res 58:427–444

Scott RF, Daoud AS, Wortmen B, Morrison ES, Jarmolych J (1966) Proliferation and necrosis in coronary and cerebral arteries. J Atheroscler Res 6:499–505

Scott RF, Morrison ES, Kroms M (1970) Effect of cold shock on respiration and glycolysis in swine arterial tissue. Am J Physiol 219:1363–1365

Smith EB (1982) Metabolism of the arterial wall. In: Born GRV, Catapano AL, Paoletti R (eds) Factors in formation and regression of the atherosclerotic plaque. Plenum, New York, pp 21–33

Solberg LA, Strong JP (1983) Risk factors and atherosclerotic lesions. A review of autopsy studies. Arteriosclerosis 3:187–198

Stange E, Papenberg J (1978) Changes in chemical and metabolic properties of rabbit aorta by dietary cholesterol, and saturated and polyunsaturated fats. Atherosclerosis 29:467–476

Stary HC (1990) The sequence of cells and matrix changes in atherosclerotic lesions of coronary arteries in the first years of life. Eur Heart J 11 [Suppl E]:3–19

St. Clair RW (1976) Metabolism of the arterial wall and atherosclerosis. Atherosclerosis Rev 1:61–118

Steinberg D, Parthasarathy S, Carew TE, Khoo JC, Witztum JL (1989) Beyond cholesterol: modifications of low density lipoprotein that increase its atherogenicity. N Engl J Med 320:915–924

Steinbrecher UP, Zhang H, Lougheed M (1990) Role of modified LDL in atherosclerosis. Free Radic Biol Med 9:155–168

Tanner FC, Noll G, Boulanger CM, Lüscher TA (1991) Oxidized low density lipoproteins inhibit relaxations of porcine coronary arteries—role of scavenger receptor and endothelium-derived nitric oxide. Circulation 83:2012–2020

Tarczy M, Heinle H, Lindner V (1981) Early changes of vascular permeability after electrical stimulation of the common carotid artery. Pflügers Arch 389 [Suppl]:R17

Thomas WA, Kim DN (1983) Atherosclerosis as a hyperplastic and/or neoplastic process. Lab Invest 48:245–255

Tries S (1990) Reaktionen der Gefäßwand unter atherogenen Reizen und therapeutischen Eingriffen: Untersuchungen zum Einfluß von Peroxidationsprodukten des LDL bzw. von Ballon-Angioplastie auf die Arteria carotis des Kaninchens. Thesis, University of Tübingen

Trimm JL, Salama G, Abramson JJ (1986) Sulfhydryl oxidation induces rapid calcium release from sarcoplasmic reticulum vesicles. J Biol Chem 261:16092–16099

Tsai AC, Chen NSC (1979) Effect of cholesterol-feeding on tissue glucose uptake, insulin-degradation, serum lipids and serum lipoperoxide levels in rabbits. J Nutr 109:606–612

Velican C, Velican D (1982) Atherosclerotic involvement of human intracranial arteries with special references to intimal necrosis. Atherosclerosis 43:59–69

Wiegel WB (1985) Aktive und passive mechanische Eigenschaften atheromatöser Proliferate der Arteria carotis bei Kaninchen. Thesis, University of Tübingen
Wissler RW, Vesselinovitsch D, Getz GS (1976) Abnormalities of the arterial wall and its metabolism in atherogenesis. Prog Cardiovasc Dis 18:341–369
Wolff SP, Jiang ZY, Hunt JV (1991) Protein glycation and oxidative stress in diabetes mellitus and ageing. Free Radic Biol Med 10:339–352
Zemplenyi T (1974) Vascular enzymes and the relevance of their study to problems of atherogenesis. Med Clin North Am 58:293–321
Zemplenyi T (1977) Metabolic intermediates, enzymes and lysosomal activity in aortas of spontaneously hypertensive rats. Atherosclerosis 28:233–246

Parallels Between Renal Transplant Arteriopathy and Atherosclerosis in Respect of Functional Morphology*

E. VOLLMER and A. ROESSNER

1 Introduction

Despite greater standardization of surgical technique and considerable progress in the postoperative management of patients who have undergone allogeneic organ transplantation, we are increasingly faced with the problem of obliterative transplant arteriopathy, particularly after kidney transplantation. In addition to interstitial and glomerular reactions within the transplant, vascular, i.e. predominantly arterial, lesions present intriguing problems to the pathologist. Many facets of the pathogenesis of renal transplant arteriopathy (RTA) are still unexplained. Judging by macroscopic and histologic analysis of the cellular pattern, the morphology of transplanted vessels shows considerable similarities with the morphogenesis of atherosclerosis (ZOLLINGER et al. 1978; CERILLI et al. 1987; MÜELLER-HERMELINK and DÄMMRICH 1989; ROESSNER et al. 1989; VOLLMER et al. 1991b).

The current interpretation of the pathogenesis of RTA focuses principally on immunologic processes that damage or alter the vascular endothelium (HRUBAN et al. 1990). The subsequent processes of activation and transformation affecting immunocompetent cells, and resulting in drastic morphologic, functional, and metabolic changes in all cells involved in the sclerotic progress, show

* This chapter is dedicated to Prof. Dr. J. Oepen, Marburg.

Current Topics in Pathology
Volume 87, Vollmer/Roessner (Eds.)

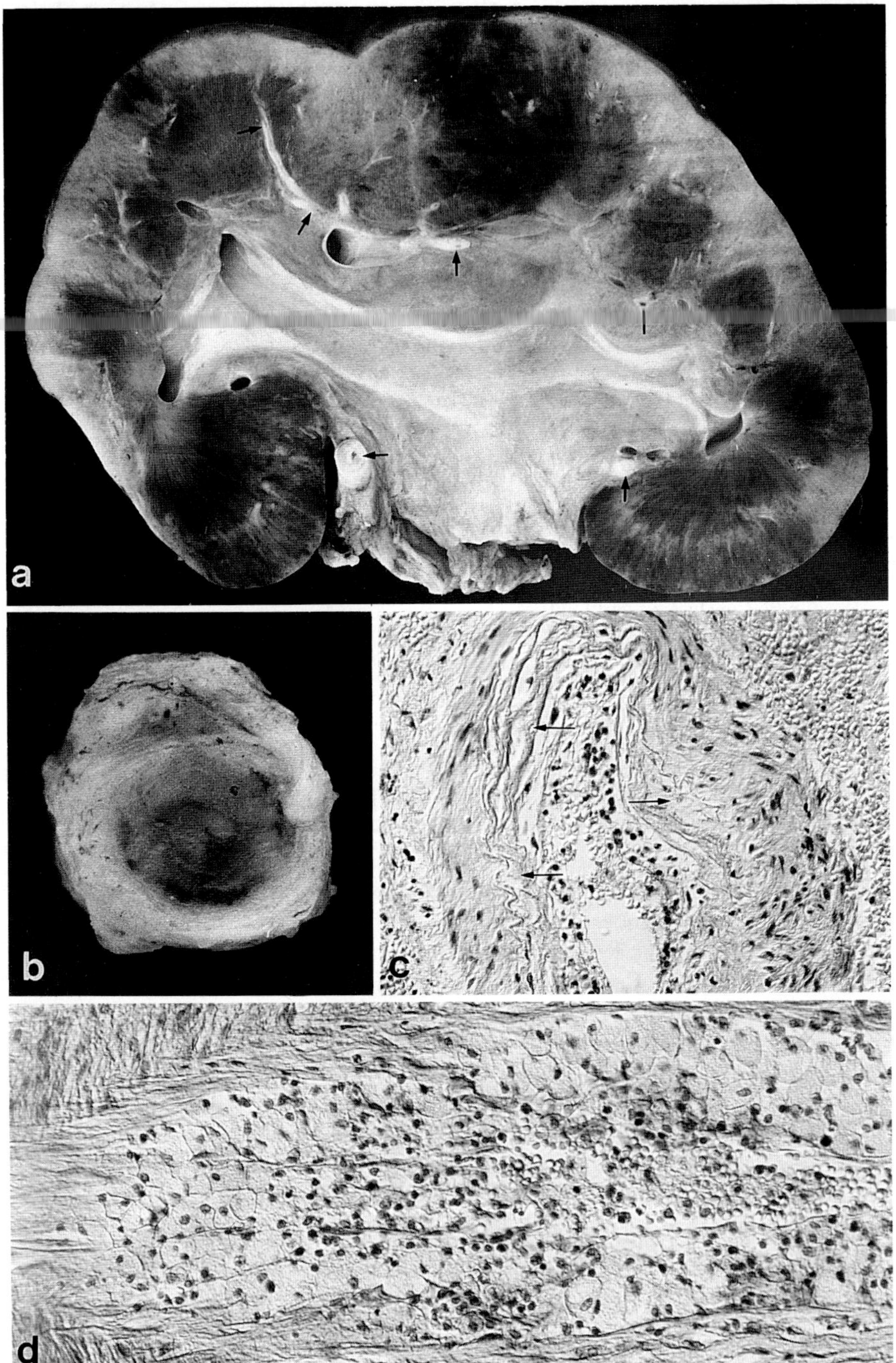
a
b
c
d

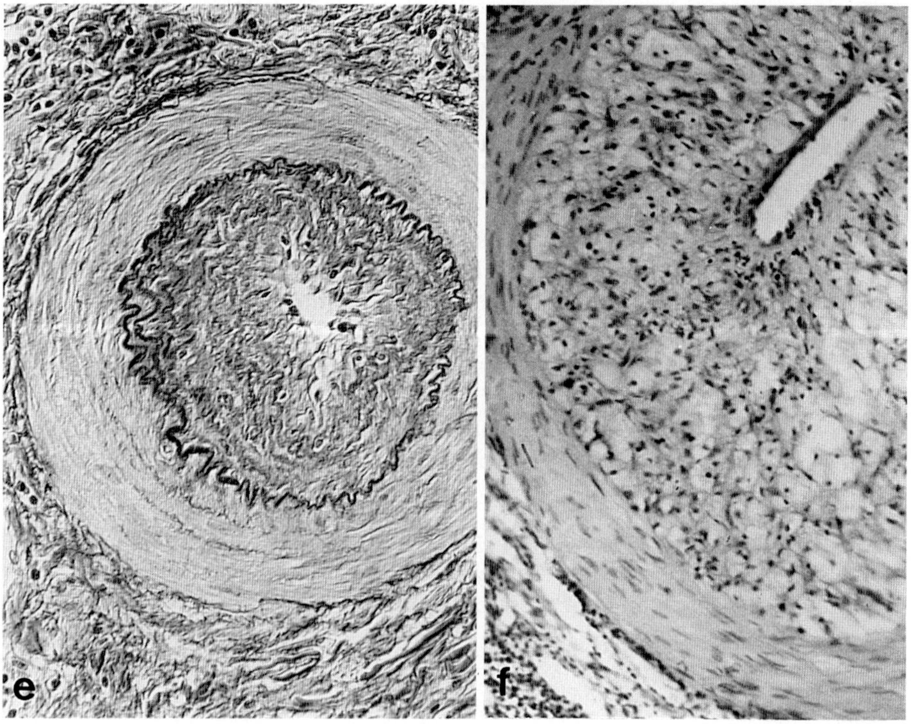

Fig. 1a–f. General morphologic pattern of RTA. **a, b** High-grade thickening of the wall and extensive obliteration in medium-sized and larger renal arteries (indicated by arrows). **c** Acute stage of RTA with edematous thickening of the arterial intima, endothelial swelling, evidence of mononuclear inflammatory infiltrates, and splitting and further loss of lamina elastica interna (*arrows*). × 160. **d** First subendothelial foam cells in the acute phase of RTA. × 220. **e** Chronic obliterative RTA with an increase in spindle-shaped subendothelial cells. × 250. **f** Intimal accumulation of numerous foam cells in chronic obliterative RTA. × 120

considerable similarity to those observed in conventional atherosclerosis (CAS). RTA predominantly affects the renal arteries with medium and smaller calibers, in particular the Aa. arcuatae and interlobulares, but sometimes the large renal arteries are also involved; arterioles are mostly spared (Fig. 1a, b).

Using light microscopy, the acute stages of obliterative RTA are characterized by endothelial swelling and edemotous widening of the intima, with the occurrence of mononuclear inflammatory infiltration (Fig. 1c); the extent of the latter is most likely dependent on the results of immunosuppressive therapy prior to explantation. There is some first evidence of subendothelial foam cells (Fig. 1d). In addition to initially subendothelial proliferation of spindle cells, there is slowly increasing proliferation of medial myocytes with splicing and continual loss of the lamina elastica interna (Fig. 1c). In the event of severe vascular damage, endothelial lesions with thrombi composed of fibrin and thrombocytes are seen. Less frequent are fibrinoid necroses of the vascular wall or of the media with additional granulocytic infiltration. In severe acute disease, the often considerable obliterations will eventually lead to focal infarction of renal tissue.

In chronic obliterative RTA, fibrinoid necroses of the vessel wall are observed less often, but an increase in subendothelial spindle cells is very evident in many cases (Fig. 1e). On the other hand, there is an intimal accumulation of foam cells (Fig. 1f), often accompanied by considerable fibrosis of the intima and also of the media, the latter with focal destruction. A sequel to chronic obliterative RTA of protracted course will be severe interstitial fibrosis. In most cases, arterial lesions predominate, but venous alterations may also occur, affecting almost exclusively the renal vein and its larger branches, and hardly ever the intrarenal veins. Here, too, the sequelae are intimal edema, loose mononuclear infiltration, and proliferation of spindly subendothelial cells, together with fibrosis.

In the following we aim to analyze the different cell types found in the vascular wall in chronic RTA by light and electron microscopy using immunologic techniques. The questions requiring clarification are:

1. Which pathomorphologic and functional changes and which cell–cell interactions are present in various vascular lesions?
2. What is the significance of these cells, and of their altering phenotypes?
3. How and to what extent does RTA represent an accelerated manifestation of CAS?

2 Materials and Methods

Our study comprised 33 nephrectomy specimens with chronic transplant rejection. The transplants had remained in the recipients for between 3 and 96 months; the age of the donors ranged from 3 to 50 years, and that of recipients from 12 to 64 years. No correlation was found between the duration between transplantation and rejection and the degree of arterial obliteration. Vascular findings ascertained by the pathologist also failed to reveal any correlation with available clinical parameters—sex, blood pressure, smoking history, original kidney disease, laboratory data regarding blood sugar and fat—or with data concerning immunosuppressive therapy.

Freshly resected material was appropriately cut and fixed in buffered 3.5% formol for 24 h, then embedded in paraffin as usual. Sections of about 3 μm were stained with hematoxylin and eosin and elastin-van Gieson. Immunolabeling was performed on paraffin sections with the APAAP technique (alkaline phosphatase/antialkaline phosphatase, modified after CORDELL et al. 1984), with staining by means of the indirect alkaline phosphatase and/or indirect peroxidase technique. If necessary, paraffin sections were subjected to enzymatic predigestion. Simultaneous labeling of several antigens was performed using the enzyme peroxidase and alkaline phosphates in sequential steps of the immune reaction. In structures supposedly present in rather small amounts, peroxidase was applied first, while the more frequent structures were labeled by alkaline phosphatase in a second step.

Unlike our light microscopic studies, those on the ultrastructural level called for the securing of fresh surgical material with absolute priority, for which we used chemical as well as physical (cryo)fixation. The first method provided insolubility of organic matrix (reducing the solubility of essential organic components). Depending upon the problem investigated, we applied glutaraldehyde or periodate-lysine-paraformaldehyde fixatives (McLean and Nakane 1974). The second method, cryofixation, was performed using a metallic mirror (Sitte et al. 1987), thereby ensuring the prerequisites for ultrastructural presentation of highly sensitive antigen binding sites that are liable to destruction under even weaker chemical fixation. Optimal cryopreparation of our samples was possible by cryosubstitution following cryofixation (Humbel and Schwarz 1989; Sjöestrand 1990), with subsequent embedding in Lowicryl resins. This method and that of ultracryosectioning (modified) after Tokuyasu 1984) using 2.3 *M* sucrose solution as cryoprotectant served to permit immunohistochemical labeling by indirect immunogold techniques. In addition, we analyzed samples in conventional Epon embedding for electron microscopy.

Our arsenal of primary antibodies comprised those against muscle-specific α- and γ-actin (HHF35, ORTHO, Heidelberg) as well as against intermediate filament desmin (DE-R-11) and vimentin (V9), and also antibodies specific for distinguishing various types of lymphocytes (UCHL1, OPD4, L26, all from DAKO, Hamburg). Other antibodies were directed against proliferating cells (PCNA-PC 10) and factor VIII (F VIII)-associated antigen and the lectin UE1 (all from DAKO, Hamburg). Antibodies specific for labeling monocytes/macrophages (27-E-10, 25-F-9, MRP8, MRP14) were kindly supplied by the workgroup of Prof. Dr. C. Sorg (Institute of Experimental Dermatology of Münster University) (Zwadlo et al. 1985, 1986, 1988), and a commercially available marker (MAC 387 from DAKO, Hamburg) was also used.

3 Results

3.1 Endothelium

In RTA the endothelium is often more detached from its base than in CAS. Denuded cell areas are frequent, and both spindle cell and cuboid cell types are evident, the latter being rather more prominent than in CAS. Association with microthrombi and mononuclear cells is seen in most cases, the cellular infiltration consisting of either monocytes/macrophages or lymphocytes (Fig. 2a–c).

Immune/lectin histochemistry reveals stronger expression of F VIII-associated antigen than of the binding site for UE1. In some places, erythrocytes

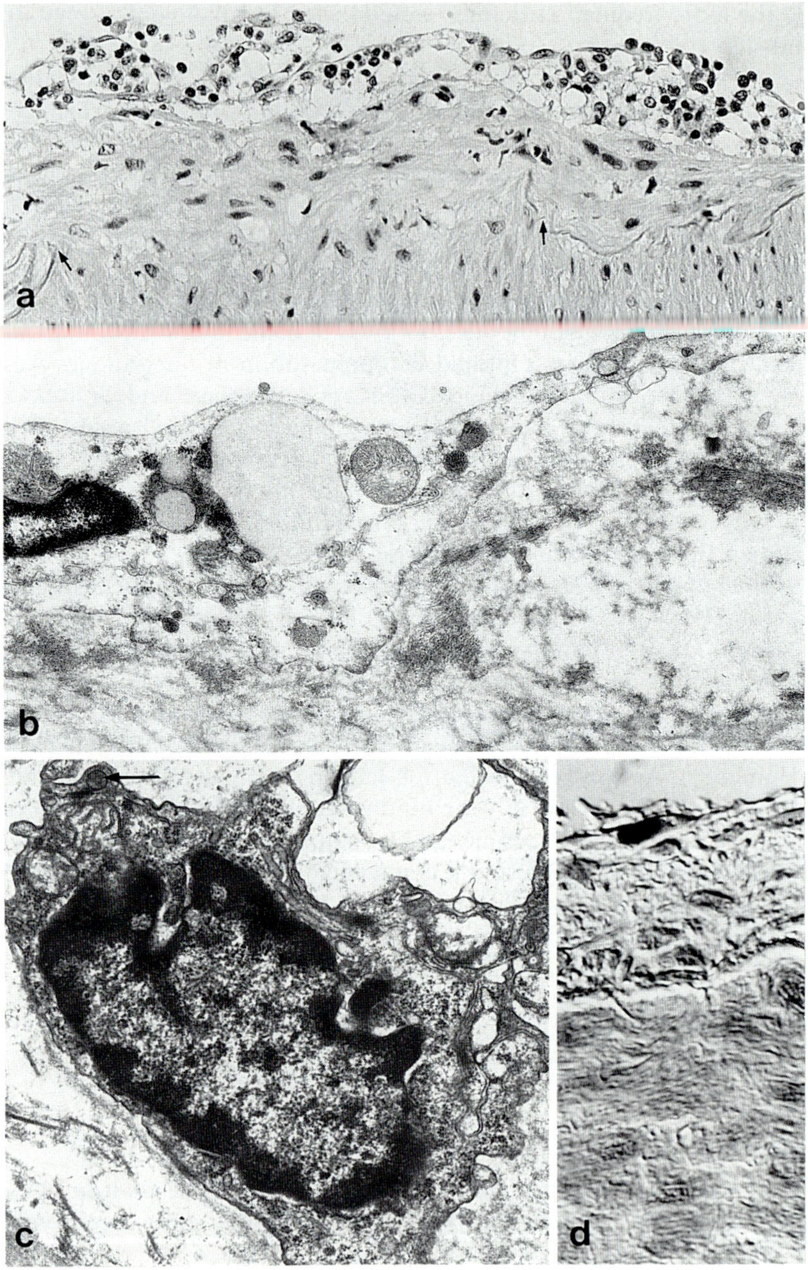

Fig. 2a–h. Endothelium. **a** Distinct, partly arched endothelial detachment with an increased number of mononucleate cells in close contact with partly spindle-shaped, partly cuboid-bulky endothelial cells. The lamina elastica interna (*arrows*) is split and somewhat defective. × 300. **b** Ultrastructural presentation of spindle-type endothelial cell in arched detachment. × 16 000 **c** Endothelial cell of cuboid type (*arrow* indicates a Weibel-Palade body). × 16 000. **d** Proliferating endothelial cell expressing PCNA. × 500. **e** Intimal presentation of F VIII-associated antigen in comparison with **f** binding site for UE1: note stronger expression of F VIII, where an apical and a basal layer of

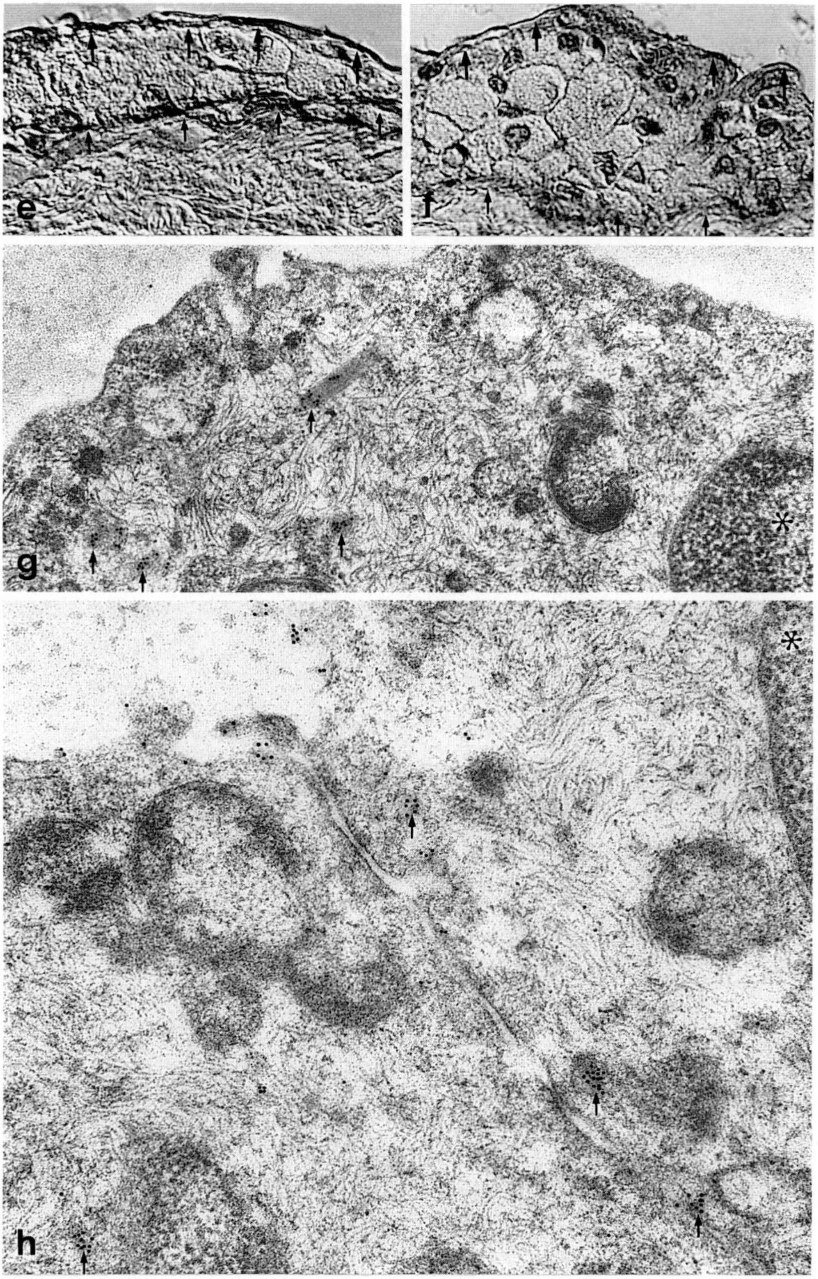

endothelia (*arrows*) are manifested, with some mononuclear cells in between, predominantly in foamy transformation. **e** and **f** × 500. **g, h** Ultrastructural demonstration of intracytoplasmic F VIII (**g**) and the UE1 binding site (**h**), the latter being visible in intracytoplasmic as well as in optically dense areas of the cell membrane surface. Note intact interendothelial junctions! (∗= nuclear sections are indicated by asterick and specific intracytoplasmic immunogold labeling by arrows; ultracryosubstitution). **9**, × 25 000; **h**, × 30 000

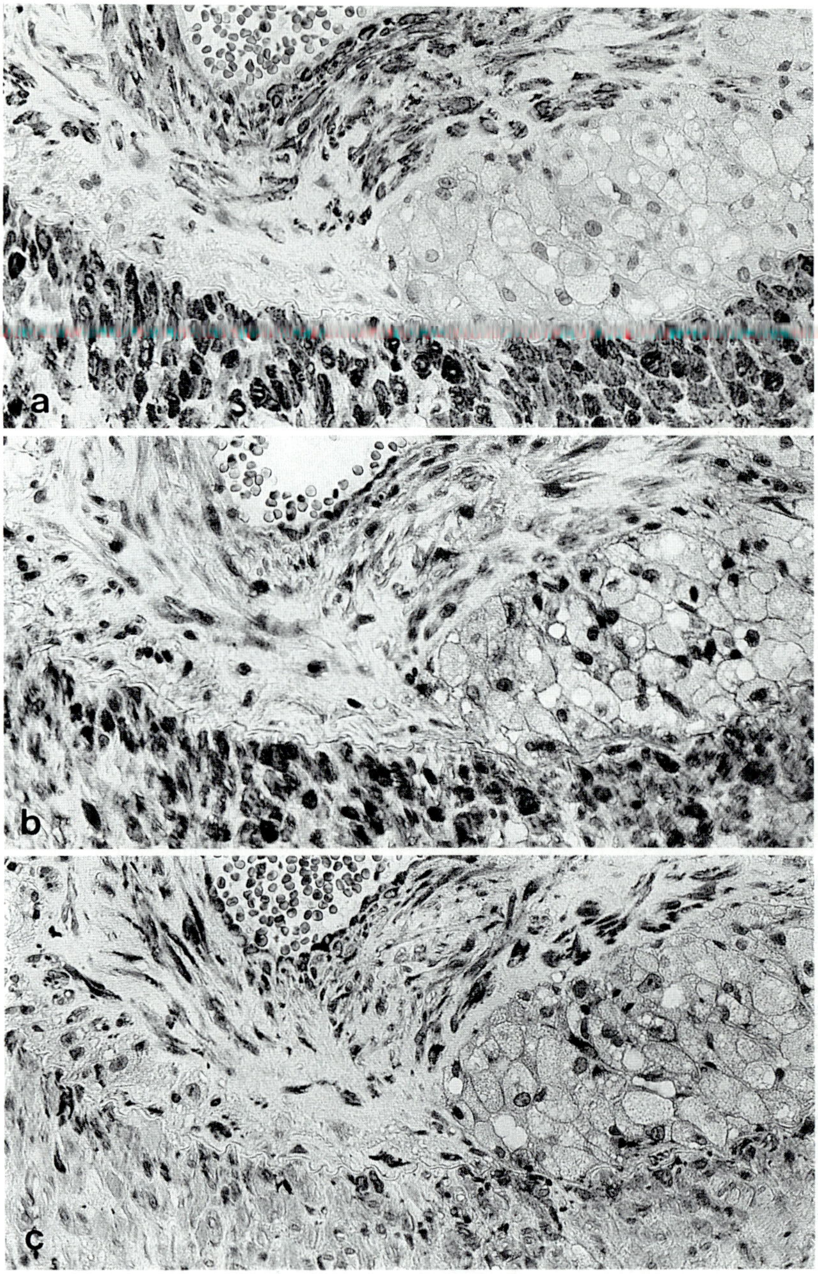

Fig. 3a–f. Smooth muscle cells: Immunocytochemical demonstration of the cytoskeleton in consecutive sections of a medium-sized renal artery with marked intimal fibrosis and a subendothelial cushion of foam cells (*center, right side*) and intact lamina elastica interna (*lower third*). **a** Strong expression of muscle-specific actin in many spindle-shaped cells of the thickened fibrotic intima and in nearly all medial myocytes. × 250. **b** Weaker expression of desmin in the intimal and medial layers. × 250 **c** Strong expression of vimentin in the intimal layer; media myocytes can be stained only in lower numbers and with weaker intensity. The vimentin filament is additionally expressed in endothelial cells (*center, top*) and occasionally in foam cells. × 250. **d** Immunocytochemical double

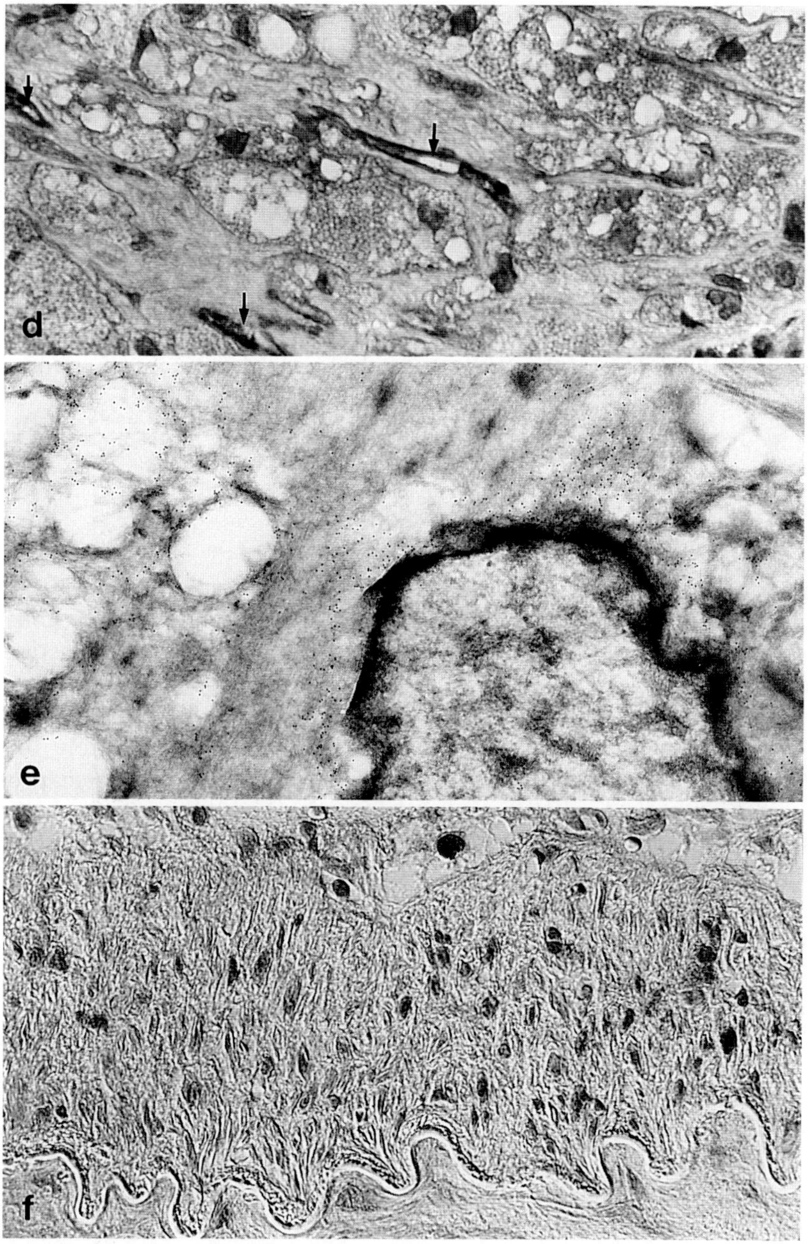

labeling with antibodies against muscle-specific actin and against macrophages reveals the predominantly histiocytic origin of nearly all foam cells; there are only a few, mostly spindle-shaped cells (*arrows*) expressing actin and thereby identifiable as myocytes. × 500. **e** Ultrastructural demonstration of vimentin in predominantly perinuclear adhesion and net-like meshwork surrounding preexisting lipid droples. × 25 000 (ultracryosection). **f** Numerous proliferating spindle cells of thickened, fibrotic intima expressing PCNA, and an equally proliferating endothelial cell of bulky-cuboid type (*top center*). × 500

are also labeled with UE1. No difference is evident between minor and major renal arteries. The frequently increased subendothelial accumulation of leukocytes, some of which are foamy, as well as the disintegration and detachment of endothelial cells in RTA can be clearly demonstrated by the endothelial markers used in our study. Quite often such mononuclear cells are well integrated into the endothelial structures, showing distinct apical and basal cell layers; the individual endothelial cells are labeled with varying intensity or not at all (Fig. 2e, f). Even the expression of PCNA is not rare in these endothelial (Fig. 2d), obviously reflecting an increased cell turnover.

Immunoelectron microscopy permits the specific in situ identification of the relevant binding sites for our endothelial markers: They appear intracytoplasmic for F VIII, while for UE1 they are located intracytoplasmically and in optically dense areas of the cell surface (Fig. 2g, h).

3.2 Smooth Muscle Cells

The intima of medium-sized renal arteries displays marked fibrosis with a myocyte-depleted center and abundant extracellular matrix. Sclerotic lesions are often less well developed in major arteries. On the whole the lamina elastica interna seems to show signs of splicing and destruction less often in RTA than in CAS.

According to our immunocytochemical analysis of the cytoskeleton, the antibody against muscle-specific actin stains most strongly in spindle-shaped cells of fibrotic intima; many cells express the intermediate filament vimentin, but hardly any express desmin (Fig. 3a–c). Whenever foam cells are evident in deeper intimal layers, they are mostly negative for these markers, expressing, if anything, only vimentin. Immunocytochemical double labeling with antibodies against macrophages (see below) and muscle-specific actin reveals the histiocytic origin of these foam cells. Only a few foam cells express actin, most of them displaying a spindly form and myocytic appearance (Fig. 3d).

Nearly all smooth muscle cells of the media (cf. Fig. 3a–c) show intense expression of the microfilament actin, and many also of the intermediate filament desmin, whereas vimentin, labeled by the appropriate antibody, revealed but minor expression in medium-sized renal arteries. The medial myocytes of the Aa. renales, however, show stronger vimentin expression. In addition to wall myocytes, endothelial cells express vimentin, and foam cells, too, occasionally may be vimentin-positive.

During the progression of sclerotic lesions, there is an ultrastructural increase in myocytes of the synthesizing type. Immunoelectron microscopy showed considerable analogy with CAS with regard to cytoskeleton expression. Among the elements also present in CAS, muscle-specific actin was fairly regularly seen in almost all myocytes, whereas desmin was expressed in varying intensity on individual myocytes. In addition to vimentin expression, often enhanced in the perinuclear region, there was often a kind of cytoskeletal meshwork encircling the lipid droplets (Fig. 3e), resembling the pattern in CAS. In some cases (especially when there was distinct intimal fibrosis), the nuclei of spindle cells presented immunohistochemical evidence of PCNA, predominantly in medium-sized renal arteries (Fig. 3f).

3.3 Monocytes/Macrophages

In kidney transplant rejection, granulocytes are found in the acute phase. Apart from these granulocytes, the main feature is mononuclear infiltration from the lumen, adhering to and penetrating the endothelium, and finally visible in the subendothelial layer. These cells, originating from the recipient, are classified as lymphocytes and predominantly as monocytes/macrophages. Initially they belong to the phenotype of blood monocytes labeled by the marker 27-E-10 (Fig. 4a). However, there are also cells labeled by the antibodies MAC 387 and, more intensely, by MRP8 and MRP14 (Fig. 4b–d). Subsequently, these monocytes/macrophages migrate into deeper layers of the vascular wall, where they turn into what we call "mature tissue macrophages"; most are transformed into foam cells and labeled with antibody 25-F-9 (Fig. 4e). Quite often some of these foam cells also express PCNA (Fig. 4f). In addition to these foam cells of histiocytic origin there may be some cells of myogenic origin (cf. Fig. 3d), as visualized by immunohistochemical double labeling.

3.4 Lymphocytes

Both the major and the medium-sized renal arteries contain, besides monocytes/macrophages, a large population of lymphocytes adhering to the endothelium or in a subendothelial position (cf. Fig. 2a). These lymphocytes, equally recipient dependent, can be stained by the antibody DAKO UCHL1 (CD45R) and belong almost exclusively to the T cell subpopulation. B lymphocytes are but poorly visualized with antibody DAKO L26 (CD20). The infiltration is often stronger in medium or minor arteries (Fig. 5a) than in the major Aa. renales (Fig. 5b–d). Consecutive sections enabled us to establish, by grossly orientating semiquantitative analysis, that about half of the T cell population belonged to the T helper/inducer subtype (CD4) that can be labeled by the marker DAKO OPD4. (So far, no paraffin-adaptable antibody is available for T suppressor/cytotoxic cells in chemical fixation.)

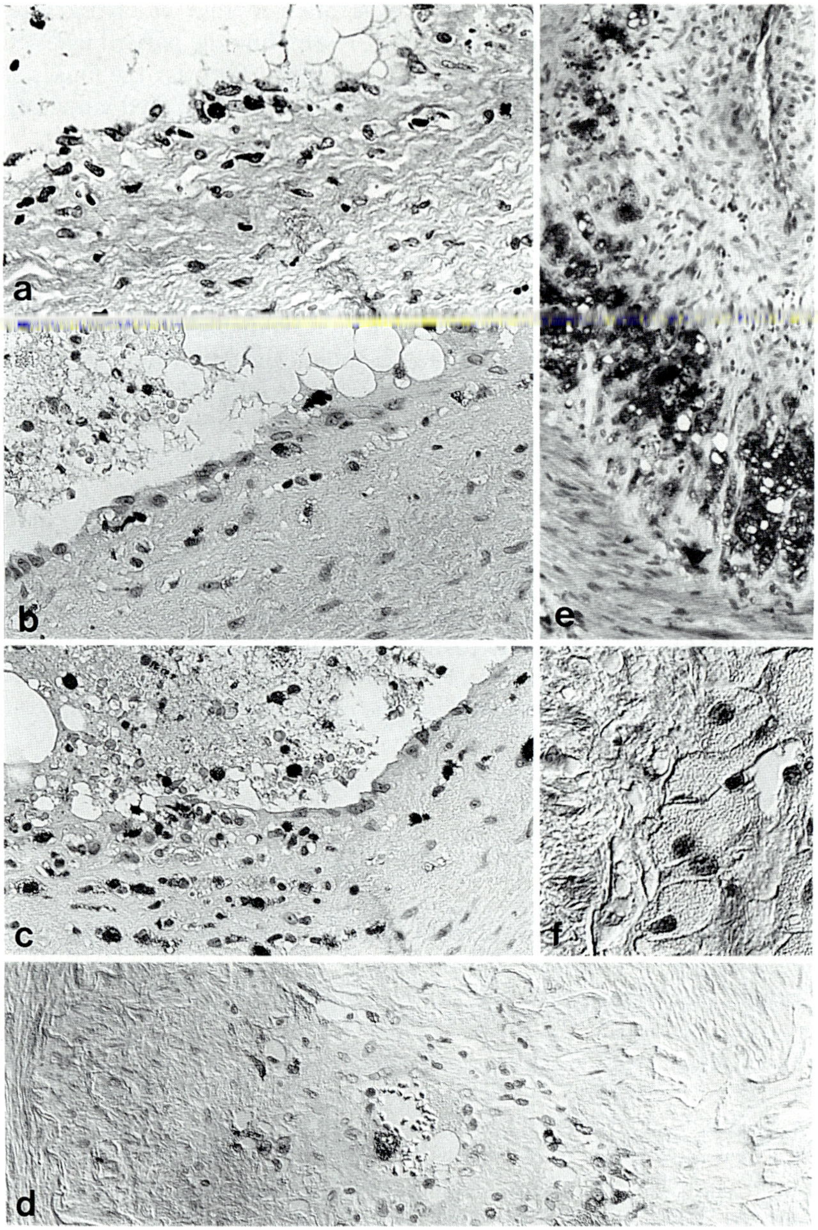

Fig. 4a–f. Monocytes/macrophages: RTA presenting various (sub) types of monocytes/macrophages: **a** 27-E-10-positive cells; **b** MRP8-positive cells; **c** MRP14-positive cells; **d** MAC 387-positive cells all in lumen and vessel wall; **e** 25-F-9-positive foam cells localized exclusively in the vascular wall; **f** proliferating foam cells expressing PCNA. **a–c**, × 250; **d**, × 200; **e**, × 150; **f**, × 500

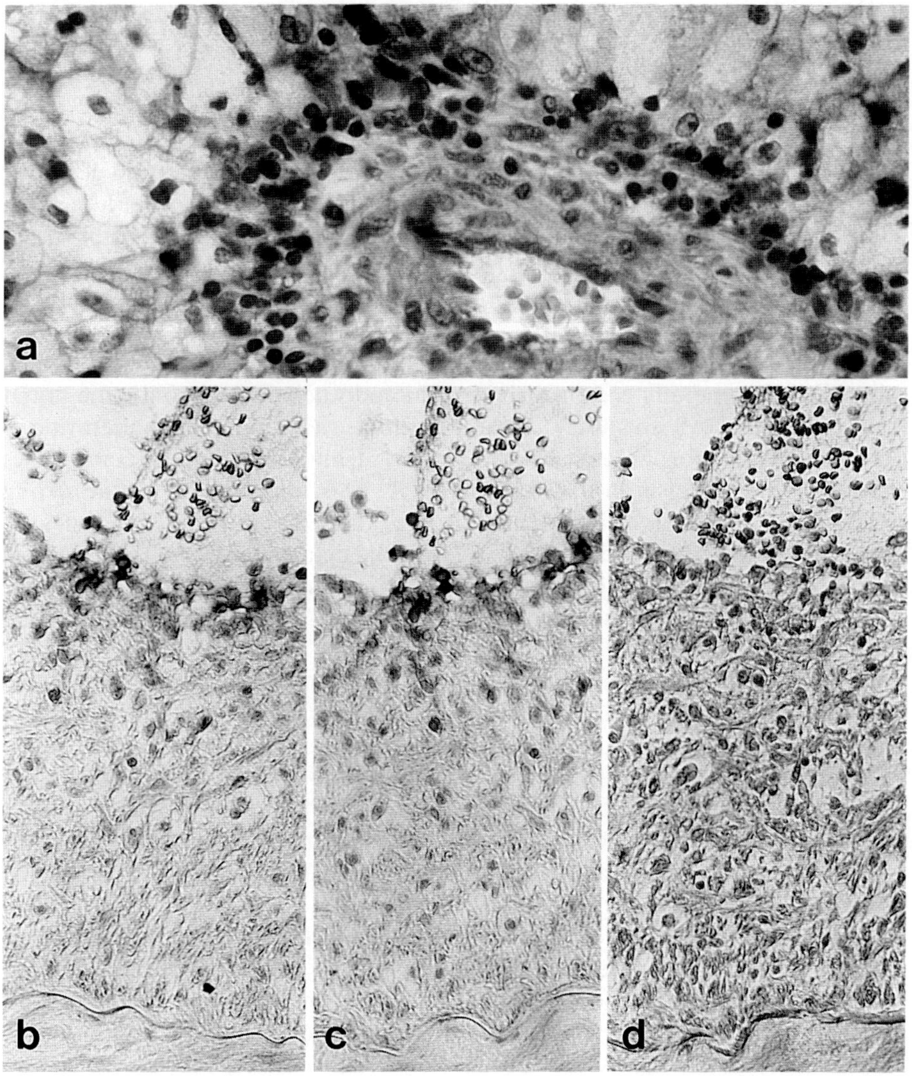

Fig. 5a–d. Lymphocytes. **a** Minor renal artery with numerous T lymphocytic infiltrates (CD45R) and intimal foam cell sheets, in contrast to an A. renalis with less lymphocytic infiltration (consecutive sections **b–d**). Demonstration of **b** pan-T-lymphocytes (CD5R), **c** T helper/inducer cells (CD4), and **d** immunohistochemically negative reaction for B lymphocytes (CD20). **a**, × 330; **b–d**, × 200

4 Discussion

4.1 Endothelium

It was a frequent finding in our analysis that endothelial cells appeared detached in arc-like fashion from the vessel wall, protruding instead into the lumen. In addition to flat, spindle-shaped endothelial cells there were also cells of rather bulging, cuboid form. According to current concepts (GERRITY 1990) these different cell forms reflect, at least in CAS, the functional status of endothelia in terms of metabolic activity. In fact, cuboid endothelial cells appear increased in those areas of vessel that are interpreted as preferentially liable to atherosclerosis. It is generally accepted today that endothelial alteration is the initial trigger of both CAS and RTA. To some extent, such endothelial alteration is associated with morphologically ascertained denudation, but in many cases endothelia are intact in both CAS and RTA. This must be due to the strong regenerative potential of endothelia (REIDY and SILVER 1985). This view is supported by the frequent evidence of endothelial detachment from the basement lamina with integration of mononuclear cells, some in foamy transformation, into the endothelial structure, and the presence of PCNA in adjacent endothelial cells.

That the alteration of endothelial cells is initiated by an immunologic mechanism is firmly established for RTA (HRUBAN et al. 1990; MÜLLER-HERMELINK and DÄMMRICH 1989). Whether this also holds true for CAS is still under discussion, although leukocyte–endothelial interactions are undisputed in this disease, too (MUNRO and COTRAN 1988; HANSSON et al. 1989b; GIMBRONE et al. 1990). Besides cellular mention must be made of humoral immune mechanisms, such as circulating immune complexes which are recognized in both RTA and CAS (WISSLER et al. 1989).

As a general truth it must be remembered that endothelial alteration, whether initiated by an immunologic, chemical, or infectious cause, will lead to arteriosclerosis. Whatever the cause, it will alter the endothelial function and so lead to the development of an atherosclerotic lesion, with or without the involvement of thrombocytes. The lesion then leads to thrombocyte aggregation in the intimal layer of the wall, and to transport of mitogenic factors secreted by these thrombocytes. These factors are eventually released into the peripheral blood via the endothelium in its altered state of permeability. There may also be some interactions with endothelia that are nonresistant to thrombosis, leading, among other things, to the secretion of growth factors (e.g., platelet-derived growth factor, PDGF) with active transport via endothelial cells into the subendothelial layers. Another source of thrombocyte-independent growth factors is from monocytes/macrophages and smooth muscle cells, and even from the endothelium proper (SCHARF and HARKER 1987). Moreover, endothelial cells possess a large number of low-density lipoprotein (LDL) binding sites. It was shown by VASILE et al. (1983) that the intimal cholesterol uptake is regulated by the vesicular transport system: Macromolecules of up to 70 nm in diameter, enclosed in vesicles, are carried via endothelial cells into the vascular wall. Obviously, high-density lipoproteins (HDL) and LDL can take part in this transcytosis without difficulty. A minor role is attributed to intercellular transport via endothelial tight junctions, which accept only particles of less than 2 nm (SIMIONESCU et al. 1986) and no macromolecules like LDL or HDL. This is in agreement with our ultrastructural results (cf. Chap. 5). With the very start of atherosclerotic changes, these conditions seem to undergo pathologic alteration, too, most likely due to increased endothelial permeability (MUNRO and COTRAN 1988). It is not only in atherosclerosis that risk factors, whatever they may be, are initially thought to augment endothelial permeability for macromolecular substances such as cholesterol-bearing lipoproteins (JELLINEK and DETRE 1986); rather in RTA, too, these factors are held responsible for the accelerated vascular changes. The alteration in endothelial cell shapes triggered by atherogenic factors may be associated with structural deformations of the cytoskeleton that are observed in parallel with the developing lesion (YOST and HERMAN 1988; GERRITY 1990). Subendothelial lipoproteins are known to exert chemotaxis on circulating monocytes, obviously by an increased supply of chemotactic adhesion factors (PRITCHARD et al. 1990).

Our study of RTA ascertained the existence of close interactions between leukocytes and endothelium, as are known to occur in CAS. The immigrating cells may release certain toxic substances such as lysosomal hydrolases, and so, by their capacity for lipid oxidation, continue to damage the affected endothelial cells, thereby assisting the progress of sclerotic lesions. In both diseases, certain cytotoxic effects from immigrating leukocytes against altered endothelial cells may also play a role. We want to mention in this context that all immigrating cells in RTA must belong to the transplant recipient, and so are directed against the transplant itself, whereas in CAS all leukocytes are of autologous origin.

Despite these speculations we have to admit that, so far, the damage to endothelial cells that is responsible for the development of the initial lesion cannot be defined in detail. The main problem lies in our imperfect grasp of the morphologic aspects of many endothelial alterations. Moreover, we are still looking for a marker capable of recognizing such altered endothelial cells, and of determining whether and when endothelial alteration will lead to arteriosclerosis.

In RTA, F VIII was found to be a better endothelial marker than the carbohydrate binding site for UE1, because the application of the anti F VIII antibody yielded nearly complete labeling of endothelial cells in the rejected transplants analyzed in our study. Ultrastructural evidence of F VIII-associated protein in the organelles of synthesis of these cells was convincingly presented in a previous publication (VOLLMER et al. 1989). The present in situ investigations, too, recorded specific, exclusively intracytoplasmic labeling for F VIII, while carbohydrate binding sites for UE1 were labeled in intracytoplasmic locations as well as in dense areas of the cytoplasmic membranes. According to current knowledge, such specific carbohydrate structures act as mediators of physiologic immune modulations in cell–cell interactions (reviewed by VIERBUCHEN 1991); various immune modulators are known for binding to specific cells such as macrophages, cytotoxic cells, natural killer cells, and even B lymphocytes. It is becoming increasingly probable that the activities of immune modulators can be specifically hindered by simple glycolipids, glycopeptides, and even simple sugars. Therefore interactions between certain lymphokines and their target cells also seem to include lectin-like reactions. We may infer that some important functions of the immunocompetent cells (including proliferation and differentiation) and of the effector molecules of lymphocytes and macrophages are in fact induced and mediated by carbohydrate recognition proteins, i.e., lectins. Admittedly, not much is known to date about the physiologic function of endogenous carbohydrate binding activities. We may assume that this is a point of difference between CAS, where endothelial labeling by UE1 is more marked, and RTA, with its stronger evidence of leukocyte–endothelial interaction.

Adhesion of circulating leukocytes to the wall of a vessel is one of the essential components in acute or chronic inflammatory disorders; RTA and CAS have to be classified, in a more general sense, in that category. The process begins with the activation of vascular endothelia by certain inflammatory stimuli leading to increased expression of leukocyte-adhesion molecules to which blood leukocytes will be attracted and bound. This transitory endothelial activation is characterized by the expression of specific surface structures on the endothelial cells proper. Several structures of endothelial adhesion have now been identified which also represent specific attractors and receptors for leukocytes. In this context, mention must be made of so-called endothelial leukocyte adhesion molecule (ELAM 1-also named E-selectin). Its expression increases in correspondence with the acuteness of the inflammatory process. Although ELAM 1 is of mainly functional importance for selective neutrophil adherence, the system may also emit signals that start the migration of monocytes/macrophages and lymphocytes. Moreover, the molecule is expressed more rapidly than other endothelial surface receptors, but its expression is transitory (SCHULZE-OSTHOFF et al. 1989; VOLLMER et al. 1989). In human CAS, neutrophil leukocytes are present in only minor quantities, but they play a considerable role in animal experiments. There is still a need for studies with a specific marker against ELAM 1 in RTA, where granulocytes are more frequent than in CAS. A recent pilot study of CAS revealed, in comparison with antibodies against UE1 and F VIII, a much lower proportion of immunohistochemical positivity when using a specific anti-ELAM marker (VOLLMER 1991).

In the recruitment of lymphocytes known to adhere to the endothelium, a certain endothelial recognizing structure identified as "vascular cell adhesion molecule" (VCAM) plays an important role. Compared to ELAM 1, this molecule shows a shifting, but continual expression on stimulated endothelial cells. In addition to these structures, the "intercellular adhesion molecules" (ICAM I and II) belong structurally to the immunoglobulin super family. These proteins are able to bind poly- and mononuclear cells via heterodimeric structures, among them the so-called integrins. ICAM I, which occurs even on unstimulated endothelial cells, is supposed to possess an unspecific stabilizing function in cell adhesion. Within 1 day it will manifest maximum endothelial expression which will continue under prolonged stimulation. In addition to the expression of adherence structures, the active coordinating role of endothelial cells is manifested in both CAS and RTA by their capacity for producing a number of signal substances influencing the immune response. Moreover, endothelial cells may express Fc and complement receptors, thereby influencing the phagocytic activity of immunocompetent cells. Another regulatory effect on inflammation is exerted by activated endothelial cells secreting various immunomodulating cytokines (COTRAN 1987).

Since arterial endothelial cells are known to express, under pathologic conditions, molecules of the major histocompatibility complex (MHC) class II, they can also act as antigen-presenting cells and may participate, like monocytes, in the cellular immune response. The expression of such antigens also has an important function in the transmigration of T lymphocytes (cf. Sect. 4.4), as identified in transplant arteriopathy (MÜLLER-HERMELINK and DÄMMRICH 1989; LIBBY et al. 1989; SALOMON et al. 1991) but also in atherosclerosis (GIMBRONE et al. 1990).

4.2 Smooth Muscle Cells

Several parallels between RTA and CAS were also established by our studies on the phenotypic characterization of myocytes at the light and electron microscopic level, using immunocytochemical techniques. In both diseases, myocyte phenotypes were found to change from the contractile to the synthesizing form as vascular lesions advanced. In most cases, the media bears numerous smooth muscle cells rich in filaments but depleted of organelles, whereas the intima contains an increasing number of synthesizing smooth muscle cells rich in organelles. These results agree well with experimental studies performed by YOSHIDA et al. (1988) in a rabbit model.

According to our immunocytochemical data, in RTA as in CAS, the modulating expression of intermediate and microfilaments in different layers of the vascular wall is of major importance for the occurrence and progression of sclerotic changes (VOLLMER 1991), a feature that is obviously independent of the initial cause.

Modulation of the smooth muscle phenotype—from myofilament-bearing contractile to filament-depleted, organelle-bearing synthesizing type—is currently seen as a prerequisite for myocytic proliferation (ROSS 1986) and so as a clue to the better understanding of arteriosclerotic changes. With proliferation kinetic studies, it has been possible to ascertain that more proliferating myocytes are present in obliterative RTA that in CAS, especially when there is marked intimal fibrosis (VOLLMER 1991; GORDON et al. 1989). With regard to CAS, these facts suggest two possible interpretations: Either there is no proliferation phase like that found in RTA, or the initial mechanisms associated with myocyte proliferation—adequately confirmed by animal experiments (ROSENFELD and ROSS 1990), especially with balloon catheterization and subsequent mechanical damage to the myothelial layer—are mostly terminated in human material and so inaccessible to immunohistochemical investigation, in contrast to the situation in RTA. Our findings in RTA are largely in agreement with those of DEMETRIS et al. (1989), who recorded marked myocytic proliferation, mainly in the intima, in ten kidney and ten heart transplants. On the whole, these data support the interpretation of RTA as a manifestation of accelerated atherosclerosis.

Obviously, the antibody against muscle-specific α- and γ-actin is better suited for the correct identification of smooth muscle cells than the antibody against desmin. In contrast, but as expected, the intermediate filament vimentin in expressed not only on smooth muscle cells but also on some inflammatory cells and endothelial cells. In RTA, only a few of the foam cells are of myogenic origin, as shown by immunohistochemical double labeling. The majority of foam cells are of histiocytic origin, like those seen in the fatty streaks of CAS (ROESSNER et al. 1987; VOLLMER et al. 1991a). Only very advanced atherosclerotic lesions will contain a larger proportion of myogenic foam cells. One of the typical features of vimentin-bearing intermediate filaments is their perinuclear concentration, as shown in ultrastructural pictures. The close association with the nucleus suggests that vimentin offers mechanical support to the cell, thereby ensuring its position in the cell (LAZARIDES 1980). More recent studies postulate a role of vimentin in the intracellular accumulation of lipid droplets: vimentin fibers are known to knit a filamentous meshwork around these drops (FRANKE et al. 1987), an observation confirmed by our own data on lipid-bearing myocytes. The initial controversy over the coexistence of vimentin and desmin in smooth muscle cells (FRANK and WARREN 1981) has now been closed by the study of FUJIMOTO et al. (1987). Having established ultrastructural proof of the coexistence of vimentin and desmin in the intermediate filaments of vascular smooth muscle cells, these authors suggested that the changing of filament expression might be due to the remodulation of existing filaments rather than to de novo polymerization.

Currently (CAMPBELL and CAMPBELL 1990; CAMPBELL et al. 1990a, b), phenotype modulation in the myocyte is seen as a result of various cell interactions and of changes in the cellular matrix, and/or as a response to other messages (e.g., from hormones). Cell culture studies have established that the biologic behavior of synthesizing smooth muscle cells differs from that of the contractile phenotype in that the former can proliferate more readily, synthesize collagen, and accumulate lipids. These faculties are essential for the formation of arteriosclerotic plaques. Why myocytes display a different phenotype in this context is not yet fully explained, but we do know that many factors are involved. An important role is attributed to the influence of monocytes/macrophages and lymphocytes on the progress of sclerotic vascular lesions (cf. Sects. 4.3 and 4.4). Thus, the phenotype modulation of smooth muscle cells must be of central significance for both RTA and CAS.

4.3 Monocytes/Macrophages

Recent morphologic studies of the pathogenesis of CAS (ROESSNER et al. 1986; STARY 1987a, b; MITCHINSON et al. 1990) have reported in extenso the particular role of monocytes/macrophages in the early stages of the lesion. According to MASSMANN (1979) the metabolic activation of this cell system is an atherogenic stimulus in itself, although the subendothelial population of monocytes/macrophages is seen as a physiologic component of the subendothelium in the larger arteries of many species and man, too. Our investigations in rejected kidney transplants have shown, in analogy to findings in CAS, a mononuclear infiltrate from the lumen clinging to the endothelium, penetrating it, and then becoming visible in the subendothelial layer. It must be an essential difference between RTA and CAS that such cells originate from the transplant recipient. The central role of monocytes/macrophages, of the growth factors formed by them (but not by them alone), and of their effect on smooth muscle and endothelial cells is thought to be an essential factor in the pathogenesis of arteriosclerotic sheets (MÜLLER-HERMELINK and DÄMMRICH 1989; ALPERS et al. 1990).

Despite many similarities with regard to morphology, cytochemistry, kinetics, and cytogenesis, the monocyte/macrophage system is composed of functionally rather heterogeneous cells (VAN FURTH 1982; RADZUN 1988). Provision of impressive evidence of this has been made possible in recent years by the development of a wide spectrum of highly specific markers for different types of monocytes/macrophages, differentiated according to (or dependent on) systemic and organic requirements, i.e., the type of organ or tissue or the functional status of such cells (VOLLMER et al. 1991c).

In the chronology of arteriosclerotic lesions, the endothelial adherence of monocytes/macrophages and lymphocytes, with eventual permeation and migration of these cells into deeper layers of the vascular wall, has an important and initiating impact. Admittedly, the true factors initiating the quasi-inflammatory infiltration of monocytes/macrophages into the arterial wall, and the formation of a lesion, are still unclear. Intensive study is presently being devoted to the molecular mechanisms of leukocyte adherence to the endothelium and of their migration (GIMBRONE et al. 1990). The so-called endothelial leukocyte adhesion molecules (cf. Sect. 4.1) are involved in both acute and chronic inflammatory diseases; in such conditions, the normally well-regulated gene expression appears disturbed. Persistent expression of surface structures may present a continuous stimulus for leukocytes to take up continual transmigration into the vessel wall. In addition to inducible cell surface adhesion molecules, endothelial cells are capable of synthesizing a number of soluble substances (the so-called mediators) that exert an influence on the interactions of monocytes/macrophages of the vascular wall. The actual mechanism of passage through interendothelial gaps, aided by pseudopodial cell protrusions, has been identified and confirmed mainly by ultrastructural studies (MASUDA and ROSS 1990a, b; HORT and BÜRRIG 1989; WATANABE et al. 1985; SCHWARTZ et al. 1985).

In many cases, monocytes/macrophages were also found in the intima and in deeper layers of the wall. The markers used in our study—27-E-10, MRP8, MRP14, and MAC 37 (ZWADLO et al. 1986, 1988)—labeled monocytes within the vascular lumen and also in lumen-adjacent layers of the wall. As expected, the monoclonal antibody MAC 387 showed weaker immunolabeling than the polyclonal antibody MRP8 directed against a similar antigen. Moreover, some of these monocytic/histiocytic cells showed vacuolated cytoplasm corresponding to the so-called foam cell picture. The foam cells were observed in the vascular wall as well as in the lumen. In contrast, foam cells staining with the marker 25-F-9 were found only in the vessel wall; this marker only labels so-called mature tissue macrophages (ZWADLO et al. 1985), while cells with monocytic properties remain unlabeled. In the lumen, there was thus no evidence of 25-F-9-positive cells. Based on these observations, it may be postulated that these cells originally must be infiltrating monocytes of the recipient which, differentiating to mature tissue macrophages in the donor kidney, take up abundant lipids and so transform into foam cells. Obviously, remigration of these fully differentiated, lipid-laden macrophages is then no longer possible. Remigration is feasible only by 27-E-10-positive macrophages and by the subpopulations positively labeled by the markers MRP8, MRP14, and MAC 387. The process of cell maturation and differentiation is paralleled by increasing, irreversible uptake of lipids resulting in foam cell formation; the monocyte-specific antigen 27-E-10 is no longer discernible in these cells, which eventually break down at the base from sheer lipid overload. Between the 27-E-10-positive cells with the pure properties of blood monocytes and adequate migration potential, and the 25-F-9-positive histiocytic foam cells appraised as mature and sedentary, there are obviously some that are labeled by other markers and may possess some other functional properties, thereby occupying an intermediate position.

Taking up excess lipoproteins from the surrounding tissue, foam cell macrophages will sometimes show, in cases of severe obliterative RTA, even the proliferation-associated nuclear antigen (PCNA). We may deduce that histiocytic foam cells, generally seen as the fully differentiated definitive form, may still be capable of proliferation, in opposition to current opinion. This idea is supported by some data in the literature. STARY (1987), for instance, reported mitotic foam cells showing the ultrastructural characteristics of macrophages in experimental atherosclerotic lesions of the monkey intima. In a rabbit model studied by simultaneous autoradiographic thymidine incorporation and immunohistology using monoclonal antibodies, ROSENFELD and ROSS (1990) found that up to 30% of proliferating cells in the vascular wall had to be appraised as foam cell macrophages, dependent on the actual stage of the atherosclerotic lesion. Other autoradiographic and electron microscopic studies by VILLASCHI and SPAGNOLI (1983) on human fibroatheromatous plaques recorded positive thymidine labeling of foam cell macrophages. In contrast to these authors' findings and to our own and DEMETRIS et al.'s (1989) data on RTA, we were never able to confirm the presence of proliferating foam cells in CAS lesions

(VOLLMER 1991). Although the proliferating foam cells found in RTA have not yet been analyzed by immunohistochemical double labeling for a possible myocytic origin, this appears rather unlikely in view of their distinct and intense staining with the highly specific marker 25-F-9, which is directed exclusively against mature tissue macrophages (ZWADLO et al. 1985). Negative confirmation is also found in the study of 15 transplanted kidneys of MÜLLER-HERMELINK and DÄMMRICH (1989), wherein all foam cells were exclusively traced back to macrophages, never to smooth muscle cells.

The (unexpected) proliferation of foam cells may reflect the fact that, in contrast to the situation in CAS, with its slow and prolonged progress, in RTA there is a failing supply of blood monocytes for dealing with the sudden necessity of lipid metabolization in maturing macrophages, and so additional mitosis is needed on the spot. This interpretation supports the view of RTA as a kind of accelerated arteriosclerosis. We have to bear in mind that in RTA, the monocytes/macrophages are always supplied by the recipient and, being directed against the heterogeneous transplant, are migrating into this alien tissue.

4.4 Lymphocytes

DUFF et al. (1957) were among the first to postulate the functional involvement of lymphocytes in the development of CAS. This idea was taken up by JORIS et al. in 1979, and substantiated by electron microscopic studies. The number of such cells rises in parallel with increasing arteriosclerosis, in both spontaneous and experimentally induced lesions (BABA et al. 1977; GEER 1965; STILL and MARRIOTT 1964; JORIS and MAJNO 1979; JORIS et al. 1983). Detailed data on an inflammatory infiltrate in human atherosclerotic lesions were published by JONASSON et al. (1985, 1986): In studies of plaques in human carotids, 11% of cells could be labeled with a pan-T lymphocyte marker, while only 1% reacted to an antibody against B lymphocytes. Among the whole population of T lymphocytes, the T helper cells dominated the suppressor cells. These findings agree with the results published by HANSSON et al. (1989a) and VOLLMER et al. (1988), but contradict those of EMESON and ROBERTSON (1988). More recent studies by SCHWARTZ et al. (1990) have identified an inflammatory autoimmune component in adventitial lymphocytic infiltrates, possibly provoked by accumulating ceroid in atherosclerosis. These authors also discussed the possibility that the inflammatory autoimmune process plays a decisive role in the development of atherosclerotic thrombosis. STRATFORD et al. (1986) had also recognized adventitial infiltration of T and B lymphocytes in approximately balanced proportions, which they interpreted as a sequel to, rather than a cause of, atherosclerotic changes. Lymphocytic infiltration in both adventitia and media was also ascertained by KOCH et al. (1990), who postulated an immune-mediated reactions as the most likely cause for the development of aneurysm. However, it was also considered possible that inflammatory infiltration might be a mere epiphenomenon. MUNRO et al. (1987) interpreted lymphocytic infiltration in fatty streaks—with a ratio of T helper to T suppressor cells of 1:2—as an inflammatory-like process underlying atherosclerosis: in multifactorial genesis, cellular as well as humoral immunologic factors must play a considerable role. Unfortunately, despite all of the above findings, it remains the case that a truly comprehensive interpretation of the immunologic mechanisms involved in the development of atherosclerosis is far from being agreed upon (KLURFELD 1983; MUNRO and COTRAN 1988; ROSS 1990).

Much more definite and detailed, in contrast, are the current concepts on the immunologic mechanisms involved in transplant rejection. After any transplantation, the recipient's lymphocytes will physiologically start to pervade and circulate through the transplanted organ. The immigrating T lymphocytes are capable of recognizing the foreign antigens of the HLA system. Sensitized by these, some of the lymphocytes acquire cytotoxic properties. Another group of lymphocytes first leaves the transplant via its efferent pathways, accumulates in regional nodes, and begins to proliferate, subsequently returning to the transplant in the role of cytotoxic lymphocytes. There is also a somewhat delayed sensitization of the B cell system. When the synthesis of specific antibodies commences, rejection reactions become increasingly complicated by humoral immune reactions; these, by way of complement activation, release of kinins, etc. will eventually lead to an antibody-dependent, cell-mediated cytotoxic reaction. The whole rather complex course of events, in which the humoral immune reactions (type II = cytotoxic, type III = immune complex reactions) and cell-mediated reactions (type IV) have a varying impact, also involves other immunocompetent cells such as monocytes/macrophages and natural killer cells. A particular role in the development and progression of the disease is attributed to the vascular endothelial cell, seen as the primary target cell for the initiation of obliterative RTA.

According to our present studies, the number of T lymphocytes markedly exceeds that of B lymphocytes in the inner layers of the vascular wall. T lymphocyte (sub)populations are generally responsible for the recognition, initiation, and regulation of an immune response. The pathologic as well as the physiologic response is initiated by antigen recognition by T lymphocytes involving the major histocompatibility complex (MHC) on antigen-presenting cells. In tissues with normal delayed-type immune reaction as well as in lesions of autoimmunologic origin, a large number of lymphocytes and of antigen-presenting cells expressing MHC class 2 will be found. It must be asked whether the lymphocytes seen in arteriosclerotic lesions recognize specific antigens or are in fact directed against these antigens. Today, two classes of HLA antigens are distinguished: Those of class I are subdivided into HLA-A, -B, and -C according to regions or specificities and can be found on all nucleated cells and thrombocytes of the organism. These antigens will be recognized by CD8-positive suppressor/cytotoxic lymphocytes. Any tissue cell expressing foreign HLA I antigens may be assailed by the cytotoxic attack of CD8-positive cells. The tissue distribution of HLA class II antigens (HLA-DR, -DP, -DQ) is much more limited than that of HLA I antigens. They are found on B lymphocytes, macrophages, dendritic cells, and Langerhans cells of the skin. HLA II are the target cells for CD4-positive T lymphocytes which, when activated, will mainly secrete cytokines. Such an activation of T lymphocytes is known to occur after the transplantation of foreign tissue, like in the kidney transplants of our study. The parallels with CAS that can be inferred from our results are rather suggestive of a similar process. It may be assumed that in CAS, CD8-positive T lymphocytes are involved in the initiation of the atherosclerotic lesion, somewhat like in RTA. The obvious damage to, or general alteration of, the endothelium at the very beginning of the atherosclerotic process has already been mentioned in Sect. 4.1. In this context, mechanical, chemical, toxic, and viral causative factors have been discussed (Hansson et al. 1989b; Müller-Hermelink and Dämmrich 1989; Munro and Cotran 1988; Virella and Lopez-Virella 1987; Emeson and Robertson 1988; Ross 1990). Nevertheless, the actual etiology is far from satisfactorily explained.

It appears possible at least, that even in CAS, as in RTA, resting CD4-positive cells are able to recognize foreign HLA via their T receptor molecule. Thus activated, the T cell would produce the T cell growth factor interleukin-2 (IL-2), simultaneously binding receptors for IL-2 on its surface. Binding IL-2 to the appropriate receptor will stimulate and secrete other cytokines in addition to IL-2. CD8-positive T cells, however, which recognize foreign HLA I, will subsequently also express IL-2 receptors. If IL-2 is supplied by activated, CD4-positive T lymphocytes, the IL-2 receptor-positive cell is also able to proliferate and to differentiate into a cytotoxic effector cell.

Thus, it appears quite feasible that CD8-positive cells are involved in the initiation of atherosclerotic lesions in parallel to RTA, but that the individual progress of the lesion may undergo a switch to a CD4-dominated immune reaction. In fact, such a switch appears all the more likely given that the only contradictory report citing an opposite ratio of T cell subpopulations in CAS (Emeson and Robertson 1988) was based on the exclusive study of vessels from children and young adults (aged 15–34) dying of acute trauma. It may be inferred that the material of that study covered only lesions at a very early stage. Further information also derives from the study by Masuda and Ross (1990a, b) on macaques with low-level hypercholesterolemia, ascertained that there was a preponderance of CD8-positive lymphocytes in the lesions.

It may be concluded that in all other studies mentioned above, including our own (Vollmer et al. 1988), despite the evidence of morphologically early stages, the functionally initial stage of CAS, manifested by the predominance of CD8-positive lymphocytes, is already over. This means that CD4-positive helper/inducer cells immunohistochemically evident in sclerotic vessels are acting in conjunction with other immunocompetent cells (e.g., monocytes/ macrophages) that are also present in abundance. The cytokines produced by these cells in the course of an immune response are able to modulate the growth and differentiation of other vascular cell elements (endothelia and myocytes) as well as the local lipid metabolism.

We may infer from our results that, although the initial mechanisms in CAS still cannot be exactly defined, certain morphologic and functional parallels can be demonstrated between the patterns of CAS and RTA. The better understanding of the latter may help to explain and verify the specific immune mechanisms responsible for the development of CAS. However, it must always be remembered that in RTA the lymphocytes studied are the recipient's own immigrating cells.

5 Summary, Conclusions, and Outlook

In this chapter we have presented the results of our studies of the cellular activities in the vascular wall in RTA and have discussed various pathogenetic aspects of RTA and CAS, comparing their functional and pathologic morphology. In both diseases, the initial and central role is attributed to the *endothelium* and its activities:

1. Immunologic cell–cell interactions with processes of activation and proliferation, including humoral and cellular mediators
2. Transformation from flat, spindle-shaped endothelial cells to a metabolically active, cuboid-bulky phenotype
3. Modulations in the expression of adherence structures and carbohydrate binding sites of endothelial cells, dependent on the development of the lesion

The phenotypic modulation of the *smooth muscle cell* is also seen as an important factor in both diseases. It seems to occur independent of the initial causation of the development and progress of arteriosclerotic lesions. The modulation is effected by:

1. Modulating the expression of intermediate and microfilaments
2. An increase in synthesizing type myocytes
3. (Ir?) reversible proliferative stimuli acting on myocytes and/or their potential migration
4. An enhanced synthesis of extracellular matrix, and a lipid accumulation in these cells (?)

In addition, we have to be aware of humoral and cell-mediated immune mechanisms and of metabolic disorders.

Besides endothelial cells and myocytes, i.e., local cells of the vascular wall, are also immigrating cells. Here the crucial difference between the disease patterns lies in the fact that in RTA, the transplant is infiltrated by *heterologous* lymphocytes and monocytes/macrophages (of recipient origin).

Nevertheless, the following similarities and differences may be established at least for the behavior of *monocytes/macrophages*:

1. Obviously, only the blood monocytes activated by various pathogenetic mechanisms (characterized by positivity for 27-E-10, MRP14, and to some

extent MRP8 or MAC 387) are capable of adhering to the endothelium and of migrating into the arterial walls.
2. In the arterial wall these cells will eventually differentiate to so-called mature tissue macrophages (25-F-9-positive) and gradually lose their originally phenotypes, with concomitant lipid uptake leading to the formation of foam cells.
3. Some of the lipid-bearing cells within the vascular wall (mainly MRP8- and MAC 387-positive) are obviously activated to effect lipid clearance with subsequent remigration into the bloodstream.
4. When this capacity is exhausted, the now sessile cells with their lipid overload (exclusively 25-F-9-positive) will "dig their own graves".
5. Since in RTA the sudden lipid influx into the arterial wall occurs in a limited period of time (unlike in CAS), the observed and sometimes increased proliferation of foam cells must be interpreted as a compensatory mechanism within the local lipid metabolism of the vascular wall.
6. In opposition to current opinion, these foam cells obviously do not bear so much metabolic overload as to suffer obligatory necrosis; remigration into the cell cycle appears possible in RTA, at least in the earlier (not yet 25-F-9-positive) stages.

As regards the many other features of monocytes/macrophages manifested during the course of the immunologic processes, and their metabolic peculiarities in each disease, a brief summation must suffice.

The results discussed above in respect of *lymphocytes* have shown that, despite differing initial causes of the vascular lesions, some remarkable immunologic parallels can be detected between CAS and RTA. In the framework of cell-mediated immune reactions of the delayed type, T lymphocytes have an important role, although it is effective only in combination with the major histocompatibility complex. Admittedly, many details of the pattern of interactions are still unclear, but a certain common pathogenetic mechanism can be identified in both diseases:

1. CD8-positive lymphocytes will recognize altered or alien HLA I, and induce HLA II on endothelium; cells expressing the latter antigen class may be subjected to cytotoxic attack.
2. HLA II-positive cells are, in turn, target antigens for CD4-positive lymphocytes which are reactivated by HLA II induction.
3. Consequently, CD8-positive lymphocytes assume a primary role in the initiation of arteriosclerotic processes; the maintenance of such pathogenetic mechanisms is effected by CD8- and CD4-positive lymphocytes in various ways.

Certain effector mechanisms of B lymphocytes are also present, e.g., antibody production, immune complex formation, and complement-mediated as well as antibody-dependent cytotoxicity. Here again it must be remembered that in RTA, the observations are always made on heterologous lymphocytes of the recipient, which are acting in and on the transplant.

Summing up our results, we conclude that the pathogenetic course in RTA proceeds in a somewhat accelerated but otherwise largely similar pattern to that in CAS. We may see the process as a suitable human "model" permitting more rapid observation of certain pathogenetic mechanisms responsible for the development and progression of atherosclerosis, and more detailed study of their highly complex interactions, than would be feasible in the slower and longer-lasting process of CAS. Clarification of the immunologically induced, obligatory reaction in (renal) transplant arteriopathy, reflected in the extreme and persistent activation of reparative processes within the vascular wall, will assist us in obtaining greater insight into the functional morphology of such lesions, and so improve our understanding of atherosclerotic vascular lesions.

Acknowledgement. This work was supported by Deutsche Forschungsgemeinschaft grant VO 386/1.

References

Alpers CE, Gordon D, Gown AM (1990) Immunophenotype of vascular rejection in renal transplants. Mod Pathol 3:198–203

Baba N, Bashe WJ, Jordan B, Liuzzi F (1977) Human coronary atheromatous plaques. Am J Pathol 86:50a

Campbell GR, Campbell JH (1990) The phenotypes of smooth muscle expressed in human atheroma. Ann NY Acad Sci 598:143–158

Campbell GR, Campbell JH, Ang AH, et al. (1990a) Phenotypic changes in smooth muscle cells of human atherosclerotic plaques. In: Glagov S, Newman WP III, Schaffer SA (eds) Pathobiology of the human atherosclerotic plaque. Springer, New York Berlin Heidelberg, pp 69–92

Campbell JH, Kalevitch SG, Rennick RE, Campbell GR (1990b) Extracellular matrix-smooth muscle phenotype modulation by macrophages. Ann NY Acad Sci 598:159–168

Cerilli J, Brasile L, Sosa J, Kremer J, Clarke J, Leather R, Shah D (1987) The role of autoantibody to vascular endothelial cell antigens in atherosclerosis and vascular disease. Transplant Proc 19(4), Suppl 5:47–49

Cordell JL, Falini B, Erber WN, et al. (1984) Immunoenzymatic labeling of monoclonal antibodies using immune complexes of alkaline phosphatase and monoclonal anti-alkaline phosphatase (APAAP complexes). J Histochem Cytochem 32:219–229

Cotran RS (1987) New role for the endothelium in inflammation and immunity. Am J Pathol 129:407–413

Demetris AJ, Zerbe T, Banner B (1989) Morphology of solid organ allograft arteriopathy. Identification of proliferating intimal cell populations. Transplant Proc 21(4):3667–3669

Duff GL, McMillan GC, Ritchie MB (1957) The morphology of early atherosclerotic lesions of the aorta demonstrated by the surface technique in rabbits fed cholesterol. Am J Pathol 33:845–873

Emeson EE, Robertson AL (1988) T-lymphocytes in aortic and coronary intimas. Am J Pathol 130:369–376

Frank ED, Warren L (1981) Aortic smooth muscle cells contain vimentin instead of desmin. J Cell Biol 78:3020–3024

Franke WW, Hergt M, Grund C (1987) Rearrangement of the vimentin cytoskeleton during adipose conversion: formation of an intermediate filament cage around lipid globules. Cell 49:131–141

Fujimoto T, Tokuyasu KT, Singer SJ (1987) Direct morphological demonstration of the coexistence of vimentin and desmin in the same intermediate filaments of vascular smooth muscle cells. J Submicrosc Cytol 19:1–9

Geer JC (1965) The fine structure of human aortic intimal thickening and fatty streaks. Lab Invest 14:1764–1783

Gerrity RG (1990) Arterial endothelial structure and permeability as it relates to susceptibility to atherogenesis. In: Glagov S, Newmann WP, Schaffer SA (eds) Pathobiology of the human atherosclerotic plaque. Springer, Berlin Heidelberg New York, pp 13–46

Gimbrone MA, Bevilacqua MP, Cybulsky MI (1990) Endothelial-dependent mechanisms of leukocyte adhesion in inflammation and atherosclerosis. Ann NY Acad Sci 598:77–86

Gordon D, Schwartz SM, Benditt EP, Wilcox JN (1989) Growth factors and cell proliferation in human atherosclerosis. Transplant Proc 21(4):3692–3694

Hansson GK, Holm J, Jonasson L (1989a) Detection of activated T-lymphocytes in the human atherosclerotic plaque. Am J Pathol 135:169–175

Hansson GK, Jonasson L, Seifert PS, Stemme S (1989b) Immune mechanisms in atherosclerosis. Arteriosclerosis 9:567–578

Hort W, Bürrig KF (1989) Endothel und Arteriosklerose. Z Kardiol 78 [Suppl 6]:105–112

Hruban RH, Beschorner WE, Baumgartner WA, Augustine SM, Ren H, Reitz BA, Hutchins GM (1990) Accelerated arteriosclerosis in heart transplant recipients is associated with a T-lymphocyte-mediated endothelialitis. Am J Pathol 137:871–882

Humbel B, Schwarz H (1989) Freeze substitution for immuno-chemistry. In: Verkleij AJ, Leunissen JLM (eds) Immuno-gold labeling in cell biology. CRC, Boca Raton, Fla., pp 115–134

Jellinek H, Detre Z (1986) Role of the altered transmural permeability in the pathomechanism of arteriosclerosis. Pathol Res Pract 181:693–712

Jonasson L, Holm J, Skalli O, Gabbiani G, Hansson GK (1985) Expression of class II transplantation antigen on vascular smooth muscle cells in human atherosclerosis. J Clin Invest 76:125–131

Jonasson L, Holm J, Skalli O, Bondjers G, Hansson GK (1986) Regional accumulations of T-cells, macrophages, and smooth muscle cells in the human atherosclerotic plaque. Arteriosclerosis 6:131–138

Joris I, Majno G (1979) Inflammatory components of atherosclerosis. Adv Inflammation Res 1:71–85

Joris I, Stetz E, Majno G (1979) Lymphocytes and monocytes in the aortic intima. Atherosclerosis 34:221–231

Joris I, Zand T, Nunnary JJ, Krolikowski FJ, Majno G (1983) Studies of the pathogenesis of atherosclerosis. I. Adhesion and emigration of mononuclear cells in the aorta of hypercholesterolemic rats. Am J Pathol 113:341–358

Klurfeld DM (1983) Interactions of immune function with lipids and atherosclerosis. CRC Crit Rev Toxicol 11:355–365

Koch AE, Haines GK, Rizzo RJ, Radosevich JA, Pope RM, Robinson PG, Pearce WH (1990) Human abdominal aortic aneurysms. Immunopathologic analysis suggesting an immune-mediated response. Am J Pathol 137:1199–1213

Lazarides E (1980) Intermediate filaments as mechanical integrators of cellular space. Nature 283:249–255

Libby P, Salomon RN, Payne DD, Schoen FJ, Pober JS (1989) Functions of vascular wall cells related to development of transplantation-associated coronary arteriosclerosis. Transplant Proc 21:3677–3684

Massmann J (1979) Mononuclear cell infiltration of the aortic intima in domestic swine. Exp Pathol 17:110–112

Masuda J, Ross R (1990a) Atherogenesis during low level hypercholesterolemia in the nonhuman primate. I. Fatty streak formation. Arteriosclerosis 10:164–177

Masuda J, Ross R (1990b) Atherogenesis during low level hypercholesterolemia in the nonhuman primate. II. Fatty streak conversion to fibrous plaque. Arteriosclerosis 10:178–187

McLean IW, Nakane PK (1974) Periodate-lysine-paraformaldehyde fixative. A new fixative for immunoelectron microscopy. J Histochem Cytochem 22:1077–1083

Mitchinson MJ, Carpenter KLH, Ball RY (1990) The role of macrophages in human atherosclerosis. In: Glagov S, Newman WP, Schaffer AS (eds) Pathobiology of the human atherosclerotic plaque. Springer, Berlin Heidelberg New York, pp 121–128

Müller-Hermelink HK, Dämmrich JR (1989) Die obliterative Transplantatvaskulopathie: Pathogenese und Pathomechanismen. Verh Dtsch Ges Pathol 73:193–206

Munro JM, Cotran (1988) Biology of disease. The pathogenesis of atherosclerosis, atherogenesis and inflammation. Lab Invest 58:249–261

Munro JM, van der Walt JD, Munro CS Chalmers JHC, Cox EL (1987) An immunohistochemical analysis of human aortic fatty streak. Hum Pathol 18:375–380

Pritchard KA Jr, Wong PYK, Stemerman MB (1990) Atherogenic concentrations of low-density lipoprotein enhance endothelial cell generation of epoxyeicosatrienoic acid products. Am J Pathol 136:1383–1391

Radzun HJ (1988) Differenzierungslinien im Monozyten/Makrophagensystem. Verh Dtsch Ges Pathol 72:50–56

Reidy MA, Silver M (1985) Endothelial regeneration. VII. Lack of intimal proliferation after defined injury to rat aorta. Am J Pathol 118:173–177

Roessner A, Vollmer E, Zwadlo G, Sorg C, Greve H, Grundmann E (1986) Zur Differenzierung von Makrophagen und glatten Muskelzellen mit monoklonalen Antikörpern in der arteriosklerotischen Plaque der menschlichen Aorta. Verh Dtsch Ges Pathol 70:365–370

Roessner A, Herrera A, Höning AJ, et al. (1987) Identification of macrophages and smooth muscle cells with monoclonal antibodies in the human atherosclerotic plaque. Virchows Arch [A] 412:169–174

Roessner A, Bögeholz J, Bosse A, Vollmer E, Buchholz E, Winde G, Bründermann H (1989) Immunhistologische Differenzierung der Zellen in der Arterienwand von Transplantatnieren. Verh Dtsch Ges Pathol 73:242–247

Rosenfeld ME, Ross R (1990) Macrophage and smooth muscle cell proliferation in atherosclerotic lesions of WHHL and comparably hypercholesterolemic fat-fed rabbits. Arteriosclerosis 10:680–687

Rosenfeld ME, Palinski W, Ylä-Herttuala S, Butler S, Witzum JL (1990) Distribution of oxidation-specific lipoprotein adducts and apolipoprotein B in atherosclerotic lesions of varying severity from WHHL rabbits. Arteriosclerosis 10:336349

Ross R (1986) The pathogenesis of atherosclerosis—an update. N Engl J Med 314:488–500

Ross R (1990) Mechanisms of atherosclerosis—a review. Adv Nephrol 19:79–86

Salomon RN, Hughes CGW, Schoen FJ, Payne DD, Pober JS, Libby P (1991) Human coronary transplantation-associated arteriosclerosis. Am J Pathol 138:791–798

Scharf RE, Harker LA (1987) Thrombosis and atherosclerosis: Regulatory role of interactions among blood components and endothelium. Blut 55:131–144

Schulze-Osthoff K, Meinardus-Hager G, Sorg C (1989) Das Endothel und seine Schlüsselrolle in der Entzündung. Jahrb Dermatologie 41–52

Schwartz CJ, Sprague EA, Kelley JL, Valente AJ, Suenram CA (1985) Aortic intimal monocyte recruitment in the normo- and hypercholesterolemic baboon (*Papio cynocephalus*). Virchows Arch [A] 405:175–191

Schwartz CJ, Sprague EA, Valente AJ, Kelley JL, Edwards EH, Suenram CA (1990) Inflammatory components of the human atherosclerotic plaque. In: Glagov S, Newman WP, Schaffer SA (eds) Pathobiology of the human atherosclerotic plaque. Springer, Berlin Heidelberg New York, pp 107–120

Simionescu N, Vasile E, Lupu F, Popescu G, Simionescu M (1986) Prelesional events in atherogenesis. Accumulation of extracellular cholesterol-rich liposomes in the arterial intima and cardiac valves of the hyperlipidemic rabbit. Am J Pathol 123:109–125

Sitte H, Edelmann L, Neumann K (1987) Cryofixation without pretreatment at ambient pressure. In: Steinbrecht RA, Zierold K (eds) Cryotechniques in biological electron microscopy. Springer, Berlin Heidelberg New York, pp 87–113

Sjöstrand FS (1990) Common sense in electron microscopy. About cryofixation, freeze-substitution, low temperature embedding, and low denaturation embedding. J Struct Biol 103:135–139

Stary HC (1987a) Macrophages, macrophage foam cells, and eccentric intimal thickening in the coronary arteries of young children. Atherosclerosis 64:91–108

Stary HC (1987b) Evolution and progression of atherosclerosis in the coronary arteries of children and adults. In: Bates SR, Gangloff ED (eds) Atherogenesis and Aging. Springer, New York Berlin Heidelberg, pp 20–36

Still WJS, Marriott PR (1964) Comparative morphology of the early atherosclerotic lesions in man and cholesterol atherosclerosis in the rabbit—an electron microscopic study. Am J Atheroscler Res 4:373–386

Stratford N, Britten K, Gallagher P (1986) Inflammatory infiltrate in human coronary atherosclerosis. Atherosclerosis 59:271–276

Tokuyasu KT (1984) Immuno-ultracytomicrotomy. In: Polak JM, Varndell JM (eds) Immunolabeling for electron microscopy. Elsevier, Amsterdam, pp 71–82

van Furth R (1982) Current view on the mononuclear phagocyte system. Immunobiology 161:178–1185

Vasile E, Simionescu M, Simionescu N (1983) Visualization of the binding endocytosis and transcytosis of low density lipoprotein in the arterial endothelium in situ. J Cell Biol 96:1677–1689

Vierbuchen M (1991) Lectin receptors. In: Seifert G (ed) Cell receptors. Springer, Berlin Heidelberg New York (Current Topics in Pathology 83:271–361)

Villaschi S, Spagnoli LG (1983) Autpradiographic and ultrastructural studies on the human fibro-atheromatous plaque. Atherosclerosis 48:95–100

Virella G, Lopes-Virella MF (1987) Infections and atherosclerosis. Transplant Proc 19/4, Suppl 5:26–35

Vollmer E (1991) Atherosklerose und renale Transplantatarteriopathie, patho- und funktionsmorphologische Parallelen. Habilitationsschrift, Faculty of Medicine, Münster

Vollmer E, Maurer T, Roessner A, Bosse A, Winde G, Böcker W (1988) Immunhistologische Untersuchungen zum Lymphozyteninfiltrat in unterschiedlichen Stadien der humanen Arteriosklerose. Verh Dtsch Ges Pathol 72:600

Vollmer E, Roessner A, Bosse A, Voss B, Goerdt S, Sorg C, Böcker W (1989) Immunoelectron microscopic investigations for the phenotypical characterization of endothelial cells. In: Hauss WH, Wissler RW, Bauch HJ (eds) Modern aspects of the pathogenesis of arteriosclerosis. Westdeutscher Verlag, Düsseldorf, p 235

Vollmer E, Roessner A, Bosse A, et al. (1991a) Immunohistochemical double labeling of macrophages, smooth muscle cells, and apolipoprotein E in the atherosclerotic plaque. Pathol Res Pract 187:184–188

Vollmer E, Bosse A, Bögeholz J, et al. (1991b) Apolipoproteins and immunohistochemical differentiation of cells in the arterial wall of kidneys in transplant arteriopathy. Pathol Res Pract 187:957–962

Vollmer E, Shimamoto F, Krieg V, Grundmann E (1991c) Macrophages/reticulum cells in early and late phases of lymphogenous metastasis. In: Grundmann E, Vollmer E (eds) Reaction patterns of the lymph node. Springer, Berlin Heidelberg New York (Current Topics in Pathology 84/2:49–79)

Watanabe T, Hirata M, Yoshikawa Y, Nagafuchi Y, Toyoshima H, Watanabe T (1985) Role of macrophages in atherosclerosis. Lab Invest 53:80–90

Wissler RW, Vesselinovitch D, Ko L (1989) The effects of circulating immune complexes on atherosclerotic lesions in experimental animals and in younger and older humans. Transplant Proc 21(4):3707–3708

Yoshida Y, Mitsumata M, Yamane T, Tomikawa M, Nishida K (1988) Morphology and increased growth rate of atherosclerotic intimal smooth muscle cells. Arch Pathol Lab Med 112:987–996

Yost JC, Herman IM (1988) Age-related and site-specific adaptation of the arterial endothelial cytoskeleton during atherogenesis. Am J Pathol 130:595–604

Zollinger HU, Mihatsch MJ, Thiel G, Harder F, Heitz P, Uebersax S, Gudat F (1978) Renal pathology in biopsy. Springer, Berlin Heidelberg New York

Zwadlo G, Bröcker EB, von Bassewitz DB, Feige U, Sorg C (1985) A monoclonal antibody to a differentiation antigen present on mature human macrophages and absent from monocytes. J Immunol 134:1487–1492

Zwadlo G, Schlegel R, Sorg C (1986) A monoclonal antibody to a subset of human monocytes found only in the peripheral blood and inflammatory tissues. J Immunol 137:512–518

Zwadlo G, Brüggen J, Gerhards G, Schlegel R, Sorg C (1988) Two calcium-binding proteins associated with specific stages of myeloid cell differentiation are expressed by subsets of macrophages in inflammatory tissues. Clin Exp Immunol 72:510–515

Subject Index

Index of Volumes 84–86 Current Topics in Pathology

Volume 84/1: Reaction Patterns of the Lymph Node.
Edited by E. GRUNDMANN, E. VOLLMER

Volume 84/2: Reaction Patterns of the Lymph Node.
Edited by E. GRUNDMANN, E. VOLLMER

E. VOLLMER, F. SHIMAMOTO, V. KRIEG, E. GRUNDMANN, Macrophages/Reticulum Cells in Early and Late Phases of Lymphogenous Matastasis

H. COTTIER, R. KRAFT, F. MEISTER, Primary Immunodeficiency Syndromes and Their Manifestations in Lymph Nodes

G. R. F. KRUEGER, D. V. ABLASHI, P. LUSSO, S. F. JOSEPHS, Immunological Dysregulation of Lymph Nodes in AIDS Patients

J. DIEBOLD, J. AUDOUIN, A. LE TOURNEAU, S. PREVOT, G. SZEKERES, Lymph Node Reaction Patterns in Patients with AIDS or AIDS-Related Complex

Volume 85: Gynecological Tumors. Edited by N. SASANO

G. DALLENBACH-HELLWEG, Endometrial Carcinomas

S. G. SILVERBERG, Mixed Müllerian Tumors

K. NODA, Cervical Intraepithelial Neoplasia and Microinvasive Carcinoma of the Cervix

R. KUDO, Cervical Adenocarcinoma

R. H. YOUNG and R. E. SCULLY, Endocrine Tumors of the Ovary

A. TALERMAN, Germ Cell Tumors

Y. TOMODA, T. ISHIZUKA, S. GOTO, and Y. FURUHASHI, Trophoblastic Disease

M. K. SIDAWY, Cytology in Gynecological Disorders

T. OKAGAKI, Impact of Human Papillomavirus Research on the Histopathologic Concepts of Genital Neoplasms

G. UEDA and M. YAMASAKI, Neuroendocrine Carcinoma of the Uterus

D. A. BELL, Flow Cytometry of Ovarian Neoplasms

H. SASANO and C. T. GARRETT, Oncogenes in Gynecological Tumors

Volume 86: The Pathology of Devices Edited by C. L. BERRY

U. LÖHRS and I. BOS, The Pathology of Artificial Joints

M. D. O'HARA and C. M. HILL, Pathology of Injected Polytetrafluoroethylene

H. H. SCHELD and W. KONERTZ, The Pathology of Bioprosthetic Heart Valves and Allografts

M. M. BLACK and P. J. DRURY, Mechanical and other Problems of Artificial Valves

A. COUMBE and T. R. GRAHAM, The Pathology of Artificial Hearts and Ventricular Assist Devices

J. COX, The Pathology of Cardiac Pacemakers

K.-M. MÜLLER and G. DASBACH, The Pathology of Vascular Grafts

C. H. BUCKLEY, The Pathology of Intra-uterine Contraceptive Devices